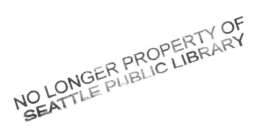

D0555849

UNHEALTHY POLITICS

Unhealthy Politics

The Battle over Evidence-Based Medicine

Eric M. Patashnik

Alan S. Gerber

Conor M. Dowling

PRINCETON UNIVERSITY PRESS

PRINCETON AND OXFORD

Copyright © 2017 by Princeton University Press

Published by Princeton University Press,
41 William Street, Princeton, New Jersey 08540

In the United Kingdom: Princeton University Press,
6 Oxford Street, Woodstock, Oxfordshire OX20 1TR

press.princeton.edu

Jacket image courtesy of Shutterstock

All Rights Reserved

ISBN 978-0-691-15881-5
Library of Congress Control Number: 2017935148

British Library Cataloging-in-Publication Data is available

This book has been composed in Adobe Text Pro and Gotham

Printed on acid-free paper. ∞

Printed in the United States of America

10 9 8 7 6 5 4 3 2 1

CONTENTS

LIST OF FIGURES AND TABLES

Figures

Tables

ACKNOWLEDGMENTS

This book has had a long gestation. It is a pleasure to express our appreciation to the many individuals who have supported our work.

We are especially grateful to the scholars who read all or part of the manuscript, including Alan Cohen, Carolyn Engelhard, David Mechanic, Jonathan Oberlander, Mark Schlesinger, and Jon Skinner, as well as to two readers for Princeton University Press (one of whom, Ann Keller, revealed her identity to us after the manuscript was accepted). Their detailed comments, incisive criticisms, and thoughtful suggestions improved the book immeasurably. We also learned a tremendous amount from interviews, conversations, written feedback, and e-mail exchanges with many other scholars, experts, and policy makers, including Tom Allen, John Appleby, Carol Ashton, Eugene Bardach, Shawn Bishop, Michael Cannon, Dan Carpenter, Carolyn Clancy, Paul Cleary, David Cutler, Ara Darzi, John Ellwood, Sherry Glied, Phyllis Greenberger, Colleen Grogan, Michael Gusmano, Jacob Hacker, Ruth Hanft, Jennifer Hochschild, Karen Ignagni, Gary Kupfer, Miriam Laugesen, Julian Le Grand, Frank Levy, Peter Littlejohns, Rick Mayes, Etienne Minvielle, Bruce Moseley, Jonathan Nichols, Bernard Patashnik, Mark Peterson, Harold Pollack, Sir Michael Rawlins, Lise Rochaix, Jill Rutter, Herman Schwartz, Topher Spiro, Kathy Swartz, Peter Swenson, Gail Wilensky, and Nelda Wray. We apologize to anyone we have forgotten to thank and wish to stress that we alone are responsible for any errors of fact or interpretation.

Our work has been supported by talented research assistants. In a class by herself is Catlan Reardon, now a doctoral student at UC Berkeley. Other graduate students and postdoctoral fellows who contributed to this project include Daniel Biggers, David Hendry, Seth Hill, and Maya Mahin at Yale University; Victoria Catanese, Kenneth Lowande, and Jesse Rhodes at the University of Virginia; Rachel Lowenstein and Aaron Weinstein at Brown University; and Nichole Gligor at the University of Mississippi. The public opinion studies presented in this book draw on several journal articles that were coauthored with David Doherty. Thank you, David, for your major contribution to this project.

One of the benefits of a long-term research project is the opportunity to share preliminary findings and arguments with diverse audiences. Especially helpful were the constructive feedback and insightful criticisms we received from people who attended workshops and symposia held at or organized by the NYU Wagner Graduate School of Public Service, Harvard University RWJF Scholars Program, Virginia Commonwealth University, University of Minnesota, University of Washington, University of Virginia School of Medicine, the Miller Center of Public Affairs, Senior Statesmen of Virginia, Institute of Governmental Studies at UC Berkeley, University of Wisconsin, University of Chicago Center on Health Administration Studies, Dartmouth Institute for Health Policy and Clinical Practice, Yale School of Medicine, and Brown University. We also benefited from presentations on panels at the American Political Science Association and the Association for Public Policy Analysis and Management.

We also wish to thank colleagues for their personal, professional, and administrative support at various stages, including Jennifer Costanza, Howard Goodkin, Pam Greene, Jed Horwitt, Greg Huber, Pam Lamonaca, Dr. Heinz I. Lippmann, Rick Locke, Jim Morone, and Carrie Nordlund. We thank the Albemarle County Medical Society for its assistance in helping us to field a pilot survey of physician beliefs.

For financial support, we extend our profound thanks to the Robert Wood Johnson Foundation Investigator's Award in Health Policy Research and to the Smith Richardson Foundation. We are grateful to Alan Cohen and Mark Steinmeyer for their patience, guidance, and encouragement during the completion of this project. We also are grateful for financial support from the Bankard Fund for Political Economy at the University of Virginia and the Institution for Social and Policy Studies (ISPS) at Yale University.

We also wish to express our gratitude to the following academic institutions: the Frank Batten School of Leadership and Public Policy at the University of Virginia, the Watson Institute for International and Public Affairs at Brown University, ISPS and the Center for the Study of American Politics at Yale University, and the College of Liberal Arts at the University of Mississippi. We especially thank David Breneman, John Bruce, Jacob Hacker, Harry Harding, Chris Ruhm, Wendy Schiller, Ed Steinfeld, and Craig Volden for creating stimulating and supportive environments in which to conduct our writing and research.

At Princeton University Press, we thank the two outstanding senior editors we worked with. Charles Myers helped us with the project's initial framing. And Eric Crahan, our primary editor during the book's writing and completion, has been a consistent source of insight, wisdom, and sound advice. We thank Ellen Foos for managing production, Kathleen Kageff for copyediting, and Steven Moore for preparing the index.

An earlier version of chapter 2 appeared as Alan S. Gerber and Eric M. Patashnik, "Sham Surgery: The Problem of Inadequate Medical Evidence," in *Promoting the General Welfare: New Perspectives on Government Performance*, edited by Alan S. Gerber and Eric M. Patashnik (Washington, DC: Brookings Institution Press, 2006): 43–73. Chapter 3 draws on earlier versions of the following articles: Alan S. Gerber, Eric M. Patashnik, David Doherty, and Conor Dowling, "Doctor Knows Best: Physician Endorsements, Public Opinion, and the Politics of Comparative Effectiveness Research," *Journal of Health Politics, Policy and Law* 39 (1): 171–208; Alan S. Gerber, Eric M. Patashnik, David Doherty, and Conor Dowling, "The Public Wants Information, Not Board Mandates, From Comparative Effectiveness Research," *Health Affairs* 29 (10): 1872–81; Alan S. Gerber, Eric M. Patashnik, David Doherty, and Conor Dowling, "A National Survey Reveals Public Skepticism about Research-Based Treatment Guidelines," *Health Affairs* 29 (10): 1882–84. Chapters 5 and 6 draw on earlier versions of Alan S. Gerber and Eric M. Patashnik, "Problem Solving in a Polarized Age: Comparative Effectiveness Research and the Politicization of Evidence-Based Medicine," *Forum* 8 (1): Article 3; Alan S. Gerber and Eric M. Patashnik, "The Politicization of Evidence-Based Medicine: The Limits of Pragmatic Problem Solving in an Era of Polarization," *California Journal of Politics and Policy* 3 (4): Article 4.

Finally, we wish to thank our family members for their love and support: Debbie Gordon and Michael and Josh Patashnik; Rachel, Eva, Miriam, Ben, and Helen Gerber; and Carey, Larkin, and Anorah Bernini Dowling.

UNHEALTHY POLITICS

Introduction

In 2002, the *New England Journal of Medicine* reported that a common operation, performed on millions of Americans suffering from osteoarthritis of the knee, "worked no better than a sham procedure in which patients were sedated" while a surgeon merely "pretended to operate."[1] The patients who underwent the real surgery got better. They had less pain and could climb stairs more easily. But the patients who received the fake surgery experienced *just as much* pain relief and improvement in joint function as those who had undergone the real operation. In sum, the benefits of the procedure were a product of the placebo effect. Leading experts stated that 80–90 percent of these procedures should not be done.[2]

We were stunned when we learned about the sham surgery study. We assumed that hard evidence *must* have existed for the knee operation's medical benefits. To our surprise, it did not. We carefully reviewed the medical literature and found that claims for the efficacy of the procedure rested on studies with weak research designs and that the theory behind the surgery was speculative at best.[3] Yet the dearth of evidence and lack of an accepted causal mechanism to explain the procedure's purported effects did not prevent the operation from diffusing widely into practice. "There's a pretty good-sized industry out there that is performing this surgery," Dr. David T. Felson of Boston University said. "It constitutes a good part of the livelihood of some orthopedic surgeons. That is a reality."[4]

The knee surgery case is not an aberration. Some experts believe that less than half the medical care in the United States is based on or supported by evidence of its effectiveness.[5] As leading health services experts Carol M. Ashton and Nelda P. Wray write,

The goal of every treatment is to make the patient's outcome better than it would have been without any intervention. Because of advances in research in the past six or so decades, clinical scientists are able to estimate with considerable precision whether a particular intervention will lead to net benefit over harm in groups of individuals possessing certain characteristics. That said, much of clinical practice lacks a supporting evidence base, and what research evidence exists is predominately of poor quality.[6]

Procedures and tests are regularly prescribed on the basis of limited scientific information.[7] Once doctors decide that a particular treatment "works," it can become "locked in." Randomized controlled trials—the "gold standard" for determining the effects of a treatment—are almost impossible to carry out on a treatment that has already diffused into practice.[8] It is common for patients in one geographic area or region to receive different medical interventions than patients with the exact same condition in another part of the country, without a reliable mechanism to learn which approaches are best and translate this discovery to patients and clinicians.[9] And when solid scientific evidence *does* emerge about the benefits and risks of a treatment, the informational uptake often proceeds slowly. Studies have found that more than a decade can pass before the evidence alters clinical practice.[10]

It is unsettling to find out that widely used treatments and tests rest on little or no evidence. Even more troubling is learning that this situation is an open secret among health care experts. Recognition of the "medical guesswork" problem (together with growing awareness of geographic variation in utilization and medical spending) has prompted calls for rationalization of health care delivery for decades. These issues have been the subject of government reports, articles in leading newspapers, and cover stories in popular magazines, such as *Businessweek*.[11]

To its credit, the Obama administration—along with prominent Republican health policy experts—recognized the benefits for patients, payers, and providers of moving toward a more evidence-based medical system. The Affordable Care Act (ACA; "Obamacare") launched a new, independent, nongovernment entity—the Patient-Centered Outcomes Research Institute (PCORI)—to fund and disseminate research on the comparative effectiveness of different interventions to prevent, diagnose, treat, and monitor health conditions. Comparative effectiveness research (CER) compares two or more health care interventions, such as a drug, diagnostic test, or surgical procedure, to determine which interventions work best for which patients. CER is distinct from cost-effectiveness analysis, which examines medical interventions through an economic lens. Cost-effective analysis asks how much an intervention costs, and whether the outcomes it produces are worth its cost.[12]

The overall mission of PCORI is to help people make informed health care decisions, and improve outcomes, by "producing and promoting high-integrity, evidence-based information that comes from research guided by patients, caregivers, and the broader healthcare community."[13] Following a contentious debate in which critics charged that CER would lead to rationing and "death panels," Congress established a narrow medical research program that left existing patterns of therapeutic authority and health care financing largely untouched. In contrast to publicly funded comparative effectiveness and health technology assessment entities found in other advanced democracies, including Australia, Germany, France, and the United Kingdom, which have linkages to policy-making bodies, PCORI's research findings may not include "practice guidelines, coverage recommendations, payment, or policy recommendations."[14] In addition, PCORI's research is not required to consider whether an intervention is cost effective.[15]

Despite its narrow research mission, PCORI has been mired in controversy. Its funding expires in 2019, and it is not clear that the entity will win congressional reauthorization. If PCORI does not survive, its death will follow a long line of failed reform initiatives. Past federal efforts to promote evidence-based practices through medical research and clinical guideline development have crumbled under pressure from doctors, drug companies, and the medical device industry.[16] Yet even if Congress unravels the insurance subsidies and Medicaid expansion under the Affordable Care Act and the United States shifts to greater reliance on an individualized system of health savings accounts, there will still be a pressing need for public funding of CER. Health markets cannot function efficiently if physicians and patients lack reliable information about the comparative effectiveness of treatment options, and the market cannot be counted on to generate the optimal level of this information without public subsidy. In sum, government has a role to play in generating evidence about what works in medicine irrespective of the organization and financing of the insurance system. We discuss the future prospects of the evidence-based medicine movement in the concluding chapter. For now, it is fair to say that PCORI has not had a major impact. The agency did not transform the everyday practice of medicine, build a durable base of political support, or solve the systemic problems we describe. All this is unsurprising given PCORI's limited power and the restrictions placed on Medicare to not consider cost and cost-effectiveness in its coverage decisions, but it is a failure of governance just the same.

Why Evidence-Based Medicine Is Important

The sluggish incorporation of medical evidence into clinical practice is a concern for three key reasons—safety, quality, and the efficiency of resource allocation. First, the delivery of unproven care can expose patients to serious risks. For example, each year 100,000 Americans undergo a painful procedure called vertebroplasty, in which their collapsed vertebras are filled with bone cement, even though according to two *New England Journal of Medicine* studies there is no clear answer to the question of whether the procedure works better than physical therapy, injections of local anesthetic, or simply just waiting to heal.[17] Second, the slow integration of evidence can lead to suboptimal outcomes for patients who receive treatments that work less well for their conditions than alternatives. Third, the failure to implement evidence-based practices encourages wasteful spending, causing the health care system to underperform relative to its level of investment. While the drive to root out inefficiency is unlikely to stir the passions of ordinary citizens, it is a key to a health care system's long-run performance.

Evidence-based medicine is also related to cost containment, but the two are not synonymous. First, better use of evidence can and should sometimes lead to *more* spending, not less. A 2003 Rand Institute study found that Americans receive just half of the recommended care for a range of medical conditions.[18] Also, the delivery of low-value care, while certainly wasteful and expensive, is not the only reason why the United States spends far more on health care than do other advanced nations. The United States also has much higher service prices and administrative costs than do other rich nations.[19]

Yet the utilization of services—that is, the amount of care delivered to patients—is still important to cost containment, especially in the Medicare program. There are two basic strategies for taming health care costs—limit how much providers can charge (control prices) or reduce the amount of low-value care (control utilization). Researchers at Dartmouth College, following the pioneering work by John E. Wennberg and Alan Gittelsohn on geographical variations in health care delivery,[20] have found more than a twofold variation in per capita Medicare spending in different regions of the country. The main driver of these regional differences in Medicare spending is not differences in poverty rates, the relative illness of patients, or differences in how much Medicare pays for services, but rather variation in *utilization*.[21] Hospitals that give more tests and treatments to their Medicare patients do not achieve consistently better outcomes than those that deliver fewer services.[22] However, spending more on *effective* treatments does produce better results, and higher quality hospitals do tend to have higher market shares and expand more over time.[23] Reducing the overuse of low-value treatments by patients over 65 could help control Medicare spending growth and federal budget deficits.

The situation is different for patients outside Medicare who obtain insurance from their employers. While Medicare uses its authority to regulate prices for hospitals, employer-sponsored plans generally pay more variable (and higher) prices than the government does. For example, hospital prices for lower-limb MRIs vary by a factor of twelve across the nation.[24] In under-65 commercial markets, prices, not utilization, are thus the driver of variations in spending levels across hospital regions.[25]

Yet there are still huge variations in utilization in under-65 private insurance markets.[26] Indeed, the correlation between what doctors do for their under-65 patients and their elderly Medicare patients is remarkably high. That is, regional utilization patterns in Medicare provide a strong predictor of utilization rates in the private insurance population.[27] To be sure, reducing unwarranted variation in treatment decisions by promoting evidence-based practices would not by itself solve the overall cost problems in American health care. It would, however, significantly improve the quality, safety and efficiency of service delivery. This is too huge an opportunity to miss.

Our Approach

Our argument blends policy analysis and political science. Our comparative advantage is to use political science methods and concepts to generate fresh answers to questions that mostly have occupied economists and health services researchers. We seek to identify the forces that sustain a political equilibrium characterized by widespread utilization of tests and treatments that are unproven and possibly useless, or, at best, produce low value for the money spent on them. In sum, we identify, analyze, and document a major national problem and ask why the solutions to this problem are not being designed, advocated for, and vigorously implemented.

The U.S. health care system is a vast topic. If we attempt to explore every facet of institutional performance, and investigate every actor who participates in the production, delivery, financing, and regulation of U.S. medical care, we will lose the forest for the trees. To keep our eyes on the fundamentals, our analysis focuses on a single performance indicator: whether credible scientific information is available on the comparative clinical effectiveness of alternative interventions, meaning evidence on what tests, treatments, and procedures work best for groups of patients with different conditions, and whether such information informs the decisions of patients, providers, and payers. In sum, our concern is whether the delivery of medical care in the United States is *evidence based*.

Evidence-based medicine (EBM) has been defined as "the conscientious, explicit, and judicious use of current best evidence in making decisions about the care of individual patients."[28] The aim of the EBM movement is to "evaluate the safety, effectiveness, and cost of medical practices using tools from science and social science and to base clinical practice on such knowledge."[29] There is sufficient consensus among medical experts to make the implementation of EBM a reasonable baseline expectation. As the National Academy of Medicine (formerly the Institute of Medicine) summarizes its work on developing the infrastructure required for CER, "Evidence is the cornerstone of a high-performing healthcare system."[30]

To be sure, there are limits to the extent to which evidence can guide the activities of actors within the health care system. There are large uncertainties in medicine, and, as we discuss, the quest for applying standardized forms of evidence to individual treatment circumstances is viewed with great suspicion by both clinicians and the public. They are not always wrong to be skeptical. Sometimes industry funding compromises the objectivity of medical studies, and research questions can be distorted by unexamined cultural biases.[31] Even if the scientific quality of research studies were assured and the production of medical evidence were much enhanced, there would still be important limits to the application of generalized rules to particular circumstances. A great deal of medical care consists of patients insisting on help when the correct pathways are not obvious.[32] In many instances, patients have different reactions to drugs or other treatments in the same class (for example, psychiatric or hypertensive drugs), and the treatment that fares best on average is not necessarily the best for the individual patient.[33] In short, there is tremendous value to having physicians who know their patients well, even if (as we argue) physician discretion is commonly exercised in ways that lack scientific grounding.[34]

In sum, we are not simplistically advocating for rule-following behavior. As Mark Schlesinger and Bradford H. Gray argue, clinical practice needs to strike a careful balance between *generalized expertise* (understanding the evidence generated though scientific research) and *particularized expertise* (applying that evidence to individual patients).[35] Our starting point, however, is that by systematically ignoring scientific evidence (or the lack thereof), the United States is *substantially* out of balance.[36] As we discuss in chapter 1, a significant fraction of the medicine that Americans consume is based on minimal scientific evidence about its comparative effectiveness. Many treatments offer only minor benefit over alternatives—and some are useless. As physician Atul Gawande wrote in the *New Yorker*: "Millions of people are receiving drugs that aren't helping them, operations that aren't going to make them better, and scans and tests that do nothing beneficial for them, and often cause harm."[37] In a national survey of primary care physicians, nearly one-half said their patients received too much medical care.[38] Overutilization does not apply to all Americans, and some patients are clearly harmed by receiving too few effective treatments.[39] By all accounts, the failure of physicians to practice evidence-based medicine is a serious problem in the United States, as it is in many other nations.

By having prevalent treatments that are inefficacious or even cause harm, patients are diverted away from other treatments that are actually effective. The United States can certainly "afford" to spend a fifth or more of national income on health care if its citizens wish to do so—but there are trade-offs. Spending money on useless (or low-value) treatments reduces the money available to spend on effective cures,[40] or on valuable social investments in education, worker training, and infrastructure. If the nation does not evaluate the comparative effectiveness of treatment alternatives to help reduce waste and improve quality, and if such evidence does not affect clinical or policy decisions, it suggests that the defects of our institutions are *first-order* concerns, not minor flaws in an otherwise high-performing system.

The failure of the American political system to represent the diffuse public interest in the generation and use of medical evidence is a political economy puzzle. Given the high level of U.S. health care spending, and the desire of patients to receive the best therapies, we must understand how a democratic political system can produce inefficient outcomes year in and year out without triggering an effective response. While existing research provides many insights, new perspectives are needed.

The political scientist James Q. Wilson noted that policies with diffuse benefits and concentrated costs are unlikely to be passed without the presence of a "political entrepreneur" who can mobilize latent public support.[41]

A policy to promote the generation and use of medical evidence to improve clinical practice and resource allocation decisions is clearly an instance of diffuse benefits and concentrated costs: the public (and taxpayers) would gain from the policy, and drug companies and medical device makers who profit from expensive but ineffective products would lose. Our work builds on Wilson's framework in two ways. First, using a survey experiment, we demonstrate the risks to members of Congress who would consider becoming a political entrepreneur in this area, showing that there are few electoral benefits to be gained. Second, we focus attention on the important mediating role of the medical profession. The professions do not play a prominent role in Wilson's theory of general-interest policy making, but we believe they should be on center stage. The Progressive tradition in America has long believed in the positive role of the professions to bring scientific knowledge and expertise to bear on societal problems and improve all collective endeavors.[42] One would hope that the concentrated interest of the medical profession in preserving its prestige and autonomy would make it a natural supporter of evidence-based medicine both to check the influence of concentrated interests such as insurers, hospitals, and drug companies and to preserve doctors' hard-earned reputation as uniquely trusted guardians of patient welfare. But as we show in chapter 2, many medical societies support evidence-based medicine in the abstract but oppose research that challenges treatments in their practice areas.

Every policy system consists of pressures pushing to maintain and challenge the status quo,[43] but there is no guarantee that the two sets of forces will be equally matched. In U.S. health policy, the forces supporting overutilization, unwarranted variation in utilization, and the suboptimal use of medical evidence to improve quality and efficiency appear as strong or stronger than the forces pushing for reform. One important force maintaining the status quo is the political influence of drug and medical device companies.

The pharmaceutical and health products industry is consistently near the top when it comes to federal campaign contributions. During the 2014 election cycle, for example, the Pfizer company contributed over $1.5 million to federal candidates, Amgen gave more than $1.3 million, and McKesson more than $1.1 million. The industry trade group Pharmaceutical Research and Manufacturers of America (PhRMA) spent over $16 million on lobbying in 2014.[44] The industry's goals include ensuring quicker approval of drugs and products entering the market. As we detail in chapter 6, the medical products industry's influence affected the organizational design of the PCORI. Recently, a top industry priority has been passage of the 21st Century Cures Act, which (besides increasing funding for research on cancer and other diseases) would permit manufacturers to submit real-world evidence to the FDA for approval of new drugs and devices and for new indications for existing products, including observational data arising from routine clinical use, rather than data from randomized controlled trials.[45] The intention is to expedite the product approval process, but some observers point out that changing the FDA's traditional standards of evidence may have "an unpredictable long-term effect on drug safety and efficacy."[46] Finally, pharmaceutical and health technology companies not only seek to influence the regulatory environment, but they also spend billions of dollars annually on marketing to both doctors and consumers. The pharmaceutical industry is a major presence at the meetings of many medical associations, and drug company representatives often seek to build personal relationships with physicians to influence clinical decisions.[47]

In short, there is tremendous pressure from powerful economic actors to maintain the health care status quo. Eliminating a dollar of waste in the health care system usually means reducing someone's income.[48] The distinctive values of the United States constitute a second force for conservatism in the health care system. As medical ethicist Daniel Callahan writes, "American health care is radically American: individualistic, scientifically ambitious, market intoxicated, suspicious of government, and profit-driven."[49] These values contribute to a political unease with explicit limits on the consumption or supply of medical technology.

Our focus in this book is not on the deep-seated economic and cultural forces sustaining the status quo. Rather, we explore why there is relatively little *opposing* pressure for meaningful reform to promote quality and evidence-based medicine, for it is the relative weakness of countervailing reform pressures, *together* with the strength of existing norms and practices, that generates the inefficient outcomes that patients, payers, and providers actually experience. To be sure, any effort to explain a "dog that doesn't bark" must be somewhat speculative. By drawing on political science models, surveys, survey experiments, case studies, and analysis of policy history, however, we hope to generate insights into why this "unhealthy politics" persists.

Rather than provide a full account of the gap between what needs to be done and what is actually happening, we investigate the incentives and behavior of just three sets of actors: physicians, politicians, and the public. Our objective is to explain how these actors interact to produce a stable system that generates large amounts of waste as a by-product, and more generally, to advance an understanding of the conditions under which a democratic polity can sustain grossly inefficient sectors seemingly indefinitely.

Our approach is somewhat selective and incomplete. As important as it is, we do not provide a detailed analysis of the antireform (medical products industry) side of the equation. Instead, we focus on how political incentives conspire to keep proreform forces relatively weak. While the importance of physicians, politicians, and the public has been recognized in existing scholarship,[50] the desire of many scholars to offer comprehensive accounts of health politics and policy have sometimes caused them to get lost in the shuffle. Our distinctive contribution is to place the actions and interaction of these actors on center stage, and to explain why reform pressures can be anemic even when the potential for social progress is great.[51]

A Preview of Our Argument

This book explores the roles of physicians, the public, and politicians in the nation's failure to take the steps necessary to promote a high-performing, evidence-based health delivery system. We focus on doctors because their beliefs always mediate (and often determine) what treatments patients receive, because the system cannot be reformed without their leadership, and because the scope and implications of the medical profession's power, despite important research on the topic,[52] has not been fully explored in the literature. We focus on the public because improving patient welfare is the objective of the medical system and because ordinary citizens influence Medicare policy making through their roles as taxpayers and voters. Finally, we examine the role of elected officials because Medicare and other government health programs shape the overall context in which medical services are funded and delivered, and government can support EBM through rules or incentives.

The delegation of authority to the medical profession rests on an implicit social contract: Doctors as a profession receive the "privilege of self-regulation" and financial rewards on the expectation that they will serve the health needs of individual patients and society.[53] If the social contract between the medical profession and society is malfunctioning, politicians need to repair it. But can they do so? *Unhealthy Politics* investigates how political forces undermine the reform of medical governance.[54]

THE MEDICAL PROFESSION: THE REPOSITORY
OF TRUST AND AUTHORITY

There is no doubt that American physicians today face much stronger external pressures than they did in the past. Their clinical decisions are routinely reviewed and sometimes questioned by third parties, and they have to justify their actions with a lot more paperwork. It is undoubtedly more stressful to be the typical doctor today than it was to be a typical physician in the 1950s.

Nonetheless, the argument that the political and economic power of physicians has eroded is arguably overstated.[55] Most U.S. doctors enjoy a relatively high degree of professional autonomy in practice as a result of the dilution of strong utilization management controls following the backlash to managed care.[56] Although insurers today may require prior authorization for certain therapies, they typically defer to physicians' judgments about what treatments are medically necessary, even if the treatments are not supported by rigorous evidence.[57] Off-label usage of treatments is commonplace. Moreover, efforts by insurers to deny reimbursement of questionable or unproven interventions have sometimes been overturned by courts.[58] As we discuss later in the book, the views of doctors and medical societies are prominent when public controversies arise over the interpretation of research studies indicating that tests or treatments are not as effective as believed. And, as health policy scholar Miriam Laugesen observes, doctors retain enormous influence in technical, low-visibility venues, such as in the panels that make reimbursement and coverage decisions under the Medicare program.[59]

Why does society delegate so much authority to the medical profession? One answer is that it represents a sensible response to "market failure." Knowledge about treatment effects is esoteric and asymmetrically distributed between doctors and patients.[60] It is often impossible for the patient (even in the Internet age) to know what treatments he or she needs. Society is better off by hiring well-trained experts to prescribe therapies and shape payment rates. The sociologist Talcott Parsons held the professions in high regard, characterizing the autonomy and privileges of the professions as a "functional exchange in which society receives, in exchange, the technical competence it needs to achieve critical ends."[61] The "social trustee" model of the professions, however, has been strongly challenged.[62] In his important book *Profession of Medicine*, Eliot Freidson argues that the social authority of organized medicine is in fact a "political commodity."[63] It was not earned as a reward for social responsibility, but rather won through political contestation and negotiation.[64] How physicians use their autonomy and privileges is thus a key issue for democratic accountability.

Some physicians and health care experts argue that the implied social contract is that physicians not only will be competent technical experts, but will also ensure an appropriate distribution of finite medical resources.[65] As the American Board of Internal Medicine (ABIM) states in its physician charter,

> Professionalism is the basis of medicine's contract with society. . . . While meeting the needs of individual patients, physicians are required to provide health care that is based on the wise and cost effective management of limited clinical resources. They should be committed to working with other physicians, hospitals, and payers to develop guidelines for cost effective care. The physician's professional responsibility for appropriate allocation of resources requires scrupulous avoidance of superfluous tests and procedures. The provision of unnecessary services not only exposes one's patients to avoidable harm and expense but also diminishes the resources available for others.[66]

However, there is always a risk that professional associations, from lawyers to professors, will begin to defend the interests of its members in addition to serving the public. The concern is that governing institutions may lack the monitoring and enforcement capacity to prevent the medical profession from abusing its delegated authority to serve its own interests. If doctors do not follow evidence-based guidelines or if medical societies use their power to discredit credible studies demonstrating that a particular treatment is not as effective as advertised, medical professionalism and self-regulation becomes a myth.

The design of the Medicare Act of 1965—the foundational statute of the U.S. health care system—crystallizes the dilemma. Medicare was created in the teeth of fierce opposition from the AMA and other medical societies.[67] As political scientist Mark A. Peterson observes, "Even in 'defeat,' however, the physicians were influential enough to dictate . . . the method of reimbursement and administration under the program, demand enhancing policies and subsidies and constraints on potentially competing providers."[68]

The nation essentially committed to funding seniors' care without government scrutiny of the details and appropriateness of medical practices, which were left to physicians to determine. Medicare is permitted to exclude coverage for care that is "not reasonable and necessary for the diagnosis or treatment of illness or injury." Attempts by Medicare administrators to read this as a requirement for cost-effectiveness have generated intense opposition from provider groups and ended in stalemate.[69] In practice, billions of dollars of tax revenue flow into Medicare without the technology supply constraints or drug price controls common in European nations. The program generated vested interests and dense networks of organizations that developed material stakes in the maintenance of existing arrangements.[70] As University of Michigan law professor Nicholas Bagley writes,

> The basic contours of the [Medicare] program—public financing, private care—were fixed in 1965. Beneficiaries grew accustomed to subsidized coverage without meaningful restrictions, and physicians, hospitals, and other providers committed themselves to the new world order in which the government would pay the bills but assert no control.[71]

To be sure, Congress has taken some steps to control Medicare spending by reducing payments to providers.[72] For example, Congress has adopted a prospective payment schedule for hospitals and a fee schedule for physicians.[73] Since 1965, however, Congress has avoided efforts to control the volume or intensity of services, creating incentives for overutilization.[74] The ACA continues this long-standing pattern. While the ACA contained a number of new financial reforms, such as accountable care organizations and bundled payments, it steered clear of reconfiguring medical governance. Medicare's failure to incorporate a cost-effectiveness—or even comparative clinical effectiveness—requirement has far-reaching implications, as many commercial insurers follow Medicare's coverage policies.[75] In sum, policy makers have layered moderate cost-control measures atop, but have not eliminated, the preexisting Medicare governance framework.[76]

Doctors remain highly influential actors in the American health system despite far-reaching changes in the economic and organizational context in which medicine is practiced; their individual and collective authority over clinical decisions, as well as resource allocation, by no means goes unchallenged, but it remains quite significant. This is not to deny that there are influential reform forces *within* the medical profession. Like progressive reformers at the turn of the twentieth century who sought to expose the chaos, inefficiency, and corruption of medical practices and promote improvements in medical education and scientific therapeutics,[77] some medical societies, leading doctors and public intellectuals such as Atul Gawande and Jerry Avorn of Harvard Medical School, among many others, are seeking to raise awareness of industry influence and the failure of many doctors to follow best medical practices. A genuine EBM movement exists today.

Nonetheless, progress has been slow, uneven, and reversible. In sum, physicians still hold a position of trust and authority, even as concerns about the scientific foundation, quality, and waste of medical services have mounted.

THE PUBLIC: MISPERCEPTIONS AND INDIFFERENCE

The public is the second key actor in our analysis. Although Americans' confidence in the medical profession has fallen over time—in tandem with the decline in public confidence in most public institutions since the 1960s—doctors remain a highly trusted group within the context of American politics. People regard their doctors as knowledgeable and trustworthy agents of their own medical care and welfare, and this trust extends to matters of health policy as well.[78]

The catch, as the distinguished medical sociologist David Mechanic writes, is that "patients may trust blindly when some skepticism is warranted."[79] There are two potential sources of public misperceptions that can lead to excessive faith in physicians. First, the public may fail to recognize that medical societies are, at bottom, trade associations. If viewed as trade associations, the primary function of medical societies would be to protect the autonomy and advance the interests of their members. One can certainly find heartening examples of efforts by medical societies to improve the quality and cost-effectiveness of care. For example, several national medical societies have recently launched a campaign called "Choosing Wisely," which highlights diagnostic tests, procedures, and treatments in their respective specialty areas that do patients little good.[80] However, medical societies participating in this effort are mostly choosing low-hanging fruit. For example, the American Academy of Orthopaedic Surgeons includes an over-the-counter supplement but no major procedures on its list.[81] The initiative also lacks an enforcement mechanism; doctors remain free to ignore the recommendations if they wish. A *JAMA Internal Medicine* study suggests that the initiative has had disappointing results thus far.[82] In short, the record of medical societies is so replete with failures of self-governance that it is reasonable to raise doubts about the centrality of their commitment to eliminating ineffective or low-value care.

Back in the 1990s, for example, the Agency for Health Care Policy and Research (AHCPR) was launched to provide evidence-based clinical guidelines that would help physicians determine which treatments are most effective. When the agency found that there was little objective evidence to support surgery as a first-line treatment for lower back pain, however, back surgeon societies complained vehemently to members of Congress. As Bradford H. Gray, Michael K. Gusmano, and Sarah R. Collins observe in an insightful study of the politics of health services research, the agency's budget was slashed, and its authority to make policy recommendations was curtailed.[83] The drawing of negative messages from the AHCPR experience helps explain PCORI's limited grant of authority. Many similar examples of medical societies reacting strongly to negative study results and being unwilling to change in the face of evidence could be cited.[84] These medical society activities fall below the radar screen for most citizens. The psychological bonds that ordinary citizens develop with their personal doctors inhibit the public from recognizing the governance role that the medical profession plays in the health system. There is a tendency for people to assume that an organization's collective behavior can be predicted on the basis of the character or behavior of the people they know who belong to the organization, and in our personal experience many doctors are truly extraordinary individuals.

The second misperception of the medical profession is subtler. The public may not perceive the existence of gaps between, on the one hand, the medical profession's evolving responsibilities to patients and society, and, on the other, its willingness and capacity to fulfill those responsibilities. Such gaps may open whenever changes in the profession's behavior and orientation fail to keep pace with changes in the wider context in which medical care is delivered. Over the past half century, there has been an explosion of scientific knowledge about health and disease, and health spending has grown dramatically as a share of the economy. These twin developments create new professional obligations for doctors under the terms of the evolving social contract. As David Blumenthal, M.D., stated in his address to the 2014 Columbia University College of Physicians and Surgeons graduation ceremony, these developments challenge doctors to "stay informed and current" as well as to "husband health care resources—to become a steward of the health care dollar—in ways never before required."[85] But it is not clear that the medical profession is developing the capacity to respond effectively to these scientific and economic challenges. Most doctors have not received extensive training in the modern research methods or the data analysis skills needed to keep up with scientific literatures on the relative benefits, costs, and risks of treatments. Yet without such training, it is difficult for doctors to make recommendations about what is best for patients. And despite concerns about the rising cost of both private insurance and public programs like Medicare, a recent physician survey found that only about a third of physicians believe they bear a major responsibility to control health care costs.[86]

(Doctors blamed rising health care costs on lawyers, insurance companies, drug and device manufacturers, hospitals, and patients.) This is a denial of the profession's collective responsibility to society, but one the public—reasoning from their positive encounters with their personal doctors—may not perceive.

In sum, previous research has argued that the public shifts its individualized trust in doctors to trust in medical societies, which has allowed the medical profession to block the drive for a universal government insurance program during the postwar era and obtain favorable financial terms when Medicare finally passed in 1965.[87] *Unhealthy Politics* considers the possibility that the consequences of Americans' trust in the medical profession are broader and even more concerning. Despite their position as a repository of public trust in a complicated policy area, doctors and their professional societies have not consistently used their authority, standing, and prestige to promote the steps necessary to root out waste, bad science, and inefficiencies in the health care system—and too often have used their political capital to fight these steps.

POLITICIANS: THE WEAK INCENTIVES FOR POLITICAL ENTREPRENEURSHIP AND CONSENSUAL PROBLEM SOLVING

Finally, we explore how politicians themselves have contributed to the persistence of the medical evidence problem. Our analysis has implications not only for an understanding of the roots of the resistance to the implementation of evidence-based medicine, but also for a more general understanding of how inefficient practices can persist in the American democratic polity. Our argument focuses on political failures at two stages: agenda setting and decision making.

The American political system is often claimed to have properties of self-correction. When governance veers dramatically off course, and the preferences of citizens are not being met, opportunities may arise for creative political entrepreneurs to frame problems, develop solutions, and "sell" their ideas to the public—to capture a political reward.[88] Yet there is no guarantee that the need for political entrepreneurship will generate its own supply. The medical evidence problem has prompted only limited investments of political entrepreneurship from members of Congress, despite the substantial costs the problem imposes on society. If the supply of entrepreneurial problem solving is too low even in a sector as important and salient as health care, it is likely to be inadequate in other sectors as well.

We develop a theory of "*zero-credit politics*" to explain the undersupply of political entrepreneurship targeted at promoting diffuse interests.[89] The incentive for lawmakers to engage in entrepreneurial activities to address a national problem may be especially weak when challenges to the policy status quo would threaten not just the incomes of business groups (such as the medical products industry) but also the autonomy and authority of trusted professionals, such as doctors. It may be an uphill battle for the political entrepreneur to convince the public that its understanding of reality is mistaken and that reform is warranted; the entrepreneur could decide to take his or her creative energy elsewhere, where there is more likelihood that such effort will be rewarded. This is not to say that there will be literally zero entrepreneurial investment in solving the problem, but that reelection incentives will induce much too little effort *relative* to the magnitude of the problem, because the risk to a reelection-minded politician of being seen as challenging doctors is too great.

A second source of failure occurs at the decision-making stage. As the political scientist Donald E. Stokes argues, policy issues typically come in two generic forms: position issues—on which voters hold conflicting preferences, such as whether taxes on the wealthy are too low—and valence issues—on which voters hold common preferences, such as whether the government should promote prosperity or fight corruption.[90] When valence issues are on the decision agenda, the electoral stakes are extremely high. No political party can afford to be seen as the "antigrowth" or "procorruption" party. In an idealized democracy, the positions of the two parties will tend to converge on such issues, and the government will make decisions that voters support. As Congress expert Frances E. Lee argues, however, in an era of partisan polarization and persistently close electoral competition, there can be strong incentives for the out party to behave strategically and block progress on what could be consensual, good government issues.[91] One tactic the minority party can use is to transform a valence issue into a position issue, creating a partisan or ideological squabble where none had previously existed by reframing efficiency into a debate about the size and role of government. While this is not an entirely new dynamic in American politics, it has become a more common one in the modern era.

And this is in fact precisely what occurred during the debate over the Obama administration's effort to identify low-value medical treatments through an investment in CER. The Obama administration was not the first to highlight the medical evidence problem. Medicare administrators in the George H. W. Bush and George W. Bush administrations, for example, had also pointed out that a large share of medical spending is wasteful and not based on sound science. One might have expected fiscal conservatives to complement the Obama administration's support for CER, since Republican health care leaders had endorsed the CER concept in the past as a way to curb wasteful spending, not to expand government's role.

But the fierce ideological competition between the two parties over the expansion of health insurance under Obamacare undermined the incentives for bipartisan technocratic consensus on "good government" reforms like CER.[92] (One Republican congressional staff member told us in an interview that Republican support for CER was a casualty of the partisan "knife fight" over the ACA; in the middle of the knife fight, he said, you don't pause to tell your opponent that you like his shirt.) The Republican Study Committee sent out an alert stating that the purpose of the initiative was to let the government ration care. To an anxious public, CER was linked with two other contentious proposals then under consideration: voluntary counseling for Medicare patients about living wills, advance directives, and other end-of-life care; and the creation of an independent commission (Independent Payment Advisory Board, IPAB) with the power to recommend ways to achieve Medicare savings without cutting benefits. These three elements swirled around and combined in the public mind to give birth to the charge that Obama was seeking to create "death panels" for seniors. CER thus morphed into a symbol of rationing of medical services and bureaucratic interference with the doctor-patient relationship. In sum, conservatives turned a valence issue (using science to learn what works in medicine) into a position issue (the role of the federal government in health care delivery). As we show, the "devalencing" of an issue undermines pragmatic decision making and elite-led social learning in a sustained era of competitive balance between the parties and polarization.

Stimulating Conversations

In the space of a medium-size book, we cannot hope to answer all the questions we raise. We will be content if our analysis stimulates three conversations.

First, we hope to give health care experts a better understanding of the political forces that permit waste and bad science to persist in the medical system. Generating fresh insights by applying some of the ideas, habits of thought, and tools of political science to this familiar problem will help experts—including economists, health services researchers, and policy makers—craft recommendations that stand a better chance of both win-ning adoption and sticking after enactment.

Second, we wish to encourage other political scientists to devote more attention to the fundamental questions of who governs, and to what ends. As Terry Moe argues, political scientists should explore the power of vested interests of *all* kinds, including those that strategically hide their special inter-ests inside a public interest package.[93] With respect to the second question, political scientists typically use two criteria to analyze policy outcomes: the responsiveness of government to public opinion, and distributional fairness. These are very important evaluative dimensions, but they have limitations as benchmarks of government performance on complex scientific issues like the efficiency of health care. The public's opinions on such issues may be either uninformed,[94] or thoughtlessly derivative of the beliefs of policy elites.[95] Similarly, a focus on distribution may be appropriate when the government targets benefits or costs at particular groups, but it is less illuminating when government seeks to provide public goods to the citizenry as a whole.

Finally, we hope our analysis encourages reflection on the capacities and limitations of modern American government as a problem-solving in-stitution. U.S. politicians continue to promote technocratic problem solv-ing in many areas. For example, the biomedical research conducted by the National Institutes of Health helps to advance understanding of diseases and epidemics and has long drawn bipartisan support. Yet what is often overlooked is that the roles of science, expertise, and enlightened public opinion in governance are mediated by the power of interest groups and professional societies, the struggle for partisan control, and the dynamics of electoral competition. Our investigation of the uses and misuse of medical evidence shows how these factors can produce an "unhealthy politics" in which pragmatic problem solving in government is degraded.

In particular, our research encourages reexamination of the assumptions of the Progressive reform tradition that has provided an intellectual founda-tion for problem solving in the U.S.[96] At the core of this tradition is a belief in the importance of expertise and delegation of many complex tasks to the professions, including lawyers and engineers, but most prominently doc-tors. Relying on the professional ethics of doctors to self-regulate was an imperfect if understandable choice that has broader implications for how we understand delegation and the role of the professions in a democracy. Our analysis suggests that just as Congress checks the president, so elite professions—including scientists, physicians, university researchers, and policy analysts—need to monitor one another's performance to ensure the primacy of citizen welfare and a commitment to a rational allocation of societal resources. Our central claim is *not* that science and expertise alone can (or should) entirely drive policy making in a pluralistic society.[97] There will always be distributional battles over "who gets what" from government, and ideological debates over the appropriate role of the state. Yet a well-functioning policy state creates adequate incentives for problem-solving activities and ensures that elite groups who enjoy public trust, such as the medical profession, are democratically accountable and responsive to public needs. The amount of space for technocratic expertise and pragmatism in policy making is not simply a by-product of the technical complexity of a policy area;[98] rather it is shaped by the incentives created by the broader political environment. We explain why the politics in the U.S. health care sector is so unhealthy, and how shifts in the behavior of the medical profession and the design of political institutions can promote sustainable reform.

The Plan of the Book

Chapter 1 defines the "medical guesswork" problem and explains how the poor integration of evidence into clinical decision making harms the performance of the health care sector. Chapter 2 makes our argument more nuanced and concrete by presenting a detailed case study of the remarkable sham knee surgery case mentioned earlier. In chapter 3, we present the results of national public opinion surveys that illuminate how ordinary citizens think about the medical evidence problem. Chapter 4 explores the institutional roots of medical professionalism in the United States. We examine why the U.S. health care system delegates therapeutic authority to individual doctors and medical societies, with little centralized oversight in programs like Medicare. The chapter also presents findings from a national survey of physicians to gauge their views on the proper role of medical societies in medical evidence controversies.

In chapters 5 and 6, our focus turns to politicians. We explore the politics of EBM, exploring why the efforts to root out waste, bad science, and extractive behavior in health care have not engendered reliable support. Chapter 6 examines the politics of the Obama administration's effort to promote CER as the scientific foundation of health care quality improvements and cost control. In the concluding chapter, we take stock of the EBM reform project. We draw on lessons from the literature on U.S. state building to develop strategies to increase the durability of medical governance reform in contemporary American politics.

1

The Medical Guesswork Problem

The Centers for Disease Control (CDC), headquartered in Atlanta, is a national treasure. Staffed by a cadre of highly trained, dedicated professionals, the CDC protects the nation against dangerous health threats by detecting new germs as they spread around the globe, uncovering the most effective ways to combat disease, and disseminating new knowledge to physicians, policy makers and communities. The CDC sits alongside other crown jewels of America's medical system, including top private and nonprofit hospitals across the nation, such as Sloan Kettering. It is no wonder that the dominant impression is that the quality of American medical care is the best in the world—"a utopia of high-tech treatments, cutting-edge research, and expeditious and effective interventions."[1]

The best American medicine is indeed excellent, and the nation is unambiguously a world leader in some areas. Yet much of the care that patients receive is not particularly effective for their clinical conditions. Moreover, the United States spends *dramatically* more per capita on medical care than do other advanced democracies and does not consistently outperform peers on quality measures or health outcomes.[2]

For reasons that remain unclear, health care cost growth has moderated since 2002. Some experts suggest that possible explanations include "the rise in high-deductible insurance plans, state-level efforts to control Medicaid costs, and a general slowdown in the diffusion of new technology, particularly in the Medicare population."[3] Yet health care costs are projected to grow at GDP plus 1.2 percent over the next twenty years, a rate high enough to cause serious pain for taxpayers and workers.[4]

As figure 1.1 shows, in 2013 per capita spending on medical care in the United States (including out of pocket costs, insurance payments, and taxes to pay for health programs like Medicare) was $8,617—nearly double the Organisation for Economic Co-operation and Development (OECD) average. The United States is wealthier than other nations, so it would be expected to spend more on medical care. Yet the United States also spends substantially more than peer nations, even though we have fewer physicians (and fewer physician consultations) relative to the population than other nations.[5] This higher level of spending does not appear to produce consistently better results on health indicators such as life expectancy. To be sure, the United States has higher obesity and poverty rates than many European countries. But multivariate analysis that controls for income, environmental quality, and lifestyle across developed nations finds little connection between spending and health outcomes.[6] Some experts believe that the U.S. medical system is distinctively inefficient.[7] As economists Henry J. Aaron and Paul B. Ginsburg write, "Whatever the reason, it is hard to avoid the conclusion that the United States is buying less health than other nations do with its high outlays."[8]

It is critical to distinguish between the total benefits of greater health spending over time and the benefits of extra health spending at the margin. Over time, new technologies are developed, and some of them are associated with substantial improvements in health outcomes. For example, the mortality rate from cardiovascular disease has declined by more than 50 percent since 1950, at least partly because of the development of better ways to treat heart disease.[9] At any given moment, however, the knowledge about how to treat different conditions is fairly similar across developed countries. The key issues are "how much the technology is used and how much is paid for it. By comparison with other countries, the United States uses technology in lower value settings and pays more for the same care."[10] This pattern likely stems from a combination of factors, including the absence of overall budgetary limits and supply-side constraints on medical capital equipment.[11] In sum, all advanced democracies struggle with the cost and efficiency of health care delivery. However, the United States faces special challenges. Our financing and delivery systems are an unusually complex, decentralized, highly commercialized admixture of public and private plans that lack both the discipline of efficient markets and the authority of government control.

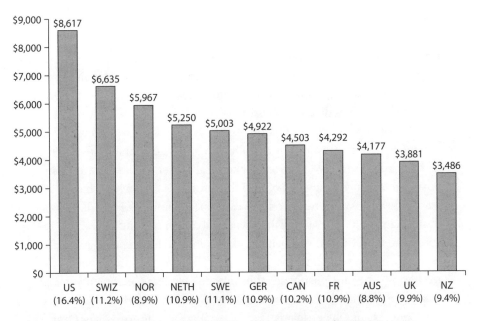

FIGURE 1.1. Health spending per capita (in US$) and as a percentage of GDP, 2013. *Source*: OECD Health expenditure and financing data (http://stats.oecd.org/Index.aspx ?DataSetCode=SHA).

Most experts agree that a substantial portion of the U.S. medical outlay is spent inefficiently, leading to little improvement in quality or outcomes. The Institute of Medicine estimates that as much as *one-third* of overall U.S. medical spending is wasted annually.[12] The United States spends $2.5 trillion annually in health care, so this corresponds to over $750 billion in waste each year—more than the budget for the Department of Defense.[13]

As health economist David Cutler argues, waste is marbled throughout the health delivery system, making it hard to cut out.[14] It comes in many forms, including excessive administrative costs, inflated prices, fraud, and—of especial concern in our analysis—overtreatment.[15] Overtreatment includes "care that is rooted in outmoded habits, that is driven by providers' preferences rather than those of informed patients, that ignores scientific findings, or that is motivated by something other than provision of optimal care for a patient."[16] According to some estimates, overtreatment added between $158 billion and $226 billion in wasteful spending in 2011.[17] No area of medicine is immune. Overtreatment exposes patients to treatments that offer little or no health benefits as well as potential harms. Sometimes entire classes of care are inappropriate, but overtreatment also arises when a given treatment is used more intensively than clinical conditions warrant. An example is using back surgery as a first-line therapy for patients with simple cases of back pain/discomfort who would benefit from much less invasive procedures, such as drugs or physical therapy.[18]

Consider this puzzling situation. According to a CDC study, every year about 60 percent of American women who have had a total hysterectomy and lack a cervix receive a Pap test for cervical cancer. While there are some posthysterectomy women who need to continue screening (such as those whose surgery was done to remove cancer), the number is small. As one obstetrician stated, "It's tough to get cervical cancer without a cervix."[19] According to the CDC, "the net benefits of screening some women, particularly women who have undergone hysterectomy . . . might be outweighed by the net harm (e.g., false-positive tests leading to needless patient anxiety and invasive procedures)."[20] The U.S. Preventive Services Task Force, the American Congress of Obstetricians and Gynecologists, and American Cancer Society all recommend against Pap tests for posthysterectomy women over the age of 30.[21] Yet despite the scientific consensus against routine screening for cervical cancer posthysterectomy, the proportion of women over 30 years of age who have had a hysterectomy and recently have been screened declined only 15 percentage points between 2002 and 2010 (figure 1.2).

Screening posthysterectomy women for cervical cancer points to a larger problem. Harvard Medical School researchers analyzed Medicare claims data, looking at 26 tests and procedures that empirical research has shown not to be beneficial for patients. They found that at least one in four—25 percent of—Medicare recipients received one or more of those services in 2009. The 26 services "are just a small sample of the hundreds of services that are known to provide little or no medical value to patients."[22] "We suspect this is just the tip of the iceberg," said study author J. Michael McWilliams.[23]

Millions of Americans receive antibiotics, MRIs, blood tests, diagnostic screenings, and surgeries they don't need.[24] Atul Gawande, a general surgeon who has been at the vanguard of the EBM movement, reports that he took a look at eight new patients who entered his clinic one afternoon. All had medical records complete enough to permit him to review their histories. Gawande found that seven of the eight had received unnecessary care. Two had expensive diagnostic tests of no value. A third patient had undergone a questionable surgery for a lump (which the surgery failed to remove).

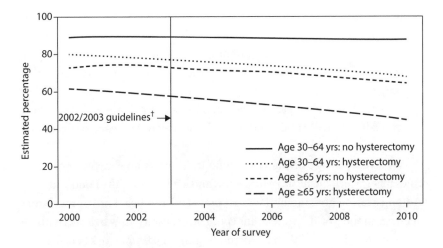

FIGURE 1.2. Percentage of women who had a recent Papanicolaou (Pap) test (within 3 years), by hysterectomy status and age group. Behavioral Risk Factor Surveillance System, United States, 2000–2010. *Note:* Even years only. All trends are statistically significant using linear test of trend [$p<0.05$]. Percentages are weighted to the noninstitutionalized, U.S. civilian population. [†]2002 American Cancer Society, 2003 American College of Obstetricians and Gynecologists, and 2003 U.S. Preventive Services task Force Pap test guidelines published. *Source*: Center for Disease Control and Prevention, 2013, "Cervical Cancer Screening among Women by Hysterectomy Status and among Women Aged ≥ 65 Years—United States, 2000–2010," *Morbidity and Mortality Weekly Report* 61 (51) (January 4): 1043–47, https://www.cdc.gov/mmwr/preview/mmwrhtml/mm6151a3.htm, accessed March 15, 2017.

Four patients "had undergone inappropriate arthroscopic knee surgery for chronic joint damage."[25] These results occurred at one of the most prestigious and sophisticated medical institutions in the world. All these unnecessary treatments not only increase costs, but they can also imperil health by exposing patients to a higher risk of side effects and medical errors.[26] "What's remarkable is how much we do with so little evidence to support what we do, especially when it comes to the patient right in front of us," said Harlan Krumholz, a cardiologist at Yale University.[27] As David Epstein wrote in an *Atlantic* magazine article, "When Evidence Says No, but Doctors Say Yes":

> For all the truly wondrous developments of modern medicine—imaging technologies that enable precision surgery, routine organ transplants, care that transforms premature infants into perfectly healthy kids, and remarkable chemotherapy treatments, to name a few—it is distressingly ordinary for patients to get treatments that research has shown are ineffective or even dangerous. Sometimes doctors simply haven't kept up

with the science. Other times doctors know the state of play perfectly well but continue to deliver these treatments because it's profitable—or even because they're popular and patients demand them. Some procedures are implemented based on studies that did not prove whether they really worked in the first place. Others were initially supported by evidence but then were contradicted by better evidence, and yet these procedures have remained the standards of care for years, or decades.[28]

We live in an age of Big Government. There is no shortage of federal rules that govern the health care sector, and agencies like the Food and Drug Administration are among the most powerful and best known regulatory agencies in the world.[29] Americans could be excused if they believe (without thinking much about it) that existing regulatory frameworks ensure that new treatments enter into clinical practice only after research has shown that they work as well as or better than alternatives, and that very expensive treatments must work at least as well as much cheaper alternatives. But this belief is mistaken.

To be sure, drugs and devices must be certified as safe and effective by the FDA before they can be marketed in the United States.[30] There are three main reasons why the FDA approval process often fails to generate the information needed to promote evidence-based medicine, curb wasteful spending, and ensure the best outcomes for patients. The first reason is that the assessment of comparative effectiveness is typically not required for FDA marketing approval.[31] Despite calls from medical reformers for greater attention to comparative effectiveness and the benefits of a new therapy over alternatives,

> the FDA has stuck with the older (and industry preferred) model of placebo studies as the gold standard by which to measure the efficacy of new products, a decision that some have argued has escalated drug costs by facilitating the introduction of expensive 'me too' drugs which offer only marginal efficacy gains, if any, over existing off-patent therapies.[32]

Clinical trials of new drugs typically compare them to alternative medications only when the manufacturer seeks to make a marketing claim that a product is superior to other treatments, "or when giving trial participants a placebo would be unethical."[33] Furthermore, the FDA's evaluations of products are often designed only to see if they are more effective than placebo on a short-term surrogate endpoint, such as a blood test, which may or may not be a good proxy for long-term clinical outcomes.[34] Physicians commonly prescribe FDA-approved drugs for "off-label" uses—that is, for uses (and types of patients) in which the drugs have not been tested in clinical trials. Most physicians are not being irresponsible in these practices; the evidence base simply does not exist for many of these uses, especially for the off-label use of drugs.[35]

A second reason why FDA review fails to generate the information needed to determine what treatments work best for what patients is that the evidentiary standards for evaluating medical devices are typically lower than for prescription drugs and biologics. Many medical devices enter the market through an expedited pathway, in which manufacturers need only demonstrate (usually without evidence from randomized controlled trials) that a new device is "substantially equivalent" to a device already being sold. As mentioned, some point out that the 21st Century Cures Act, intended to expedite the approval of new drugs and devices, could affect the quality of evidence used by the FDA to evaluate new products and new uses for existing ones.[36] In sum, federal regulation of medical products has been crafted to protect safety by keeping dangerous drugs and devices off the market, not to ensure that patients get the treatments that work best for their conditions.

The third gap in the FDA review process, less well known than the other two reasons but perhaps more important, is that many medical procedures undergo no rigorous evaluation at all. While the FDA does review devices *used* in medical procedures, it generally does not regulate the efficacy of the procedures themselves. This means that a doctor who invents a new kind of surgery can generally begin performing it without extensive evidence that it works better than less invasive alternative treatments. As Ashton and Wray observe, "Paradoxically, surgical innovations, generally costlier and riskier than pharmaceutical agents, can enter clinical practice with a much weaker evidential base than drugs and devices."[37]

The weaknesses of the FDA are compounded by the federal government's incapacity to promote efficiency in programs like Medicare and Medicaid. While all advanced nations are struggling to eliminate waste in health care, the United States is somewhat of an outlier when it comes to the use of evidence to shape coverage and reimbursement decisions. Australia, France, Germany, and the United Kingdom, for example, all have CER entities with greater authority than PCORI. These organizations differ in their roles and responsibilities, but all focus "their priorities, design, generation, and implementation of CER evidence on the explicit objective of informing health care policy decisions on the use of and payment for clinical services."[38] In comparison, CER entities in the United States have been given fewer tools to influence how health care resources are allocated.[39]

In contrast to the agencies that administer public health insurance programs in other advanced nations, the Center for Medicare and Medicaid Services lacks the ability "to actively review the vast majority of new technologies that are adopted into clinical practice and to restrict coverage for those that lack sufficient evidence of effectiveness."[40] Since its enactment in 1965, Medicare has focused primarily on clinical effectiveness, and covered any treatment that it deems "reasonable and necessary." It has not sought to constrain or limit patient choice about treatment options.[41] Medicare delegates most coverage decisions to regional contractors, who generally defer to the clinical judgment of physicians. Even when national coverage policies are developed (which applies to only a small fraction of medical services), the lack of high-quality outcomes data means that "the vast majority of new technologies and services bypass any meaningful review."[42] Medicare has not been a regular sponsor of clinical trials to address gaps in the medical evidence base, although on some occasions Medicare has sought to link the coverage of a new service to providers who participate in a prospective data collection activity by a process known as "coverage with evidence development." While Medicare has sometimes limited payments for a service to the rate paid for the "least costly alternative,"[43] Medicare reimbursement levels in the vast majority of cases are linked to the "underlying cost of providing services."[44] Administrations of both parties have sought to rationalize Medicare's coverage policies to give greater weight to the costs and benefits of services, but reforms have been elusive. In the early 1990s, the George H. W. Bush administration proposed a Medicare coverage rule that would have included a limited cost-effectiveness analysis requirement for certain technologies.[45] However, the proposal was opposed by the medical device industry, physician associations, and hospitals.[46] Members of Congress and disease-advocacy groups argued that cost-effectiveness analysis would lead to rationing, and the proposed rule was buried before the 1992 elections.[47]

Some state Medicaid agencies do use comparative effectiveness data to inform their drug formulary decisions. The innovator in this area has been Oregon. In 2003, under former governor and emergency room physician John Kitzhaber, M.D., Oregon created the Drug Effectiveness Review Project (DERP), an independent, university-based collaborative to evaluate clinical evidence on the relative safety and efficacy of different drugs in the same class.[48] More than a dozen state Medicaid programs are now involved with DERP,[49] which conducts systematic literature reviews; it does not fund major new clinical trials. While Medicaid is a major state budget item, the fact that the federal government has historically paid most of the program's total expenses has attenuated the incentive of states to identify and eliminate less effective treatments, since states would have recouped only a portion of the savings.[50]

Taken together, these governance failures contribute to a variety of problems:

- Although estimates vary, some experts believe that *less than half* of all medical care is based on adequate evidence about its effectiveness.[51]
- When there are two treatments available for the same condition— such as surgery versus medication—doctors often do not know which one works best. Consequently, "decisions about what treatments to use often depend on anecdotal evidence, conjecture, and the experience and judgment of the individual physicians involved."[52]
- Many common surgical procedures, such as spinal fusion for back surgery, rest on little evidence.[53] There have been cases where thousands of patients have undergone extremely risky operations (e.g., high-dose chemotherapy with bone marrow transplants for breast cancer) that were later determined to be ineffective when properly evaluated.[54]
- The *Dartmouth Atlas of Health Care* has identified large regional variations in utilization and spending in the Medicare program that cannot be fully explained by differences in population structure or patient illness, and that are not consistently related to health outcomes.[55] For example, regional variations in hip and knee replacement for Medicare patients were four times higher in some regions compared with others in 2005–6.[56] A recent study found that utilization changes significantly when Medicare patients move from one area to another (that is, from a high utilization area to a low one, or vice versa), and that 50 to 60 percent of the variation in utilization is due to place-specific factors, such as the practice styles and beliefs of local physicians.[57]
- It can take decades for medical research findings to enter clinical practice.[58] A Rand study reported Americans only receive 55 percent of the recommended preventive, acute, and long-term health care.[59] For example, although the benefits of Beta blockers in acute myocardial infarction (heart attack) was established in the 1980s,

Beta blockers remained widely underused, and there was still wide variation in their use as recently as 2005.[60] The failure to deliver recommended care is due not only to slow diffusion, but also to consumer resistance to many preventive interventions, a lack of medically valuable treatments that are remunerative, and the fact that many practices are not set up to do these things efficiently.

The tripartite problem of missing evidence, overutilization, and unexplained regional variation in the Medicare program has generated a massive volume of health economics and health services research.[61] The problem is so widespread that the mainstream media has taken notice. There have been many articles in the *New York Times* and *Washington Post* about the overuse of everything from cardiac stenting and Mohs surgery to CT scans, ear tubes, elective induction of labor, and antibiotics.[62] A number of important books about the problem have also appeared in recent years. Their titles tell the story: *Overdiagnosed: Making People Sick in the Pursuit of Health*;[63] *Hope or Hype: The Obsession with Medical Advances and the High Cost of False Promises*;[64] *Overtreated: Why Too Much Medicine Is Making Us Sicker and Poorer*;[65] *Overdosed America: The Broken Promise of American Medicine*;[66] *Flatlined: Resuscitating American Medicine*;[67] and *Taming the Beloved Beast: How Medical Technology Costs Are Destroying Our Health Care System*.[68] These books are riveting, but they are not screeds. Their detailed, highly informative analyses help explain why American medicine costs so much—and delivers so little.

The essence of the problem described in these books can be captured in a graph created by health economists Amitabh Chandra, Anupam B. Jena, and Jonathan S. Skinner.[69] Figure 1.3 shows a "production possibility frontier" in health care. The graph maps the relationship between factor inputs, which includes all the labor and capital used to produce medical care (e.g., physicians, nurses, hospital beds, medicines, x-ray machines, etc.) and health outcomes (survival/quality of life). A well-functioning health care system would be operating at a point somewhere *on* the curve (not inside it). That is, given its factor inputs, the health system would obtain the best possible outcomes for the overall health of the population. The goal of research on the comparative effectiveness of different treatment options is to help society reach a point on the curve (such as point B or C) by giving patients and providers the sound evidence they need to choose the treatment with the best health outcome for each clinical indication.[70] Unfortunately, the U.S. health care system is represented by point A, *inside* the production possibility frontier, due to wasteful costs, lack of effective care, or overtreatment.

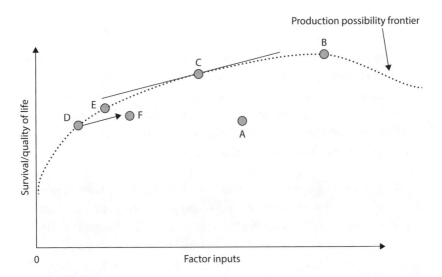

FIGURE 1.3. Cost-effectiveness and comparative efficiency in a health care production function. *Source*: Copyrighted and published by the American Economic Association as figure 1 in Amitabh Chandra, Anupam B. Jena, and Jonathan S. Skinner, 2011, "The Pragmatist's Guide to Comparative Effectiveness Research," *Journal of Economic Perspectives* 25 (2): 27–46. The published article is archived and available online at https://www.aeaweb.org/journals/jep.

That is, the United States is operating below potential. The nation could be doing much better, given the factor inputs we are allocating to the health care system, if patients received the most effective treatments for their conditions, as suggested by the examples in Chandra, Jena, and Skinner. Additional studies, such as Perlroth, Goldman, and Garber, suggest "CER could save up to $3 billion annually by establishing that for prostate cancer patients, prostatectomy ($7,300 cost) yields results as good as brachytherapy or radiation seeds ($19,000) and radiation therapy ($46,900)."[71]

There are three reasons why everyone should be concerned about a situation in which the nation finds itself far inside its "production possibility frontier." First, given what we spend, millions of people—spouses, parents, and children—are *less healthy* than they could be if medicine were more evidence based. Second, the foregone health benefits—the losses in quality of life or survival—are not inevitable. Incentives to generate and use scientific information, if missing, can be supplied. Norms supporting the practice of EBM, if weak, can be strengthened. Insurance rules that encourage overtreatment can be changed. Finally, the current situation should spark outrage because it reflects in part efforts by powerful economic interests to gain profits through deceptive practices, as noted by Ashton and Wray:

We know how to generate high-quality evidence about the benefits and harms of clinical interventions. But evidence can make winners and losers of parties [such as pharmaceutical companies] that have a stake in the decisions that will flow from the evidence. Consequently, though this flies in the face of scientific objectivity, medical ethics, and the high ideals of methods and ethics of human subjects research, parties will try to manipulate the design and conduct of research so that the process yields answers favorable to their interests.[72]

Medical evidence is generated in part to satisfy FDA review, but the data-generation system requires government monitoring and enforcement to maintain its credibility and effectiveness. Consider the rosiglitazone story. Rosiglitazone is an antidiabetes drug marketed under the name Avandia and sold by the British drug maker GlaxoSmithKline (GSK). After years of civil and criminal investigations that featured allegations of efforts to intimidate scientists, GSK agreed to pay a $3 billion fine in part for failing to report certain safety data to the FDA, including certain postmarketing studies, as well as studies conducted to address policy makers' concerns about the drug's cardiovascular safety risks.[73]

But it isn't only big drug companies that can fail to protect patient welfare. Doctors and medical administrators themselves bear responsibility. In his book *Unaccountable*, Johns Hopkins hospital surgeon Marty Makary provides detailed stories about how patients who are candidates for minimally invasive procedures are sometimes not told of their options and receive extensive surgeries, increasing their exposure to medical error.[74]

A common concern about CER is that some patients may benefit more from a treatment than others. A study that focused on the benefits for the "average patient" could miss substantial benefits for a particular subgroup of patients, such as racial or ethnic minorities. This is an important concern. While knowing the average effect of a treatment is clearly "better than the status quo of having no . . . knowledge about the effectiveness of a treatment,"[75] it is true that clinical studies focusing on average effects do not always generate the information needed to identify the best treatments for patients.[76] People vary in many ways, including their genomics, and metabolic systems, and these differences are sometimes relevant for clinical decision making. But there are viable solutions to this concern, including performing a large enough study to permit subgroup analysis so that we learn what strategies truly work best for whom and under what circumstances. Also, the results of CER studies do not have to be used to deny coverage; they can be used to inform patient and physician decisions or (if cost-effectiveness is a concern) to design payment systems that preserve freedom of choice but encourage patients and doctors to use high-value, evidence-based options.[77] A related concern is that CER threatens "personalized medicine." However, as Alan Garber and Sean Tunis note, a key "obstacle to the adoption of personalized approaches, such as genomic testing . . . is the lack of adequately designed studies assessing their clinical utility. Often there is little consensus about the best way to design and implement such studies. . . . These are precisely the kinds of issues that CER is designed to address."[78] In sum, the best answer to therapeutic uncertainty about the effectiveness of a treatment is not to fall back on medical guesswork, but more and better science to generate the information needed by physicians and patients.

Why would doctors perform tests and procedures in the absence of solid evidence about their benefits for patients? Why would some Medicare patients receive painkillers and physical therapy for back pain while other patients who are suffering from identical symptoms receive back surgery? How much of the overtreatment and regional variation problems in the United States can be explained by fee-for-service payment? By fear of malpractice suits? By supply-induced patient demand? By physician preferences or the practice norms of particular localities?

These are important questions to which health services researchers have devoted considerable attention, but resolving them is not this book's central objective. As political scientists, our major focus is *not* on the reasons why the U.S. health care sector is characterized by bad science, inconsistency, and waste. *Rather, our primary focus is on why the massive inefficiencies of the U.S. medical sector (especially in the Medicare program) have failed to stimulate a more effective political and policy response.*

A Political Puzzle

The raw power of the medical products industry clearly helps explain the pressure to maintain the status quo. There are big industry profits at stake in the current regulatory and financial environment of U.S. health care— and the industry obviously wishes to protect them. Yet if a significant fraction of Medicare dollars is being wasted on useless (or low-value services) and millions of Americans are harmed because of lack of good evidence on common treatments and the slow uptake of research findings, a serious institutional breakdown is occurring. The U.S. political system is not known for its speed, but its performance is not always this dismal. In many policy sectors, government performs quite well.[79] Further, there are many examples of public policy responding to expert recognition of societal problems, leading to reforms that opened up sectors once dominated by powerful interests. For example, when a consensus emerged among economists that inefficient regulation of the transportation sector was imposing huge costs on consumers, the trucking and airline industries were deregulated, despite howls of protest from the airlines and Teamsters.[80] When experts pointed out that America's schoolchildren were falling behind international peers, the federal government required states to put in place standardized tests and accountability mechanisms.[81] While some of these reforms have been more effective and sustainable than others,[82] all were predicated on expert identification of a major social problem and the opportunity for socially beneficial change in the face of powerful organized interests seeking to maintain existing arrangements. In sum, the U.S. system does have a capacity to address problems, at least at times. Why has the U.S. medical sector been far more resistant to reforms to improve the quality of care and the efficiency of resource allocation decisions?

The puzzle only deepens when one recognizes that other advanced nations have created robust agencies or programs to conduct health technology assessment and synthesize the evidence base to inform coverage and reimbursement decisions.[83] For example, England created the National Institute for Clinical Excellence (later renamed the National Institute for Health and Care Excellence, NICE) in 1999 to provide national guidance on health technologies and procedures to ensure that treatment decisions would be based on the best available clinical evidence. France created the National Health Authority (Haute Autorité de Santé, HAS) in 2004 "as an independent agency to advise the Ministry of Health and public health insurers about the clinical value of services, goods, and procedures. It also audits and accredits health care professionals and firms."[84] And Germany established the Institute for Quality and Efficiency in Health Care in 2004 to evaluate the quality, effectiveness, and efficiency of health services. Other nations like Australia and Canada have also built up bureaucratic capacity in this area.

To be sure, there is no evidence that health technology assessment in the U.K. (or other European nations) has constrained health care spending growth, although it has likely increased the average cost-effectiveness of covered treatments.[85] This should not be too surprising, however, since the main function of these efforts is to *rationalize* care, improve quality, and promote value for money, not to cut costs.[86] Well-done evidence synthesis and technology assessment moves a nation's health care system out to the production possibility frontier (figure 1.3). Many factors affect the growth of health care spending in any given nation, including the willingness to impose system-wide controls on prices and wages. Better generation and use of evidence may not lower the growth rate by itself, although politicians may embrace evidence generation and technology assessment in the hope they will. Indeed, despite the creation of NICE, overall health spending increased significantly in the U.K. between 2002 and 2010. NICE took advantage of a much more accommodating fiscal climate by allocating the funds to new technologies, which it would presumably be less able to do in a more constraining budget environment. As Corinna Sorenson writes,

> In the case of NICE, its guidance has most likely been cost-increasing, in the order of £1.65 billion per year in additional NHS investment. This is not surprising since most interventions that are deemed cost-effective are more expensive than their comparator interventions. The French HAS also claims that any adoption of cost-effectiveness analysis would not be used to save money (by reducing services), but attain more efficient use of resources.[87]

But there are complications. Disentangling the cost impact of health technology assessment in Europe is rather difficult since the counterfactual (what would have happened if guidance had not been issued?) is unknown.[88] It is clearly misleading to estimate the cost impact of assessment simply on the basis of the number or scope of coverage denials, since firms may price their goods in anticipation of the reviews. There is anecdotal evidence that NICE may encourage companies to lower their prices and offer deeper discounts in the hopes of securing NICE approval by getting a better QALY (quality-adjusted life year)/£ result.[89] For example, NICE originally did not recommend the cancer drug ibrutinib for routine NHS use. However, following a reduction in price, NICE approved the therapy as cost-effective.[90] The effect could also be to promote the introduction of new, more expensive treatments into the system, which could lead to higher (but perhaps *cost-effective*) spending.[91]

As we discuss later, the creation of the Patient-Centered Outcomes Research Institute under the Affordable Care Act brought the United States a bit closer to the international norm on public support for CER, but major differences remain between the United States and other nations. The failure to create a clear linkage between PCORI's research and Medicare, coupled with the fragmentation of U.S. health care delivery and financing, left formidable barriers to the routine integration of evidence into clinical decisions and policy outcomes.

The lack of an effective and politically sustainable response to the medical evidence problem—and this is a sad indictment of the U.S. political system—would be somewhat less surprising if the medical evidence problem harmed "only" politically marginalized groups, such as the poor.[92] But *all* Americans, including wealthy patients covered by generous insurance plans, suffer if doctors don't follow best practices or if evidence does not exist about, for example, the best way to treat prostate cancer or back pain. The pathologies of the U.S. medical system thus cannot be attributed to distributional bias in an otherwise high-performance system; these inefficiencies and performance breakdowns are widespread and systemic.

To explain this puzzle, we develop an extended argument about how interactions among physicians, politicians, and the public have created the present equilibrium. Before we flesh out this argument, however, it is instructive to look at how the system responds to the emergence of evidence that a common procedure does not work as advertised, which is the subject of the next chapter.

2

Sham Surgery

A CASE STUDY OF THE USE
OF MEDICAL EVIDENCE

In an ideal health care system, doctors would operate on patients only when there is a strong medical basis for doing so. Researchers would use rigorous methods to evaluate whether specific operations are safe and effective for specific conditions. If there is compelling evidence that a surgical procedure might not work as expected, physicians and medical researchers would investigate. Once the truth about the benefits of the operation is discovered, the information would be disseminated. Clinical guidelines would be revised, and physician behavior would rapidly change. In sum, treatments would be based on the best available scientific evidence, and progress would be continuous, uniform across regions, and swift.

Unfortunately, this is not how the American medical system always works. A large body of research leaves little doubt that sizable gaps exist between these aspirations and real-world performance. As chapter 1 discussed, new tests and procedures are often widely adopted before they are rigorously evaluated, and practice norms often do not change quickly and consistently in response to credible evidence. Doctors in some regions of the country may continue to perform discredited procedures long after providers elsewhere have abandoned them. Table 2.1 displays recent examples of the uneven translation of comparative effectiveness research into outcomes

TABLE 2.1. Recent Comparative Effectiveness Studies and Their Translation Outcomes

Study	Results	Dominant Practice	Translation Outcome
ALLHAT (Antihypertensive and Lipid-Lowering Treatment to Prevent Heart Attack Trial), 2002	Thiazide diuretics were superior in preventing cardiovascular disease events and less expensive than calcium channel blockers, ACE inhibitors, and alpha-adrenergic blockers.	Trend toward greater use of calcium channel blockers and ACE inhibitors	No change in practice
CATIE (Clinical Antipsychotic Trials of Intervention Effectiveness), 2005	Conventional antipsychotics were as effective as atypical antipsychotics in patients with schizophrenia.	Use of atypical antipsychotics	No change in practice
COMPANION (Comparison of Medical Therapy, Pacing, and Defibrillation in Heart Failure), 2004	Compared to optimal medical therapy, both cardiac resynchronization therapy (CRT) and CRT plus defibrillator use improved survival, reduced hospitalization rates, and improved functional status in patients with moderate to severe heart failure.	Optimal medical therapy (underuse of CRT)	Some evidence of slow adoption of CRT (with and without defibrillator)
COURAGE (Clinical Outcomes Utilizing Revascularization and Aggressive Drug Evaluation), 2007	Optimal medical therapy combined with percutaneous coronary intervention had similar survival benefit and angina relief, compared with optimal medical therapy alone in patients with stable coronary artery disease.	Use of PCI before optimal medical therapy	Little or no change in practice
SPORT (Spine Patient Outcomes Research Trial), 2008	Surgery for lumbar spinal stenosis had better outcomes than nonsurgical treatment, according to the cohort study analysis.	Surgical treatment	No change in practice
Philadelphia Bone Marrow Transplant Group, 2000	Compared with maintenance chemotherapy in conventional doses, high-dose chemotherapy plus bone marrow transplantation did not improve survival in women with metastatic breast cancer.	Trend toward greater use of bone marrow transplantation	Rapid abandonment of bone marrow transplantation

Source: Copyrighted and published by Project HOPE/ *Health Affairs* as exhibit 1 in Justin W. Timbie, D. Steven Fox, Kristin Van Busum, and Eric C. Schneider. 2012. "Five Reasons That Many Comparative Effectiveness Studies Fail to Change Patient Care and Clinical Practice." *Health Affairs* (Millwood) 31 (10): 2168–75. The published article is archived and available online at www.healthaffairs.org.

from Timbie and colleagues.[1] Many reasons have been suggested for the failure of evidence to alter clinical practice, including financial incentives, ambiguity of study results, local practice norms, and cognitive biases in the interpretation of new information.[2] These broad explanations are convincing, but they do not address the role of key organizational actors—including physicians, medical societies, and policy makers—in the uptake of clinical evidence. To gain a feel for how things work (or fail to work) on the ground, it is useful to take a detailed look at the production, use, and nonuse of evidence in a particular case.

Here, we examine the use of arthroscopic surgery to treat osteoarthritis (OA) of the knee. By the mid-1980s, arthroscopies became a preferred method of treatment for knee OA. It was believed that debridement and lavage resulted in less pain and postoperative swelling than other surgical procedures and helped patients avoid the need for a total knee replacement.[3] The use of knee arthroscopy was encouraged by the growing use of MRIs, which allowed doctors to view structural abnormalities inside the joint. More than 650,000 debridement and lavage procedures were performed annually in the early 2000s, at which time the procedures cost roughly $5,000.[4] About half of all knee OA patients typically said they felt better after their arthroscopies, but some experts doubted that the operations were beneficial. In the mid-1990s, a medical research team led by J. Bruce Moseley, a board-certified orthopedic surgeon at Baylor College of Medicine and the team physician of the Houston Rockets and of the 1996 U.S. Olympics Basketball "Dream Team," and Nelda P. Wray, a physician and health services researcher at the Veterans Administration in Houston, decided to test whether the surgery was effective. The Moseley-Wray team conducted a rare randomized placebo-controlled clinical trial of a surgical procedure, in which some patients underwent fake operations designed to mimic the real interventions. Patients assigned to the placebo arm received only incisions while they were asleep. Tests of knee function showed that patients who received the real operation did not outperform those who received the placebo on physical tasks and reported no more pain relief than those who received only the placebo incisions.[5] *In short, a surgical procedure performed on millions of patients to ease the pain of arthritic knees worked no better than a fake operation.*

On the surface, the widespread use of an operation that works no better than a fake operation is easy to "explain." A patient has knee pain and doesn't know the best treatment owing to the uncertainties and information asymmetries of medical care,[6] and his or her doctor says, "You will benefit from surgery." The patient receives "care" when he or she undergoes the surgery. That intervention produces an effect, albeit a placebo effect, but the typical patient would not know this. Moreover, if the knee surgery is the standard in the profession, even shopping around for different treatment options, which is rare, wouldn't help. There is little in the interaction between doctor and patient that would lead the patient to conclude that a safer and less disruptive treatment might have been available.

But this account, accurate as it may be, evades the really important questions. How did this situation arise? Why were doctors performing a procedure without scientifically demonstrated benefits? What was the state of the medical evidence base before the publication of the Moseley study? How did the medical and public policy communities react when the study came out? How much and how quickly did clinical practices change afterward? These are among the questions this chapter explores.

The U.S. medical system does respond to evidence. When credible research is published in a top-flight medical journal suggesting that a common treatment does not work as believed, as occurred here, the results are widely discussed. However, the uptake of evidence by clinicians is often slow, inconsistent, and variable across communities. The generation, use, and translation of evidence are technical tasks, but they are carried out through decision-making and resource allocation processes that are shaped and constrained by the economic, political, and organizational interests of health sector actors, including doctors. There are no mechanisms in programs like Medicare to ensure that important gaps in the medical evidence base are expeditiously identified and systematically filled to protect the interests of patients and taxpayers. When the effectiveness of a treatment is challenged by a gold-standard study, medical societies do not always behave in ways that put patient interests unambiguously first. Rather than using the emergence of credible evidence that an expensive, invasive procedure works no better than safer alternatives as a welcome opportunity to take a hard look at the conceptual and empirical support for existing treatment protocols, medical societies may give the narrowest possible constructions to research findings. They do so for many reasons, including a desire to maintain professional autonomy and minimize government and insurance industry interference with existing clinical practices. The evidence translation process—turning research findings into better clinical decision making and improved outcomes for patients—sometimes moves at a glacial pace and does not establish an expectation that other therapies (even related interventions in the same practice area) will satisfy higher evidentiary thresholds before diffusing into wide use. Indeed, as we will see later in this chapter, after debridement and lavage were discredited and coverage changes occurred, the number of these operations did begin to decline. However, the number of knee surgeries for tears of the meniscus cartilage of the knee increased dramatically. Many were probably not at all surprised when yet another randomized controlled trial found that the latter procedure *also* worked no better than sham surgery.[7] Arthroscopic surgery on the meniscus is still the most common orthopedic procedure in the United States, performed about 700,000 times a year at an estimated cost of $4 billion.[8] Experts agree that the procedure is appropriate under some circumstances, especially for younger patients and for tears from sports injuries. But the vast majority—as many as 80 percent—of tears occur in older patients owing to wear and aging. Some experts believe surgery in those cases is often not appropriate.[9]

The knee case is illustrative of systemic problems in the promotion of evidence-based medicine. While the involvement of more than 50 medical societies in the "Choosing Wisely" campaign to eliminate low-value, wasteful services is a positive step, the initiative thus far has had little impact. A study in *JAMA Internal Medicine* found that for seven treatment and testing services listed by the Choosing Wisely campaign as usually unnecessary, use of only two had declined. Use of the other five services either had not changed or had increased.[10] Clearly, many medical societies are failing to take seriously their professional responsibility to deliver evidence-based care to patients and ensure that the nation does not squander scarce health care dollars on treatments of dubious worth.

The remainder of the chapter is organized as follows. First, we describe how the orthopedic community mostly ignored clear warnings that the arthroscopic surgery for OA of the knee might not be effective. Next, we review the Moseley-Wray study's findings and describe the less than optimal responses they prompted from medical societies and policy makers. Finally, we briefly look at the debate surrounding another procedure for knee OA (arthroscopic partial meniscectomy) that has grown in popularity despite a lack of evidence, and identify signs of the same performance pathologies.

Arthroscopic Surgery for OA of the Knee

About 12 percent of those aged 65 and over experience frequent knee pain from OA.[11] When anti-inflammatory medication and physical therapy fail to relieve symptoms, doctors may recommend two forms of arthroscopic knee surgery: lavage or debridement with lavage. Lavage (derived from the

French "laver," meaning "to wash") is a procedure in which the knee joint is thoroughly washed out. Debridement (derived from a French word related to "debris") "cleans up" the knee by cutting away loose tissue, trimming torn and degenerated meniscus (the shock-absorbing cartilage in the knee joint), and smoothing out the remaining meniscus. These procedures originated in the medical practices of the 1930s and 1940s but did not take off until the development of fiberoptics in the 1970s.[12] By the mid-1980s, arthroscopy for OA of the knee had become extremely popular. Arthroscopies are typically performed under general anesthesia and require a recovery period during which the patient experiences pain and decreased mobility. Although serious complications from the procedure are rare, debridement may have a negative effect on the outcomes of a subsequent total knee replacement.[13]

THE WEAK EVIDENTIARY BASIS OF THE PROCEDURE

The spread of arthroscopic surgery for OA began as surgeons reported their experiences with arthroscopic surgery at scientific conferences and in journal articles. Colleagues became excited about the procedure and started performing it on their patients. These clinical experiences, rather than scientifically rigorous evaluations or a sound theoretical understanding of the mechanism behind alleged treatment effects, provided the basis for the widespread adoption of the procedure in the United States.

A review of the relevant medical literature before the 2002 Moseley study highlights the weak evidentiary basis of this surgery. Although there had been reports on operations similar to lavage and debridement several decades earlier, the first modern study of arthroscopy for OA of the knee was published in 1981. Norman F. Sprague III debrided the joints of patients for whom other therapies had failed.[14] The outcome measures were subjective assessments of pain and functioning. About fourteen months after the surgery, patients were asked to compare their current level of pain and functioning to their recollection of what they had experienced before the operation.[15] Approximately 75 percent of the patients said their pain and functioning had improved or stayed the same. This early study had two major design weaknesses that persisted in research for two decades. First, the research design did not permit the effect of the surgery to be distinguished from the natural history of the disease or from a placebo effect. Placebo effects are especially common when a subjective measure, such as pain, is the target of the treatment. Second, the assessment was not "blinded." Those conducting the evaluations knew what procedures individual patients had received. Sprague's study was actually based on patients' self-reported experiences, though a similar problem would arise if third-party evaluators knew each patient's treatment history, as unblinded assessment is an established source of bias.

At least twenty-five additional studies evaluating the effectiveness of lavage and debridement with lavage were published during the next twenty years.[16] Like Sprague, most of these follow-up studies relied on retrospective evaluations of the surgery using either patient charts or follow-up interviews—methodologies vulnerable to producing biased results. In a typical example, Yang and Nisonson evaluated 105 postoperative knees by using a 12-point scale that included both subjective measures and measurements of range of motion. Sixty-five percent of patients scored 9 or higher, the cutoff the authors selected to determine which knees should be labeled "good" or "excellent." The 65 percent "success rate" was taken as supportive of the use of arthroscopic surgery. However, the Yang and Nisonson study lacked a control group against which to measure the benefit from the intervention, and the physician who conducted the case evaluations knew whether individual patients had been operated on (i.e., the study was not blinded).[17]

The pre-Moseley literature did contain some randomized trials. A few well-designed randomized clinical trials were conducted to gauge the effectiveness of one of the two arthroscopic surgeries, lavage without debridement.[18] In contrast to most of the case series evidence, these studies failed to produce convincing evidence that lavage was effective in reducing arthritis severity as measured by outcomes such as function or stiffness. With a much larger number of case histories reporting positive effects from the procedure, however, these negative findings were downplayed. No randomized trial prior to Moseley and colleagues evaluated debridement versus a placebo version of the operation.[19]

DOUBTS ABOUT THE EFFECTIVENESS OF THE PROCEDURE

Some physicians did question whether or how arthroscopy benefited patients with OA. If there is a strong theoretical argument for how an operation produces benefits, the need for empirical support is lessened. There was, however, no broadly accepted theoretical mechanism to explain how arthroscopic surgery helped patients. Several hypotheses were offered to explain the positive findings reported in the typically nonrandomized, unblinded clinical studies. Some researchers pointed out that the arthritic joint contains irritating debris and enzymes. It was suggested that flushing out these sources of irritation might reduce pain.[20] Debridement was said to reduce pain by reducing mechanical problems of the knee such as "catching" or "popping" and improving the distribution of weight on joint surfaces.[21] These explanations were recognized as speculative. Many studies reporting positive clinical findings were at a loss to explain them. In one review article generally supportive of the surgery, for example, Hanssen and colleagues acknowledged that "the mechanism of pain relief following arthroscopic treatment of osteoarthritis is obscure."[22]

Questions about the use of arthroscopy for patients with knee arthritis were raised at medical conferences and in professional journals. In a symposium ("Uses and Abuses of Arthroscopy") conducted at the 1992 annual meeting of the American Academy of Orthopaedic Surgeons (AAOS) and an article reprinted in one of the leading journals in the field, practitioners and researchers openly discussed both the state of knowledge regarding arthroscopic surgery and how the financial incentives of the health care system might distort the decision to recommend surgery. The symposium was noteworthy for its blunt language regarding a common orthopedic procedure. Dr. John Goodfellow, a former president of the British Orthopaedic Association, mocked the use of arthroscopic surgeries for OA and suggested they might be "pseudotreatments." He commented that "no one has performed the double-blind controlled trial that would be necessary to distinguish between the placebo effects of any operation and the direct benefits of debridement."[23] Despite the obvious and recognized need for rigorous investigation to determine whether the procedure worked, there was no sense of urgency. The lack of hard evidence for the procedure's effectiveness was apparently more a regrettable condition than a pressing problem for physicians and researchers to solve.

This troubling situation—in which the lack of hard evidence for the use of a procedure is a poorly kept secret among practitioners—is not unusual in American medical practice. Many popular surgical procedures rest on weak evidence, including certain procedures done to relieve lower back, neck, spine or neurological pain, tendonitis, and impingement in the shoulder.[24] Questions have been raised about vertebroplasty, a procedure in which a form of bone cement is injected into the broken spinal bones of patients with OA. A 2009 randomized, double-blind trial found no beneficial effect compared to a sham procedure in which needles were inserted into the back without injecting cement.[25] Two years after the study's publication, the procedure was still being performed, and insurance coverage was unchanged.[26] Another example of a questionable operation is "spinal fusion surgery," in which a bone graft is used to fuse together two vertebrae in an attempt to relieve lower back pain from degenerated discs. The operation, which has been increasingly popular in the United States, can have serious side effects, including blindness and paralysis. As use of the surgery grew, evidence that spinal fusion surgery works well for its most common indications remained unclear, according to Deyo and colleagues.[27]

A WIDESPREAD PROBLEM

The problems we observe in the production of evidence in the case of arthroscopic surgery have long been known to experts. An article in *Science* magazine in 1978 noted that, although new drugs and devices must satisfy federal regulations that require rigorous testing in animals followed by carefully controlled testing, "new surgical operations may or may not be tested in animals, may be introduced as human therapy with or without review by a human experimentation committee and with or without a formal experimental design, and may or may not be evaluated by long-term follow-up observation."[28] A 1975 commentary in the *Journal of the American Medical Association* pointed out that a double standard exists for surgery. Drugs must undergo Food and Drug Administration (FDA) review—a requirement that is not costless but is almost certainly socially appropriate. Yet no agency has been created to protect the patient from harmful and ineffective operations. This same double standard exists among journal editors and reviewers, "who regularly reject inadequately controlled medical trials and regularly publish inadequately controlled surgical trials."[29]

What accounts for this double standard and for the poor state of scientific knowledge about surgical procedures more generally? Some argue that ethical considerations limit the use of rigorous, placebo-controlled clinical trials to study surgical interventions. Although it is morally acceptable to use placebos when evaluating a new drug, it is sometimes thought unacceptable to do so when studying a new operation, even though this research approach has produced startling results on the occasions it has been used.[30] Opponents of sham surgery trials argue that it is too difficult to design an operation as inert as the usual sugar pill used as a placebo in drug trials.

Proponents of placebo arms in studies of surgical procedures argue that such research designs are ethically sound.[31] Ethical reservations about sham surgery, proponents claim, confuse the ethics of clinical research with the ethics of personal medical therapy. According to bioethicist Franklin G. Miller, "Clinical trials routinely administer interventions to patients that carry risks that are not compensated by medical benefits to them, but are justified by the anticipated value of scientific knowledge accruing from their use. For example, invasive procedures such as blood draws, lumbar punctures, and biopsies are often administered to measure trial outcomes."[32] If there is no consensus among the medical community on the benefits and use of a procedure, if the scientific need for blinding is compelling, if participants are informed about the risks to the placebo control group, and if the risks to subjects in the control group are minimized, then sham surgery trials may be ethically appropriate, as the American Medical Association (AMA) has acknowledged.[33]

The ethical argument against sham surgery studies can easily be turned on its head. As physician David H. Spodick wrote,

> The omission of adequate standards for surgical therapies should be especially surprising, since even the most essential operation involves inevitable trauma—physical, metabolic, and psychic—not to mention the risks of anesthesia. Indeed, when evaluated under comparable conditions against the outcome of alternative treatments or of no treatment, a new operation resulting in net loss to the patients, or in the same degree of recovery that would have occurred spontaneously, might be fantasized as a well-intended "assault."[34]

Following Spodick's line of reasoning, if ethics were decisive, one might reasonably expect placebo-controlled arms to be *more* prevalent in the evaluation of surgery than in the evaluation of any other kind of medical intervention.

Pioneering Sham Surgery Study

The publication of the landmark study "A Controlled Trial of Arthroscopic Surgery for Osteoarthritis of the Knee," in the July 11, 2002, issue of the *New England Journal of Medicine*, presented the findings of a study that subjected a questionable procedure to rigorous scientific analysis. The article reported the results of a double-blind clinical trial in which Houston Veterans Administration hospital patients were randomly assigned to receive lavage, debridement with lavage, or "sham surgery." For patients in the debridement with lavage group, the joint was lavaged, "rough articular cartilage was shaved (chondroplasty was performed), loose debris was removed, all torn or degenerated meniscal fragments were trimmed, and the remaining meniscus was smoothed to a firm and stable rim."[35] One of the study's lead authors, surgeon J. Bruce Moseley, had long been skeptical of debridement and lavage. "I just didn't quite understand why people were reporting so much benefit when seemingly there wasn't very much done," he said.[36] Nelda Wray, the coleader of the research team, thought the placebo effect might be responsible for patients feeling better after the operation. The two researchers agreed that a sham surgery clinical trial was the best way to test whether the procedure had any benefit beyond a possible placebo effect.[37]

Participants in the trial were told that they might receive only placebo surgery and had to give their informed consent. The researchers created a placebo arm that mimicked the sight and sound of the actual procedure and included both sedation and an incision. For ethical reasons, patients in the sham surgery group were not placed under general anesthesia (they instead received a short-acting tranquilizer that caused them to fall asleep). Special care was taken to ensure that patients understood that they might receive sham surgery; subjects were required to transcribe the informed consent form prior to signing it. Subjects receiving the real procedures and those receiving the fake operations were equally likely to guess they were in the placebo group.

Moseley performed all the procedures himself and did not know whether the patient would receive a real or fake operation until he opened a sealed envelope when patients were wheeled into surgery. The effects of the procedures were assessed through subjective measures of pain and function as well as through objective measures of function, such as the amount of time it took for patients to walk thirty meters and climb up and down a flight of stairs. Measurements were obtained at several points throughout a two-year follow-up period. Evaluators did not know whether patients were in the treatment or control groups. The results suggested that the surgeries were no better than the placebo operations. At no point during the two-year period did either of the actual surgery groups report a statistically significant improvement in pain or function versus the placebo group. The average outcome measures produced by the placebo group were statistically superior to the surgery groups at two weeks. At all other time periods, the outcomes were statistically equivalent.

Although many scientific breakthroughs receive little attention from broader publics, the study's novel research design and provocative results made for arresting news copy. The study was praised in the lead editorial of the *New England Journal of Medicine* and produced extensive, if short-lived, media coverage.[38] Front-page articles appeared in major national newspapers.[39] The study's finding that a major procedure worked no better than a fake operation was something of a bombshell, but the results were probably not shocking to many experts. As one leading evidence-based medical research organization stated on its web site, "The results of the [sham surgery study] should not be a surprise based on the evidence from the literature. There never was any good evidence that lavage or debridement were useful things to do."[40]

STRENGTHS AND LIMITATIONS OF THE STUDY

The Moseley study was a significant advance on previous research. Whereas most prior investigations in orthopedics were retrospective case-series studies in which surgeons simply reported their experience with a procedure, the Moseley study was a double-blinded, placebo-controlled randomized trial—the "gold standard" in research medicine. Of course, even the best scientific studies have limitations. There were some features of the research design that might cast doubt on the validity or generalizability of the findings. An understanding of the scientific basis of the criticisms is therefore necessary to assess the reactions the study generated from interested parties.

One limitation of the study's research design is that it could not determine whether the benefits of the sham surgery intervention were due to some active placebo effect (such as some psychological benefit from receiving a physician's attention) or to the natural history of the patient's disease. If the decision to have surgery follows a period of unusually severe symptoms, simple regression to the mean might produce improvement over time in the absence of any medical intervention. Although there are reasons to believe the placebo effect was responsible for the improvement in patients' conditions, the issue cannot be resolved because of the study's lack of a natural history arm in which patients received neither a real nor a sham procedure.[41] However, whereas assigning the improvement in the placebo arm to its sources would be an important research finding, it has no implications for whether the arthroscopic procedures are superior to the sham surgery.[42]

A potentially more important criticism is the claim that the study used a flawed method for selecting patients for inclusion in the clinical trial. To gain entry into the trial, patients had to report knee pain. Critics argued that prior to the Moseley study the orthopedic community already recognized that patients who present with pain only are unlikely to benefit from the surgery, but that there are subgroups of patients with knee arthritis for whom the procedure is efficacious, including patients with early-stage arthritis and those with mechanical symptoms, such as joint "locking," "giving way," "popping," or "clicking."[43] The implication is the sham surgery study selected the wrong patients as subjects and that its findings should not fundamentally reorient orthopedic practice.

This argument is unconvincing for several reasons. First, it appears to be based on a crude misreading of the study design. The study did include patients on the basis of a pain measure but excluded patients only if they had a severe deformity or a meniscal tear that were observed preoperatively.[44] Almost all the patients included in the trial had both pain and mechanical symptoms. Mechanical problems of the knee are ubiquitous among patients with OA. In older patients with joint pain, it is nearly always possible to find some kind of mechanical symptom.[45] In follow-up correspondence appearing in the *New England Journal of Medicine*, the authors reported that 96 percent (172 out of 180) of the patients in the study had at least one mechanical problem.[46] The study results therefore suggest that neither lavage nor debridement with lavage is an effective treatment beyond placebo for patients who present with pain and one or more mechanical problems.

In addition, the sham surgery performed as well as the actual operations on the entire sample. If there was in fact a subgroup of patients for whom the operation was effective, it might be expected that the average improvement for the treatment groups, which consist of a mix of "appropriate" and "inappropriate" patients, would be attenuated but not entirely absent; there was, however, no consistent pattern of relative improvement by the treatments versus the placebo group. Third, although there were assertions about the criteria used for patient selection for surgery prior to the Moseley study, no empirical evidence was presented regarding actual patient selection practices. One study that examined the ability of doctors to anticipate which patients were likely to benefit from arthroscopy found they performed only slightly better than chance.[47] Finally, it should be noted that even if the Moseley study can be cast aside completely, the state of the evidence merely reverts to the pre-Moseley state; and, prior to Moseley, there is no methodologically convincing evidence that arthroscopic surgery works for the subgroups identified by the Moseley critics.[48]

To summarize: Moseley found no evidence that arthroscopic surgery relieves pain or improves function any better than a placebo operation for patients with knee arthritis. If there *were* any large beneficial effects, the study very likely would have found them. "Despite their current popularity, lavage and debridement are probably not efficacious as treatments for most persons with osteoarthritis of the knee," editorialized the *New England*

Journal of Medicine.[49] A leading expert stated that he believes the study's findings mean that 80 to 90 percent of the arthroscopies that have been performed on patients with arthritic knees should not have been done.[50]

Medical and Policy Community's Reactions to Moseley's Findings

At first glance, the knee surgery case might seem to illustrate the U.S. research and policy-making enterprise working at its best. Moseley, Wray, and their colleagues performed a first-class study that used powerful scientific methods to address a substantively important question. The study was conducted at a Veterans Administration hospital and paid for by federal research grants. It was published in the *New England Journal of Medicine*, and its results were disseminated to the public by media outlets. Contrary to the argument that large, bureaucratic organizations are hidebound and slow to react, key federal agencies, including the Centers for Medicare and Medicaid Services, altered their coverage policies in direct response to the study's findings.

But these first impressions are misleading. If we probe more deeply into the case, the system's performance appears troubling. After the publication of the Moseley study, the orthopedic medical societies pressured the government to adopt a very narrow interpretation of the study's findings, which preserves surgeons' clinical autonomy and minimizes the need to revise prior medical practices. The coverage decisions of federal health agencies were largely in line with the associations' position. That the sham surgery trial was conducted in the first place depended on individual initiative. Although doubts about the efficacy of arthroscopic surgery for knee arthritis had been raised at least since the early 1990s, the value of the procedure might never have been rigorously tested if the Moseley-Wray team had not fortuitously come along to conduct a critical sham surgery test. There were no institutions in place to make detection and investigation of questionable procedures a routine matter.

SURGEONS AND PROFESSIONAL SOCIETIES

We suspect that many individual orthopedic surgeons found it hard to believe Moseley's stunning finding that the surgery had no advantage over the placebo. What orthopedic surgeons *knew*—saw with their own eyes—is that their patients clearly improved after the operation. "I've done thousands of these in people with osteoarthritic knees, and they really are better," said surgeon Robert W. Jackson, a fierce defender of the procedures.[51] These surgeons may have failed to recognize that the study did not claim the procedure had no impact, only that the observed benefits are due to the placebo effect or natural history of the disease rather than the surgeon's skill.

The major initial reaction to the study from professional associations was not confusion but opposition. The professional associations defended the practices of their members and argued that Moseley's findings should not discredit use of the procedure for patients with OA. Professional groups like the American Association of Orthopaedic Surgeons (AAOS) argued that Moseley had failed to examine the benefits of the procedure for various subgroups, such as those with mechanical symptoms and normal alignment, and asserted that responsible surgeons already practiced proper patient selection.

At one level, the resistance to Moseley and colleagues' findings from the specialty associations reflects a difference in professional norms and orientations. As study coauthor Nelda Wray told us in an interview, "I speak the language of science, and the orthopedists do not."[52] In addition, the study was a direct economic threat to the specialists, observed David T. Felson, a leading physician who coauthored a *New England Journal of Medicine* editorial about the sham surgery study.[53]

Some surgeons who questioned the use of arthroscopy for patients with knee arthritis insisted it was vital to preserve insurance coverage and maintain professional autonomy. "I'm both a patient and a physician," said AAOS chief executive Dr. William J. Tipton Jr., explaining to a *New York Times* reporter that he has osteoarthritis. "My knee is buckling now, but I'm not going to have arthroscopy done. I recognize that it's not going to help." But Tipton said he would hate to see insurers refuse to pay on the basis of the Moseley study. If that occurs, he said, surgeons will complain. "This is where eyebrows are going to be raised," he said. "There's going to be a certain group of physicians who are very upset. This is another example of managed care at its lowest, with payers calling the shots. I think it's not good medicine."[54]

FEDERAL AGENCIES AND PRIVATE INSURERS

The federal government pays for a significant share of health care provision through Medicare and other programs and influences coverage decisions in the private sector. When a state-of-the-art medical study finds that an expensive medical procedure works no better than a fake operation for most

people with a common medical condition, if there is not convincing coun-
terevidence, this should be reflected in health policy decisions. Yet federal
health officials have traditionally treaded uneasily on physicians' professional
autonomy, especially with respect to clinical judgments about what services
patients require. The founding premise of the Medicare program is that the
clinical autonomy of participating physicians would be protected. Over time,
the federal government's efforts to control health care costs, along with the
growth of managed care in the private sector, has resulted in some degree of
erosion of physicians' autonomy, but the presumption remains that doctors
can best judge what treatments patients need.[55]

Federal bureaucrats are often faulted for being slow to act in the face of
new information, but federal health agencies began reviewing their coverage policies immediately after the publication of the Moseley study. The
final decisions of these agencies, however, followed a questionable, narrow
reading of the study's findings preferred by the professional associations.
Although the Veterans Administration initially recommended that arthroscopies for knee arthritis not be performed absent "clear clinical evidence of
significant derangement," it subsequently announced that the Moseley study
would not change the standard of practice at VA hospitals after all. Both an
internal review by VA officials and an expert panel on orthopedic surgery
concluded that the findings of the sham surgery study were not sufficient
to limit or prohibit knee arthroscopy within the VA. The main reason given
for the decision not to limit coverage was that outside experts asserted that
surgeons rarely perform arthroscopy solely for pain associated with OA.[56]
The federal Centers for Medicare and Medicaid Services (CMS) also made
policy decisions that were largely in line with the position of the orthopedic
associations.

Following the publication of the Moseley study, which CMS analysts believed was so important that it simply could not be ignored, the agency began
a careful review of the scientific evidence to determine whether arthroscopic
surgery for patients with arthritic knees should be nationally covered under
Medicare.[57] The agency met with Dr. Wray, spoke with Dr. Moseley on the
phone, and then held two separate meetings (in November 2002 and January
2003) with representatives of key professional associations.

The AAOS, the Arthroscopy Association of North America (AANA),
the American Association of Hip and Knee Surgeons, and affiliated groups
prepared a joint report to "provide CMS with clinical and scientific information" about arthroscopic procedures for patients with arthritic knees.
The major conclusion of the report was that many patients with OA of the

knee, especially those with early degenerative arthritis and mechanical symptoms, can be significantly helped with arthroscopic surgery.[58] All the research studies cited in support of this conclusion, however, suffered from the basic methodological problems characterizing the research literature prior to the Moseley study. These problems were not acknowledged. The report also did not address Moseley and Wray's response that 172 of 180 subjects in their study had mechanical symptoms nor did it indicate that the orthopedic groups should (and would) seek to generate hard evidence to support their claims about the benefits of the procedure for population subgroups by sponsoring replications of the study.

In July 2003, the CMS concluded that coverage should be changed in response to the Moseley study and the subsequent review of the evidence.[59] The agency concluded that there was no evidence to support lavage alone for OA patients and that the procedure would henceforth be nationally non-covered. With respect to debridement, CMS determined that the procedure would be nationally noncovered when patients presented with knee pain only or with severe OA. CMS decided, however, to maintain local Medicare contractors' discretion to cover the surgery if physicians requested it for patients with pain and other indications (for example, mechanical symptoms). This policy was subsequently echoed in the coverage decisions of major private insurers.[60]

CMS was unable to present solid evidence in support of its decision to maintain coverage of debridement for the vast majority of patients with arthritic knees (mechanical symptoms being ubiquitous in the OA population). Indeed, the agency deemed the available medical evidence on the issue to be "inconclusive because of methodological deficiencies." Including the Moseley and Wray investigation, there were only four studies that addressed debridement in patients with mechanical symptoms as the indication for surgery, but three of them were case series without random assignment to control groups and using nonvalidated assessment scales. The CMS acknowledged that the level of evidence supporting the usefulness of the procedure was "suboptimal" and that case series studies in general are considered methodologically weak in their ability to minimize bias. Nonetheless, CMS continued to pay for debridement. It argued that the three case series "consistently" pointed to improvements in outcomes. The CMS coverage analysis acknowledged the unusually high quality of the Moseley study, calling it the only "large-scale, well-designed" randomized clinical trial in the pool of evidence, but argued that the study failed to "specifically address the issue of reduction of mechanical symptoms." The fact that virtually all the patients in the Moseley study had one or more mechanical symptoms, as the authors reported in follow-up letters to the *New England Journal of Medicine* and other professional journals, went unmentioned. Although CMS's official policy is to take into account the scientific quality of medical evidence, in practice its coverage decision process weighs most heavily the findings of studies published in peer-reviewed journals, even if the methodological quality of a study is problematic.[61] CMS's coverage review process is thus based on a high degree of trust in the medical profession's ability to determine appropriate medical practices and to self-regulate.

The AAOS welcomed the CMS's coverage decision: "The coverage decision parallels the position of the musculoskeletal societies. CMS recognized that arthroscopy is appropriate in virtually all circumstances in which the orthopaedic community now employs this technology," an association newsletter stated.[62] In fact, CMS did not perform an empirical investigation of actual surgical practices regarding patient selection for OA of the knee and consequently could not provide assurances regarding current surgical practices. The societies recognized that the CMS decision left key coverage decisions in the hands of local Medicare contractors. The implementation process would therefore be critical. The AAOS promised its members that the organization would provide carriers with "specific and detailed instructions to implement the coverage decision appropriately. The instructions should clearly reflect the limited applicability of the policy decision."[63] Moseley moved on to other endeavors, and no interest group exists to balance the messages that Medicare contractors would hear about the indications for arthroscopy from surgeons.[64]

CMS was in a difficult political position because a decision to deny coverage for a procedure will create cases where CMS judgments substitute for those of a patient's doctor. The fact that CMS initiated the coverage review of arthroscopy in the first place reflects well on the agency and its staff. To go further, and deny coverage of both lavage and debridement, would likely have caused the agency to come under withering attack from orthopedists and other medical specialties. The critical policy failure is not that CMS continued to pay for a procedure for a (large) population subgroup in the absence of solid data in one specific case, but that as a result of existing law and decades of precedent the agency *routinely* makes coverage and reimbursement decisions without taking into account the comparative effectiveness of treatments.[65] The creation of a new CER institute under the ACA is unlikely to solve this problem. More fundamental shifts in Medicare payment approaches will be required.[66]

MEDICAL RESEARCH: ABSENCE OF REPLICATION STUDIES

It is interesting to take note of what did *not* happen after the publication of the landmark *New England Journal of Medicine* sham surgery study. This development did not lead the medical research community to immediately carry out new clinical trials to repeat this research design to check the robustness of the findings, even though many prominent orthopedic specialists called for just this to occur. The medical societies did not demand an immediate study to address the "supposed" methodological issues they maintained were the source of their skepticism of the Moseley-Wray study. Replication studies would have allowed any lingering concerns about the stunning finding that arthroscopy works no better than a placebo to be addressed in a scientifically valid way. At the same time, a carefully designed replication study would have allowed researchers to investigate whether the procedure works for a specific subgroup, such as those with mechanical symptoms or a meniscal tear.

Since the Moseley study, only one other randomized controlled trial focusing on the efficacy of arthroscopic debridement and lavage on pain and function has been published. Kirkley and colleagues at the University of Western Ontario, Canada, randomized patients with moderately advanced OA either to debridement plus a standard physical therapy (PT) regimen or to the PT regimen alone. While the surgical group had an initial improvement in pain or functional status compared to the PT group at the three-month follow-up visit, there were no clinically meaningful or statistically significant differences in improvement between the two groups at any subsequent visits. Thus, the Kirkley study failed to find evidence for the clinical benefits of debridement over and above standard PT. An important methodological limitation of the Kirkley RCT, however, is that it did not include a placebo arm.[67]

IMPACT ON PRACTICE

If the U.S. health care system were working well, the stunning evidence from the Moseley study would have triggered a dramatic decrease in the number of arthroscopies performed for patients with knee OA, especially because there was no good evidence that the procedures worked in the first place. There are signs that the use of debridement has indeed begun to decline, but the decrease in utilization has been gradual. A large gap remains between what research indicates and what doctors do.[68] Certainly the belief of experts like Felson that 80–90 percent of these arthroscopic procedures should no longer be done has not been matched.[69] Not only has the decline in utilization been slower than would be predicted if medical practices were fully responsive to changes in the evidence base, but the timing of the decline suggests that the revision in Medicare coverage policy was a key driver, not just the emergence of better evidence. Further, it is difficult to determine how much of the observed trend of declining utilization reflects a real change in physicians' behavior that resulted in fewer arthroscopies actually being performed on patients with knee OA. As discussed below, other possible causes of the observed trend are changes in how doctors diagnosed patients and coded procedures for purposes of insurance reimbursement and payment.

There is no national system to track the medical procedures performed on patients with knee OA. There have been several attempts, however, to measure the changes in the number of debridement and lavage procedures for knee OA patients using available databases. For example, Sunny Kim and colleagues used the U.S. National Ambulatory Surgical Database and found that the number of knee arthroscopies performed for OA patients declined by 18 percent from 1996 to 2006.[70] Howard and colleagues examined ambulatory surgery data from Florida "and found that the number of [these procedures] per 100,000 adults declined 47 percent between 2001 and 2010."[71] Utilization declined after the 2002 Moseley study and then again after the 2004 CMS coverage change and the 2008 Kirkley study. Despite the observed decline in utilization, some experts questioned how much physician behavior really changed. In 2008, Moseley told the *New York Times*, "What happened after our study was that organized orthopedics rallied the troops to try and discredit our study as much as possible. People continued to practice the way they practiced."[72]

There are several reasons why trends of declining usage may not accurately measure the actual impact of evidence on physician behavior. First, some doctors could have kept performing the procedures as before, but altered what they said was patients' main problem, giving diagnoses other than OA. After the Moseley study, AAOS clinical guidelines recommended against debridement and lavage for patients with a primary diagnosis of symptomatic OA of the knee. This guideline did not apply, however, to "patients who had a primary diagnosis of meniscal tear, loose body, or other mechanical derangement, with *concomitant* diagnosis of osteoarthritis of the knee (emphasis added)."[73] Meniscal tears are highly prevalent among people with knee arthritis, including among patients not experiencing pain. (Tears are also common among the general population.) Having a meniscal tear and knee pain does not mean that the tear is the cause of the pain; knee pain arises for many reasons.[74] The increasing use of MRIs has therefore produced many incidental findings of meniscal tears that are not the cause of symptoms.[75]

Second, some doctors that had previously debrided OA patients could have begun performing a closely related procedure, arthroscopic partial meniscectomy (APM). An indication for this procedure is symptomatic meniscal tear.[76] As noted above, meniscal tears are ubiquitous among the OA population. The key question is whether "surgeons simply used different codes (such as meniscal tear) when performing arthroscopy for OA, or actually performed fewer of these procedures in the OA population."[77] This question is difficult to answer. Over time, the number of procedures done for OA has declined, and the number done for meniscal tears has increased. The number of procedures done for OA is small in relation to the number of arthroscopies done for other indications, making it difficult to discern whether or not the former's declining utilization has contributed to the growing utilization of other procedures. There is a clear possibility that orthopedic surgeons have been "unmoved by the pivotal trials . . . and are still scoping the same patients and their knees, yet possibly coding the procedure differently," wrote Järvinen and colleagues.[78]

Déjà Vu All Over Again? The Case of Arthroscopic Partial Meniscectomy

When a strong body of research demonstrates that a common procedure does not work as advertised, the finding should cause the medical community to take a hard look at the effectiveness of other widely used treatments in the relevant practice area that rest on the same fundamental evidence base to see if use of these other treatments should also be reevaluated. The cumulative evidence about the lack of demonstrated effectiveness of the procedures examined in the Moseley-Wray study should have raised serious doubts that arthroscopic surgery would be useful for patients who have symptomatic meniscal tears in the setting of OA. Although the focus of the Moseley and Kirkley studies was on OA, there were participants in these studies who had mechanical problems and/or meniscal tears, and if the procedures were very beneficial for these subgroups, the data would likely have revealed signs of it. Still, it is understandable (indeed desirable) that surgeons would want to see evidence from studies specifically focused on the question of whether APM helps patients who have meniscal tears along with OA. As in the lavage and debridement case, however, the research designs of the early studies were poor. Then, when well-done studies, including Sihvonen and colleagues' sham-controlled randomized trial,[79] demonstrated that APM does not work as advertised, the orthopedic community again responded in ways that raise questions about its responsiveness to evidence.

By 2006, around 700,000 APM procedures were being performed annually in the United States.[80] These interventions rested on a weak evidence base. The first studies demonstrating the benefits of APM were nonrandomized studies with generally small samples.[81] The case for performing these procedures weakened further with the publication of two important randomized controlled trials in the *New England Journal of Medicine* in 2013. The first demonstrated that APM combined with physical therapy provides no better relief of knee symptoms than physical therapy alone in patients with a meniscal tear and OA.[82] The second—which echoed the power and elegance of the Moseley study of debridement and lavage—showed in a double-blind, sham-controlled randomized trial that APM works no better than a fake operation for people with a degenerative meniscal tear and no knee OA.[83] The Sihvonen study deliberately recruited knee patients *without* OA because these are the patients who were "most likely to have a good response," and if APM cannot work under the best circumstances (e.g., on those with a meniscal tear but no OA), it follows that the procedure won't be effective in "less optimal routine settings."[84]

Despite the lack of evidence for the clinical efficacy of APM relative to nonsurgical alternatives, the orthopedic community continued to resist the obvious conclusion from well-designed research studies; namely, that APM does not have demonstrated clinical benefits compared to cheaper and less invasive alternatives. Noting that the 700,000 APM procedures performed in the United States generate $4 billion in direct medical spending, one of the authors of the sham surgery study predicted that the research findings "will not be welcomed with open arms."[85] At a packed session at the annual meeting of the AAOS, the conclusions and methodology of the study "were heavily criticized by notable orthopedic leaders."[86] Criticisms from the orthopedic community were also raised in letters to the *New England Journal of Medicine*. Many of the concerns raised against the APM sham surgery study were similar to the kinds of criticisms directed at the earlier Moseley study, including the alleged exclusion of patients with mechanical problems. In fact, 47 percent of the participants in the Sihvonen study had preoperative mechanical symptoms.[87]

The most pointed criticism of the APM study, however, was not patient selection. Rather, it was that the sham used in the study was not a "true" sham but in fact *lavage*, and lavage is (according to a letter to the

New England Journal of Medicine written by three physicians critical of the study) "an accepted surgical procedure."[88] A University of Maryland surgeon quoted in a newspaper article said: "If you scope the knee (without touching the cushion), that will often help even if you don't completely address the torn-meniscus issue," he said. When fluid is injected, "you're taking out the junky, thick, irritating fluid that can give a lot of people their pain."[89]

We see where we are. According to leading orthopedic surgeons, the negative results of the most rigorous study of the benefits of APM should not be believed. And the *key reason* the study should not be believed is because the patients in the placebo arm received an injection of fluid—an intervention found equivalent to a placebo intervention in the 2002 Moseley-Wray study. In sum, several doctors claimed that APM should not be discredited because the study providing evidence of its lack of effectiveness was built on the findings of an earlier study that showed that lavage works no better than fake irrigation.

This episode shows the broader value of examining reactions to the Moseley-Wray study since the case makes subsequent developments very recognizable. Patterns repeat with surprisingly little variation over time. The problems we have documented regarding the medical system's uptake of evidence are deep-seated and widespread, rather than the result of minor performance failures in one part of an otherwise well-functioning system.

3

Doctor Knows Best

THE INFLUENCE OF PHYSICIAN LEADERSHIP ON PUBLIC OPINION

In American democracy, public recognition of societal problems often requires prompting from elites. To be sure, voters do not need to be told that traffic congestion in their neighborhoods is getting worse, the major local employer has gone bankrupt, or gas prices are rising. They can see tangible evidence of such problems with their own eyes. But the more complex, subtle, or remote from daily experience problems are, the less likely voters are to discern them on their own. A key question for the performance of U.S. political and economic institutions is whether the policy elites who are in a position to educate the public about the existence of important but less readily apparent problems will do so, or, alternatively, whether they will permit citizens to remain uninformed.

When it comes to public understanding of the "medical guesswork" problem and the large costs it imposes on both patients and the nation, no set of opinion leaders is more important than doctors. In this chapter, we draw on the results of five national surveys we carried out between 2009 and 2011 to explore how public confidence in doctors and the medical profession affects public support for proposals to improve the evidence base.[1] The surveys had sample sizes between 1,100 and 3,600,[2] and they were representative of the general U.S. population on a variety of characteristics, including gender, income, race, and health insurance status.[3]

The surveys demonstrate that doctors possess the influence, prestige, and standing to play a leadership role in educating the public about the inefficiencies and waste of the U.S. health care system. The public views doctors as more honest and hardworking than other professional groups. Americans believe that doctors are experts who are empathetic and concerned about helping people, and do not see economic incentives as a primary driver of doctors' behavior. Because most Americans believe "doctor knows best," they tend to have confidence in the advice of doctors, not only about individual medical problems, but also about broader health care reform issues. As Mark A. Peterson has persuasively argued, the trust that patients have in their doctors as medical healers leads to a broad-based social trust in doctors as policy experts and faithful representatives of the public's welfare in policy debates.[4]

Our surveys also reveal that Americans are naturally wary of health care reform proposals they fear could constrain physician discretion, such as requiring doctors to follow evidence-based clinical guidelines. The public's anxieties about proposals to make medicine more evidence based, however, *can* be overcome. Using survey experiments, we demonstrate that physician endorsements of such reforms significantly alleviate public fears. Our survey results suggest that if doctors *were* to become forceful advocates for reform, their reputations as trusted, well-motivated experts position them to shape the views of ordinary citizens. In sum, we argue not only that doctors have the professional responsibility to exercise public leadership on improvements to the health care system, but also that they have an opportunity to do so.

An Agency Model of Doctors' Persuasive Influence

The tendency of the public to defer to doctors for guidance both on personal medical problems and broader health reform issues[5] can be understood if the relationship between doctors and patients is considered from the perspective of principal-agent theory. "Agency" relationships are ubiquitous in a complex modern economy. They arise whenever a "principal" enters into a contract or agreement with an agent in which authority is delegated to the agent to perform a task on the principal's behalf or to make decisions that affect the principal's well-being.[6] For example, people hire financial advisers to recommend stocks, lawyers to draw up wills, and doctors to cure their ills;

such delegation makes people better off. However, problems can occur in an agency relationship when, as is often the case, the agent has more information than the principal. An agent could take advantage of the principal's trust by engaging in behavior that is costly for the principal to detect. For example, a car mechanic could recommend a costly repair to fix a part that is not really broken. When such information asymmetries arise, the challenge is to align the interests of the agent with those of the principal. A variety of mechanisms can be used to mitigate this problem, from contractual safeguards and warranties to government oversight and the creation of social norms against opportunistic behavior and self-dealing. The ethical norm of medical professionalism, licensure, and self-regulation can all be seen as responses to the agency problem in medicine.[7] How well these mechanisms are currently working in the U.S. health care system, however, is debatable. Indeed, the evidence we present in this book suggests that these arrangements often fail to protect patients' interest in receiving appropriate treatments for their conditions grounded in the best possible scientific evidence. From the standpoint of understanding the sources of doctors' persuasive influence on ordinary citizens, however, the crucial consideration is how the public *perceives* its agency relationship with physicians, not whether the relationship is actually working optimally.

The foundation of persuasive communication in a principal-agent framework is that the agent (the doctor) possesses expertise and either naturally shares the interests of the imperfectly informed principal (the patient) or has adequate incentives to act in the principal's interest.[8] Beyond seeing doctors as charismatic figures who offer emotional support, patients, who are typically ill-informed about both medicine and health care policy, may regard doctors as trustworthy experts who are motivated to protect their well-being. If so, this would promote the public's willingness to accept cues regarding the desirability of health policies from doctors and medical associations. Our survey results suggest that these two conditions are easily satisfied. The American public generally believes that doctors are (1) technically proficient and (2) their allies.[9] That is, the public believes doctors not only *know* best, but are also strongly motivated to *do* the right thing for patients.

Public Beliefs about the Motivations of Doctors and Medical Societies

That the public has bedrock trust in doctors is an easily overlooked feature of the U.S. health care system. Many studies have documented a decline in the public's confidence in the medical profession and its leaders over time.[10] For example, 73 percent of Americans "said they had a 'great deal of confidence in the people in charge of running medicine' in 1966. In 2010 only 34 percent expressed that level of confidence."[11] The decline in confidence in medicine may reflect not only a general decline in public confidence in government and other major institutions over the past several decades,[12] but also broad changes in the political economy of health care. In the 1960s, patients had relatively few treatment options, the health sector made up a small share of the economy, and organized medicine possessed an issue monopoly over health policy. Today, concerns about rising medical costs, increasing premiums and deductibles, and government budget deficits have sparked debates about the value of dollars spent and created a more open and contentious health politics.[13]

But these important developments should be kept in perspective. Although the medical profession may not enjoy the same absolute level of confidence as it once did, what also matters from a political standpoint is the status and influence of doctors *relative* to other actors in the health care arena such as elected officials, drug companies, and health insurance companies. Many Americans recognize that the health care system does not always serve the interests of patients, but most blame actors other than doctors for the system's flaws. Despite the secular decline in confidence in the medical profession, Americans view doctors as being honest and generally trust doctors to recommend the right thing for the country on health care.[14] In a 2008 Gallup survey, 64 percent of Americans believed doctors had very high or high ethical standards, up from 56 percent in 1976.[15] In contrast, on a separate nationally representative survey that we conducted, 68 percent of the public agreed that "drug companies keep cures for some serious medical conditions secret from the public to protect the profits they get from their current products." Despite the erosion of medical authority in American politics since the 1960s,[16] the public continues to display remarkable faith in physicians compared to other groups.[17]

In one survey, we randomly assigned respondents to evaluate one of four professions: doctors, lawyers, grade school teachers, or members of Congress. We asked respondents to rate their agreement with a series of six statements about the motivations of individuals from their randomly assigned profession. For example, those in the "doctors" condition were asked how much they agreed with the statement: "Doctors are interested in helping people." We measured responses on a five-point scale ranging from "strongly disagree" (1) to "strongly agree" (5).

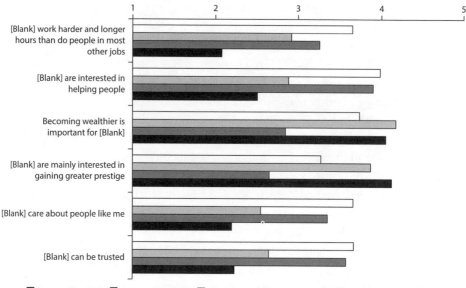

FIGURE 3.1. Beliefs about the motivations of doctors compared to other professions. *Note*: Mean responses to the question: "How much do you agree with each of the following statements?" Responses were measured on a five-point scale ranging from "strongly disagree" (1) to "strongly agree" (5). *N* represents the number of respondents randomly assigned to evaluate each profession. All the differences in the public's assessment of doctors compared to other professions are statistically significant at $p<.05$, two-tailed, with the exception of the differences between doctors and school teachers on the "interested in helping people" ($p=.26$) and "can be trusted" ($p=.25$) items. *Source*: February 17–23, 2011, YouGov/Polimetrix survey. A version of this figure was originally published as figure 1 in Alan S. Gerber, Eric M. Patashnik, David Doherty, and Conor M. Dowling, 2014, "Doctor Knows Best: Physician Endorsements, Public Opinion, and the Politics of Comparative Effectiveness Research," *Journal of Health Politics, Policy and Law* 39 (1): 171–208. Copyright 2014, Duke University Press. All rights reserved. Republished by permission of the publisher. www.dukeupress.edu.

Figure 3.1 displays mean responses to these six items for each profession. The results indicate that respondents view doctors as harder workers, more interested in helping people, more trustworthy, and as caring more ("about people like me") than each of the other professions.[18] To be sure, the public does not view doctors as exclusively altruistic,[19] but it does view doctors as being less driven by a desire to gain greater wealth and prestige than members of other elite professions, such as lawyers and members of Congress.

Although people interact most directly with their personal doctors, medical societies have a substantial influence on public policy. They take positions on proposed changes to federal rules and make recommendations for coverage and reimbursement decisions under Medicare that affect program beneficiaries and taxpayers.[20] When studies are published about the effectiveness of a common treatment—as in the knee arthroscopy case discussed in chapter 2—medical societies may issue statements about the research methodologies used and the significance of the study findings.[21] Our national physician survey (discussed in chapter 4) shows that most doctors want their medical societies to take an active role in critiquing studies that challenge the benefits of treatments in their practice areas. The statements of medical societies about the effectiveness of treatments are often quoted in the media and may in turn shape public beliefs about not only the perceived benefits of particular medical services, but also about the overall quality and efficiency of the U.S. medical system. In adopting positions that mold public opinion and influence public policy, at least, medical associations exist in large part to advance the economic interests of their members and are similar to other organizations, such as unions, trade associations or industry groups. But does the public believe doctor associations share the same motivations as other economic organizations?

To find out, we asked respondents to evaluate the importance of several factors in explaining why various groups make policy recommendations. We randomly assigned each respondent to evaluate the motivations of one of four groups: medical associations, unions, business organizations, or health insurance organizations. We investigated the importance of the following five motivations: (1) maintaining high income for group members; (2) preserving the group's influence over policy makers; (3) promoting the health of patients (for medical associations and health insurance organizations) or workers (for business organizations and unions); (4) ensuring that new laws and regulations help their industry; and (5) protecting doctors from malpractice suits (for medical associations and health insurance organizations only). We measured responses on a five-point scale ranging from "not at all important" (1) to "extremely important" (5).

Figure 3.2 displays the percentage of respondents that chose either of the top two response categories: "very important" or "extremely important." The results show that the public sees the desire to maintain high incomes for group members and to preserve group influence over policy makers as being weaker motivations for medical associations than for unions and business organizations. Only 45 percent of respondents stated that "maintaining high incomes" was either very or extremely important to medical associations, whereas 60 percent and 55 percent said the same for unions and business organizations. The public also perceives medical associations as being more concerned about promoting patient health (65 percent selected very or extremely important) than health insurance organizations (56 percent), and

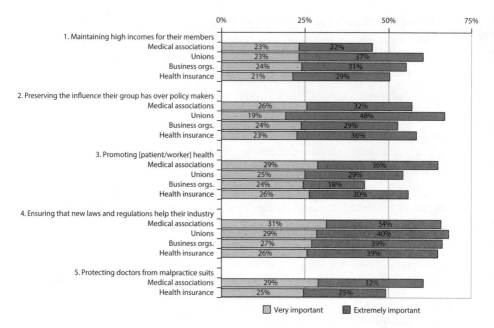

FIGURE 3.2. Beliefs about the motivations of medical associations compared to other groups. *Note*: Responses to the question: "When developing their recommendations, how important do you think each of the following considerations is to these groups?" Number of observations for each randomly assigned group were 348 (medical associations), 352 (unions), 370 (business organizations), and 342 (health insurance organizations). Responses were measured on a five-point scale ranging from "not at all important" to "extremely important." The figure displays the percent who responded that the consideration was "very important" and "extremely important" (the top two response categories). *Source*: February 17–23, 2011, YouGov/Polimetrix survey. A version of this figure was originally published as figure 2 in Alan S. Gerber, Eric M. Patashnik, David Doherty, and Conor M. Dowling, 2014, "Doctor Knows Best: Physician Endorsements, Public Opinion, and the Politics of Comparative Effectiveness Research," *Journal of Health Politics, Policy and Law* 39 (1): 171–208. Copyright 2014, Duke University Press. All rights reserved. Republished by permission of the publisher. www.dukeupress.edu.

more concerned about promoting patient health than unions (54 percent) and business organizations (43 percent) are concerned about promoting worker health. The public does, however, see the desire to protect doctors from malpractice suits as being a stronger motivator for medical associations (61 percent) than for health insurance organizations (49 percent).

The Public Fears Interference with Physician Discretion

One problem that can arise in an agency relationship is that the agent may lack the expertise needed to serve the principal's interests. As medicine becomes more complex, it becomes increasingly difficult for even diligent doctors to keep up with the latest scientific evidence about what works best for different conditions. As Austin Frakt observes,

> In 2014 alone, more than 750,000 additional medical studies were published. Granted, a physician might need to keep up only with the evidence in her specialty, but even at a fraction of this rate, it is unrealistic to expect even the best physicians to assimilate every new development in their fields. In cancer alone, 150,000 studies are published annually.[22]

Research suggests that, in certain areas of medicine, physicians whose practice styles deviate significantly from the statewide norm established in teaching hospitals for that year have much worse patient outcomes.[23] But while many experts argue that doctors should be required to follow evidence-based guidelines when caring for patients in order to improve care, reduce medical errors, and curb wasteful spending, respondents are skeptical of proposals that might narrow the ability of doctors to exercise their professional discretion to choose the treatments they receive.[24] One reason why people may be uneasy with guidelines is the belief that treatments help some people but not others and that one's personal doctor knows if a given treatment will work for them. A majority (52 percent) of respondents agreed with the statement, "If a treatment only helps some patients who get it, your doctor knows whether you will be among those for whom the treatment is effective."

Our surveys show that advocates who hope to build public support for evidence-based guidelines will need to overcome a variety of public concerns. We asked respondents how convincing they thought four arguments for and five arguments against evidence-based guidelines were, randomizing whether respondents read the block of "pro" or "con" arguments first as well as the order of arguments within each block.[25] Figure 3.3 shows that most respondents found each of the "pro" and "con" arguments to be convincing, but overall they were more likely to rate the "con" arguments as either somewhat or very convincing. They were also more likely to find the "con" arguments to be *very* convincing, relative to the "pro" arguments. No fewer than 55 percent of respondents were somewhat or very convinced by each of the four arguments in favor of treatment guidelines: economic incentives may cause doctors to give patients unnecessary care (63 percent); guidelines would improve care for most patients (57 percent); doctors can become out of touch with the latest research (55 percent); doctors follow local standards of care and may be unaware of better treatments being used elsewhere (55 percent). However, just 12–20 percent of respondents found these arguments in favor of guidelines to be *very* convincing.

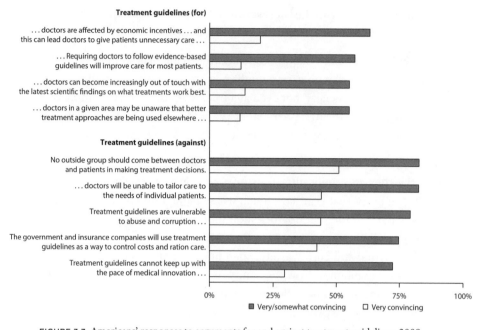

FIGURE 3.3. Americans' responses to arguments for and against treatment guidelines, 2009. *Note*: Responses to the question: "Here are some arguments people have given [for/against] requiring doctors to follow treatment guidelines. After each statement, please tell me how convincing the reason is." Responses were measured on a four-point scale ranging from "not at all convincing" to "very convincing." The figure displays the percent who responded that the argument was "very convincing" and "somewhat" plus "very convincing." *Source*: November 5–December 31, 2009, YouGov/Polimetrix survey. A version of this figure was originally published by Project HOPE/*Health Affairs* as exhibit 1 in Alan S. Gerber, Eric M. Patashnik, David Doherty, and Conor M. Dowling, 2010, "A National Survey Reveals Public Skepticism about Research-Based Treatment Guidelines," *Health Affairs* (Millwood) 29 (10): 1882–84. The published article is archived and available online at www.healthaffairs.org.

In general, respondents found the arguments against guidelines more persuasive. At least 70 percent of respondents were somewhat or very convinced by each of the five arguments against treatment guidelines. In fact, more than eight in ten respondents were convinced that forcing doctors to follow guidelines would prevent them from tailoring care to individual patients and that no outside group should come between doctors and patients. More than seven in ten respondents believed that guidelines are vulnerable to corruption and abuse, will be used to ration care, and will not incorporate the latest scientific breakthroughs. Moreover, the proportion of respondents finding each of these arguments to be *very* convincing ranged from 29 to 51 percent. The details of these results could reflect nuances in how the persuasive messages were crafted, but the substantial differences in response and the strong response to the antiguideline arguments suggests important areas of public concern.

The Public Wants Consumer Information, Not Mandates

Will the public embrace proposals to make American medicine more evidence based? Many experts believe that a significant proportion of the care that patients receive does little to improve health.[26] This conclusion reinforces the view that the U.S. health care system is wasteful, and that the adoption of evidence-based medicine might promote better patient outcomes and a more efficient allocation of resources. The general public, however, places tremendous faith in the curative power of modern medicine. Nearly 80 percent of respondents in our survey agreed with the statement that "the most recent medical innovations are more effective than treatments that were introduced 10 or 20 years ago," and over 55 percent agreed that "modern medicine can cure almost any illness [with] advanced technology and treatment." Many citizens assume that more medicine is generally better and that evidence-based guidelines limit the ability of doctors to provide appropriate care.[27]

To be sure, a segment of the public does recognize that a great deal of medicine is not based on solid evidence. We found that 50 percent of the public agreed with the statement that half or less of the care they received is evidence based.[28] The public's recognition that not all medical care is based on evidence does not, however, automatically translate into strong support for the use of research studies to mandate changes in clinical practices or the allocation of health care resources. Figure 3.4 shows that the public supports the use of CER to provide information to health care consumers, such as creating warning labels for treatments that are not supported by strong scientific evidence, but that the majority of the public does not support the use of research findings to mandate treatment decisions, determine which groups of patients should be protected from budget cuts in Medicare, or charge patients more to get a treatment that research has not shown to be effective if the patient's own doctor recommends the treatment.

Public Fears Are Easily Stoked—but Can Be Overcome with Doctor Support

Public opinion on some issues (such as the price of gas) reflects personal experience. Other issues (such as views on abortion) reflect deeply held moral

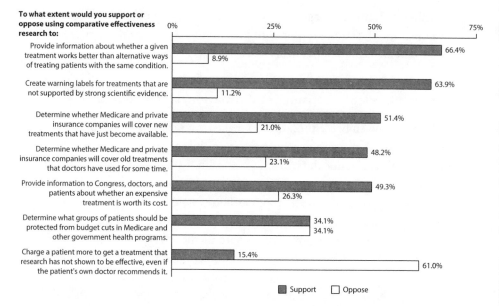

To what extent would you support or oppose using comparative effectiveness research to:

Provide information about whether a given treatment works better than alternative ways of treating patients with the same condition. — Support 66.4%, Oppose 8.9%

Create warning labels for treatments that are not supported by strong scientific evidence. — Support 63.9%, Oppose 11.2%

Determine whether Medicare and private insurance companies will cover new treatments that have just become available. — Support 51.4%, Oppose 21.0%

Determine whether Medicare and private insurance companies will cover old treatments that doctors have used for some time. — Support 48.2%, Oppose 23.1%

Provide information to Congress, doctors, and patients about whether an expensive treatment is worth its cost. — Support 49.3%, Oppose 26.3%

Determine what groups of patients should be protected from budget cuts in Medicare and other government health programs. — Support 34.1%, Oppose 34.1%

Charge a patient more to get a treatment that research has not shown to be effective, even if the patient's own doctor recommends it. — Support 15.4%, Oppose 61.0%

■ Support   □ Oppose

FIGURE 3.4. Americans' support for uses of comparative effectiveness research, 2010. *Note*: Responses to the question: "To what extent would you support or oppose using comparative effectiveness research to:" Responses were measured on a five-point scale ranging from "strongly oppose" to "strongly support." The figure displays the percent who responded that they somewhat/strongly supported and somewhat/strongly opposed; the remaining (unreported) respondents selected "neither support or oppose." *Source*: May 21–24, 2010, YouGov/ Polimetrix survey. A version of this figure was originally published by Project hope/*Health Affairs* as exhibit 2 in Alan S. Gerber, Eric M. Patashnik, David Doherty, and Conor M. Dowling, 2010, "The Public Wants Information, Not Board Mandates, from Comparative Effectiveness Research," *Health Affairs* (Millwood) 29 (10): 1872–81. The published article is archived and available online at www.healthaffairs.org.

views. On such issues, ordinary people are able to form their opinions without the influence of elites. In contrast, evidence-based medicine is a highly technical issue on which public opinion is likely to be more susceptible to the influence of opinion leaders.[29] We performed two survey experiments to explore the relative persuasiveness of arguments made in elite discourse about the pros and cons of comparative effectiveness research in a manner that simulates the back and forth of a political debate. In each experiment, participants were presented with one argument in favor of CER and one argument opposed to it.

In the first experiment, we assessed baseline support for government funding of CER (that is, whether respondents would support using taxpayer money to pay for medical research on the relative effectiveness of different treatments for a given medical condition), using a 0–100 sliding scale. We then randomly assigned respondents to be presented with one of two arguments in favor of CER and one of three arguments against (described below). The order of the pro and con arguments was also randomized. After reading the pair of arguments, respondents were again asked about their support for CER (using the same 0–100 sliding scale), allowing us to assess whether exposure to a stylized debate about CER moved opinion.

We used two common pro arguments. The first was that CER "will improve health care outcomes by giving patients and doctors the information they need to identify the most effective treatments." We paired this *improve outcomes* argument with one of three counterarguments that CER would: (1) lead to *one-size-fits-all* medicine ("the government and insurance companies will use the research to tell doctors how to practice medicine. They will force doctors to follow one-size-fits-all treatment guidelines rather than being able to use their knowledge and expertise to tailor care to each individual patient"); (2) serve as an excuse to *ration care* ("the government and insurance companies will use the research findings as an excuse to ration care and deny coverage of effective but expensive treatments"); and (3) *waste taxpayer money* ("government spending on comparative effectiveness research would waste taxpayer money because doctors already know what treatments work best").

The second pro argument was that CER "will help reduce the budget deficit by allowing the government to cut wasteful spending on ineffective treatments without lowering the quality of medical care." We pitted this *reduce deficit* argument against three counterarguments: (1) *one-size-fits-all*, (2) *ration care*, and (3) that CER would *reduce innovation* ("cutting medical spending for any reason reduces companies' financial incentive to develop new drugs and medical devices and that will be bad for patients in the long run"). We focus on the net effects of each of the six argument pairs on support for CER (i.e., average change in support for CER from the baseline question to the same question asked after the experiment). Table 3.1 presents a summary of the results of this experiment.

The key finding from this experiment is that exposure to the debate over CER generates concerns among the public. The net effect of seeing each of the argument pairings was to lower respondents' support for government funding of the medical research. For example, respondents who were exposed to the *improve outcomes/one-size-fits-all* pairing reduced their support for CER by 10.0 points on the 100 point scale. Respondents who were exposed to the *improve outcomes/ration care* pairing reduced their support by

TABLE 3.1. Net Effects of CER Debate—Predicted Change in Support by Condition

		Pro Argument	
		Improve Outcomes	Reduce Deficit
Con Argument	One-size-fits-all	−10.01 (343)	−9.90 (321)
	Ration care	−6.86 (367)	−8.03 (320)
	Waste taxpayer money	−4.23 (316)	
	Reduce innovation		−3.02 (333)

Note: Cell entries are weighted mean changes in support for government funding of CER by condition (with the number of observations in parentheses). The measures of support used to calculate changes each range from 0 (strongly oppose) to 100 (strongly support). For example, the −10.01 in the "Improve Outcomes" / "One-size-fits-all" cell indicates that respondents who viewed that argument pair reduced their support for government funding of CER by 10 points on the 0 to 100 scale. All weighted mean changes are significantly different from zero ($p<.05$).
Source: July 30–31, 2010, YouGov/Polimetrix survey.

6.9 points and those exposed to the *improve outcomes/waste taxpayer money* pairing reduced their support by 4.2 points. When paired with the *reduce deficit* pro argument, the *one-size-fits-all*, *ration care*, and *reduce innovation* counterarguments resulted in 9.9, 8.0, and 3.0 points less support for CER, respectively.[30] This experiment thus underscores that the public will need to be reassured that evidence-based medicine reforms like CER won't have negative consequences.

But what arguments in support of CER would the public find most persuasive? To answer this question, we performed a second experiment in which we examined the effectiveness of rebuttals to the strongest anti-CER argument, that CER will lead to *one-size-fits-all* medicine. We randomly assigned respondents to receive one of four pro-CER arguments tailored to rebut the con argument: (1) CER is supported by doctors (*doctors want it*), (2) the *one-size-fits-all* argument is a *scare tactic*, (3) that it is important to learn what *works best for most* patients, and (4) that research studies *can incorporate group differences* and are not limited to studying average treatment effects.[31] After they read both arguments, we asked respondents whether they found the pro or con argument to be more persuasive using a sliding scale ranging from 0 (con argument) to 100 (pro argument). Values on the response scale greater than 50 indicate that respondents found the pro-CER argument more persuasive. As table 3.2 shows, on average, people rated the

TABLE 3.2. Rebutting Arguments against CER—Mean Rating of Persuasiveness of Various Pro Arguments against "One-Size-Fits-All" Con Argument

Doctors want it: Many doctors' groups and medical associations are calling for comparative effectiveness research because the research will give doctors the information they need to identify the best treatments for their patients.	65.80 (293)
Can incorporate group differences: Medical studies can be designed not only to identify which treatments work best for the average patient, but also which work best for patients with different medical conditions and backgrounds.	59.86 (276)
Works best for most: It is unrealistic to expect doctors to view every patient as completely unique. Instead it is important to provide doctors with scientific evidence about what works best for most patients with a given medical condition.	52.39 (299)
Scare tactic: The argument that this research will lead to one-size-fits-all medicine is just a scare tactic. Doctors will be free to treat patients in the way they think is best.	51.27 (289)

Note: Cell entries are weighted mean ratings of the relative persuasiveness of the pro argument by condition (with the number of observations in parentheses). Scale: 0=con argument more persuasive; 100=pro argument more persuasive.
Source: July 30–31, 2010, YouGov/Polimetrix survey.

tailored rebuttal as either equally or more persuasive than the argument against CER in each condition.

We found that the most effective rebuttal is that *doctors want it*. This rebuttal was substantially more persuasive than the *one-size-fits-all* argument (mean score of 65.8 on 0–100 scale). This finding points to the tremendous credibility and weight that people attach to doctors' opinions. Only one of the other three rebuttals (*can incorporate group differences*; mean score of 59.9) substantially moved opinion away from the midpoint of 50.[32]

The Influence of Doctors and Politicians on Public Opinion

The findings discussed above suggest that the public can be persuaded by arguments both in support of and in opposition to evidence-based medicine reforms. However, research also suggests that the *identity* of the actors making the arguments may prove just as important.[33] Does it make a difference if the groups endorsing or opposing the proposals are doctors, elected officials, or other political elites? We explored this question by performing two complementary survey experiments.

The design of the first experiment allows us to assess how public support for a generic proposal to "help reduce the amount we spend on health care" is affected by the support or opposition of a physicians' group (the American Medical Association) as well as the positions of "political" groups (congressional Democrats, congressional Republicans, and a bipartisan commission on deficit reduction). We randomly assigned these support and opposition *cues* across respondents. The cues were designed to mimic common elements of the political debate over health care cost control.[34] We did not give the proposal any substantive content beyond indicating that it would help constrain health care costs because cost control is the dimension of CER that has been most controversial. We tested the influence of the position of the AMA (as opposed to the stance of other medical societies) because we believe it is the physician group best known to the general public. Further research could examine whether our findings generalize to other physician groups.

In order to determine if the AMA's position matters, and to whom, we manipulated two dimensions of the experiment. The first dimension varied the AMA's position. One-third of the sample was told that the AMA endorsed the proposal; another third was told that the AMA opposed the proposal; the AMA's position on the proposal was not mentioned for the remaining one-third of the sample. The second dimension of the experiment examined the effects of political cues. Each respondent saw a statement that described the proposal as (a) "supported by congressional Democrats but opposed by congressional Republicans," (b) "supported by congressional Republicans but opposed by congressional Democrats," (c) "supported by congressional Democrats and Republicans" or (d) "supported by a bipartisan commission on deficit reduction." An additional group was randomly assigned to receive no political cue. These five conditions were randomly assigned with equal probability independently of the AMA cue treatment.

In sum, we presented some respondents with the position of a single group (e.g., AMA endorsement or endorsement from a bipartisan commission) while we presented others with both a political cue and the position of the AMA. (No respondents were assigned to the condition in which neither a political cue nor the AMA cue was provided.) The outcome measure was respondents' assessments of how the particular cue (or cues) would affect their own support for the proposal and was measured using a five-point scale ranging from "much less likely to support" (-2) to "much more likely to support" (2).[35]

For each of the 14 experimental conditions, table 3.3 reports the average (weighted mean) for the outcome measure with standard errors in parentheses. The table also reports the average for each political cue condition, collapsing AMA conditions (in row 4), and the average for each AMA

TABLE 3.3. Results of AMA and Political Cues Experiment

	A No Political Cue (N=203)	B Democrats Support (N=299)	C Bipartisan Commission Supports (N=318)	D Both Parties Support (N=294)	E Republicans Support (N=298)	F All Political Conditions, with "No Political Cue" (N=1,412)	G All Political Conditions, without "No Political Cue" (N=1,209)
1 No AMA Cue (N=444)	N/A	0.01 (0.11)	0.23 (0.09)	0.18 (0.08)	−0.20 (0.13)	0.06 (0.05)	0.06 (0.05)
2 AMA Support (N=477)	0.24 (0.08)	0.25 (0.13)	0.27 (0.09)	0.32 (0.10)	0.38 (0.10)	0.29 (0.05)	0.30 (0.05)
3 AMA Opposition (N=491)	−0.05 (0.09)	−0.09 (0.12)	−0.18 (0.11)	−0.29 (0.11)	0.11 (0.13)	−0.10 (0.05)	−0.11 (0.06)
4 All AMA Conditions (N=1,412)	0.12 (0.06)	0.04 (0.07)	0.11 (0.06)	0.06 (0.06)	0.09 (0.07)	N/A	N/A

Note: Cell entries are weighted means with standard errors in parentheses. Total N=1,412. Complete question wording: "A variety of public policies have been proposed to help reduce the amount we spend on health care. Suppose you learned that a proposal was [Three AMA Treatment Conditions: none / supported by the American Medical Association / opposed by the American Medical Association] [IF AMA Treatment <> none and Political Treatment <> none then "and"] [Five Political Treatment Conditions: none / supported by congressional Democrats but opposed by congressional Republicans / supported by congressional Democrats and Republicans / supported by a bipartisan commission on deficit reduction]. Would this make you more or less likely to support the proposal?" Outcome measure ranges from −2 ("much less likely to support") to +2 ("much more likely to support").

Source: February 17–23, 2011, YouGov/Polimetrix survey. A version of this table was originally published as table 1 in Alan S. Gerber, Eric M. Patashnik, David Doherty, and Conor M. Dowling. 2014. "Doctor Knows Best: Physician Endorsements, Public Opinion, and the Politics of Comparative Effectiveness Research." *Journal of Health Politics, Policy and Law* 39 (1): 171–208. Copyright 2014, Duke University Press. All rights reserved. Republished by permission of the publisher. www.dukeupress.edu.

condition, collapsing political cue conditions (both including the "no political cue" cases [in column F] and not including those cases [in column G]).

Focusing on column G, we find that respondents who received the AMA support cue (row 2) were more likely to say this cue would increase their support for the proposal (mean=.30), while respondents who received the AMA opposition cue (row 3) were more likely to say it would decrease their support for the proposal (mean=−.11). This net difference between receiving AMA support or opposition cues of .41 is statistically significant ($p<.001$). In concrete terms, only 24 percent of the people who received the AMA opposition cue said they were (somewhat or much) more likely to support the proposal, while 38 percent of the people who received the AMA support cue said the same. Only 14 percent of those who received the AMA support cue said they were (somewhat or much) less likely to support the proposal, while 30 percent of those who received the AMA opposition cue did so.[36]

We also expected the position of a bipartisan commission on deficit reduction to affect public opinion, but the results suggest it did not. Collapsing the AMA conditions (row 4 of table 3.3), we find that in the absence of a political cue, average support for the proposal is .12 (column A). When the bipartisan commission cue is given, average support is approximately .11 (column C).[37] These results imply that endorsements from bipartisan political committees are unlikely to increase public support for proposals to reduce health care spending.[38] Aggregate support for the proposal is also not significantly affected by the other political cues. The differences between the bipartisan commission and the other political cue conditions in row 4 are not statistically significant ($p>.10$ for all pairwise comparisons). Collapsing across AMA conditions (row 4), there are no statistically significant differences between any of the other political cues and the group that received no political cue or between the other political cue experimental conditions ($p>.10$ for all pairwise comparisons).

We expected the political cues to have different effects depending on subject partisanship, however. Although a relatively small sample limits our ability to draw reliable inferences, we do find that partisans differ substantially in their responses to directional partisan cues (see table A3.2).[39] Republican respondents who were presented with an endorsement cue from congressional Republicans and an opposition cue from congressional Democrats were more likely to say the information would increase their support for the proposal (mean=.95, $p<.001$ for difference between no political cue); among Democratic respondents, this informational condition substantially decreased support for the proposal (mean=−.57, $p<.001$ for difference between no political cue). Conversely, Democratic respondents who received an endorsement cue from congressional Democrats and an opposition cue from congressional Republicans were more likely to say the information would substantially increase their support for the proposal (mean=.71, $p<.05$ for difference between no political cue), while this combination of cues considerably decreased support among Republican respondents (mean=−.67, $p<.001$ for difference between no political cue).

In summary, the results from this experiment suggest that the AMA's position may significantly influence public opinion. Although respondents who identified with a political party were strongly affected by directional cues from their party, the effects of Democratic and Republican partisan cues are largely offsetting given the aggregate distribution of partisan preferences in the overall population (see table A3.2). Only the position of the AMA influenced the attitudes of the public as a whole.[40] Neither the positions of a bipartisan commission nor a cue indicating that both parties support a proposal significantly influenced public opinion—even among Independents. These results underscore the public influence of doctors' groups. Even without giving respondents specific reasons why a proposal would be good or bad for patients, the position of doctors has the potential to significantly increase public support or opposition.

To see whether these results persist when the proposal specifically involves an effort to use research on the comparative effectiveness of treatments as a tool to control costs, we conducted a follow-up study in which the endorsement or opposition cue explicitly referenced CER. In addition, instead of the AMA, we simply referenced "leading doctors" (and also compared their effect to those of other groups, such as patient advocacy groups and drug companies). The complete details of this follow-up experiment are described in the appendix to this chapter. The findings broadly corroborate the results of the original experiment—"leading doctors," much like the AMA, had a significant effect on public acceptance of the CER cost-control proposal, underscoring the distinctive capacity of doctors' groups to shape public opinion in this policy arena.

———

Overall, our public opinion surveys suggest that physicians and medical associations have a distinctive capacity to influence public support reforms to control costs and improve the efficiency and evidence basis of medicine.[41]

No other actors in the health care system—not politicians, drug companies, or patient advocacy groups—enjoy this level of persuasive power. Our findings suggest that there is an opportunity for the medical profession to use its delegated authority to cultivate an informed public opinion and promote problem solving and social learning.

The Limits of Professional Self-Regulation

FINDINGS FROM A NATIONAL PHYSICIAN SURVEY

As chapter 3 showed, the American public believes "doctors know best" when it comes to the use of medical evidence and the allocation of resources within the health care system. But what do doctors think about these issues? In the second half of this chapter, we report the results of a national survey of physicians. What actions would doctors like their medical societies to take when high-quality studies challenge the efficacy of treatments in their practice areas? Do doctors support bringing colleagues who deviate from evidence-based protocols to the attention of disciplinary boards? How well informed are doctors about indicators of wasteful spending, such as regional variation in the Medicare program? These issues are key to explore not only because doctors are opinion leaders on health care reform, as the previous chapter showed, but also because medical societies are frequently at the center of controversies over the use of medical evidence. Consider the debate over prostate cancer screening.

In 2008, the United States Preventive Services Task Force (USPSTF), an independent panel of experts in evidence-based medicine, recommended that healthy men ages 75 and older should no longer receive a prostate-specific antigen (PSA) blood test to screen for prostate cancer because the harms of routine screening and treatment outweigh any potential benefits.[1] The PSA test produces many false positive results, and most of the prostate cancers discovered through tests are so slow growing that they are unlikely ever to become harmful, especially in older patients. Autopsy studies show that three-fourths of men over age 85 have prostate cancers, most of them clinically unimportant.[2] Prostate cancer is commonly treated through radiation or radical prostatectomies, which may cause pain and lead to serious complications such as urinary incontinence and impotence, with little or no survival benefit.[3]

Many urologists did not heed the call to stop routinely screening men 75 and older for prostate cancer. Although the American Cancer Society and American Urology Association (AUA) discouraged prostate cancer testing in men whose life expectancy was a decade or less, a study conducted four years after the USPSTF recommendation found that 43 percent of men ages 75 or over were being screened.[4] Some experts believed that the 2008 USPSTF recommendation did not go far enough to curb unnecessary screening. Professor Richard Ablin, research professor of immunobiology and pathology at the University of Arizona College of Medicine, who discovered PSA in 1970, wrote an op-ed in the *New York Times* on March 9, 2010:

> The test's popularity has led to a hugely expensive public health disaster. . . . The test is hardly more effective than a coin toss. As I've been trying to make clear for many years now, P.S.A. testing can't detect prostate cancer and, more important, it can't distinguish between the two types of prostate cancer—the one that will kill you and the one that won't. . . . I never dreamed that my discovery four decades ago would lead to such a profit-driven public health disaster. The medical community must confront reality and stop the inappropriate use of P.S.A. screening. Doing so would save billions of dollars and rescue millions of men from unnecessary, debilitating treatments.

Ablin stated that the test was still being used because it was being pushed by drug companies and advocacy groups. "Shamefully, the American Urological Association still recommends screening, while the National Cancer Institute is vague on the issue, stating that the evidence is unclear," he said.[5]

In 2012, the USPSTF updated its 2008 guidance. Based on five well-controlled clinical trials,[6] the task force now recommended against routine prostate screening for men of all age groups. The taskforce concluded that the unreliability of PSA test results, coupled with the test's inability to distinguish clinically insignificant from aggressive tumors, meant that a substantial number of men would be overdiagnosed and overtreated for prostate cancer.

Many urologists rejected this recommendation and continued to defend PSA testing. "The AUA is outraged and believes that the Task Force is doing men a great disservice by disparaging what is now the only widely available test for prostate cancer, a potentially devastating disease," the association stated.[7] The group said that it was "inappropriate and irresponsible to issue a blanket statement against PSA testing, particularly for at-risk populations, such as African American men."[8] Prominent physicians also spoke out against the recommendation. Dr. Peter Schlegel, chairman of urology at New York–Presbyterian/Weill Cornell Medical Center in New York City, stated, "Death rates from prostate cancer have dropped dramatically in the U.S. despite an aging population, which suggests evaluation and early treatment of prostate cancer is valuable in saving lives." Referencing high-risk patients, such as African Americans, who face a higher prostate cancer risk, Schlegel added, "There will be more people who die of prostate cancer because of the application of these study results."[9] This concern was a valid one, but many of the statements of the medical community failed to acknowledge the potential harms of excess screening or confront the trade-offs for public health in a scientifically responsible way.

Yet the mounting scientific evidence against routine screening put the urologists' association on the defensive. In 2013, the AUA issued new guidance of its own, stating that the association no longer recommended routine screening for men 40 to 54 years of age who are at average risk of developing prostate cancer, and also no longer recommended the test be administered to men 70 and older. The AUA's updated position indicated that men 55 to 69 should discuss the benefits and harms of PSA testing with their doctors. Some prostate experts said that the AUA "risked losing credibility" if it did not change its position, and that the new guidelines might preserve testing by favoring more moderate use.[10] In 2017, the USPSTF issued a draft recommendation (based on new evidence published since 2012) that moved its stance closer to the position of physicians. The draft maintained the recommendation against the PSA screening for men age 70 years and older, but recommended that "clinicians inform men ages 55 to 69 years about the potential benefits and harms of PSA based screening for prostate cancer."[11]

Did the 2012 USPSTF guidance against routine PSA screening for men of all ages shift practice? Yes, but not in the way many experts hoped. A 2015 *Journal of Clinical Oncology* study found that screening rates among

40 to 49 year old men did not significantly change between 2010 and 2013, but that rates did decline significantly among men over age 50.[12] However, a large fraction (about one-third) of men over 75 continued to undergo screening despite the recommendation against it.[13] A previous study, using claims-based measures of screening rates rather than patient self-reports, also found that 40 percent of men ages 75 and over continued to receive PSA tests.[14] "While we weren't surprised to see a decline in screening, we were disappointed to see the way these declines have occurred," said Michael W. Drazer of the University of Chicago Medical Center. "Instead of observing large declines among older, less healthy men who are the highest risk for overdiagnosis and overtreatment, the steepest declines in screening were observed among younger, healthier men."[15]

The PSA screening case is illustrative of several important patterns in the politics of health policy making in the United States. First, a scientific consensus that a treatment or test is not associated with better outcomes for certain patient groups may lead to public controversies in which medical societies and leading physicians take center stage. The PSA case is hardly unique on this score. There have been similar controversies over breast cancer screening and other diagnostic tests and medical interventions.[16] The American public watches these controversies unfold with considerable interest. Compared to Europeans, Americans seem to have higher expectations for medicine and are more likely to consider themselves very knowledgeable about new medical technologies.[17] Second, the positions of medical societies in these controversies reflect not only the state of medical evidence, but also a desire to preserve professional authority. When evidence emerges that common interventions are less useful than advertised, doctors and medical societies often defend current practices, at least for a time. Multiple factors—cultural, psychological, and organizational, as well as financial—explain why doctors' groups often adopt this posture.[18] The key point for our purposes is that rather than assuming a proactive, public leadership role to promote evidence-based care and the elimination of low-value services, many physicians strongly defend tests and treatments that evidence suggests have clear trade-offs for patients.

We explore the beliefs that help sustain these patterns through a national survey of physicians. The survey suggests that many doctors lack familiarity with key features of current debates over the quality and efficiency of health care delivery. For example, when asked about the existence and causes of regional variation in Medicare spending—one of the major pieces of evidence adduced to support the claim that there is vast inefficiency in health care utilization—only one in five physicians indicated that they were very or somewhat familiar with the existence of this research finding. When asked about the causes of geographic variation, doctors emphasized systemic factors such as the malpractice environment but were skeptical of the importance of physician practice style, a pattern of beliefs that is in contrast with recent research emphasizing the role of physician practice style and beliefs in driving variation in Medicare spending. In sum, although the tradition of professional autonomy places the physician at the center of the U.S. health care system, our survey evidence suggests that physicians do not recognize the important role their own beliefs (and potential misconceptions) about what constitutes good medical practice play in contributing to the problems of overutilization and inefficiency. We also find that doctors generally want their medical societies to forcefully defend treatments challenged by research. At the same time, the survey uncovers notable differences among the views of physicians based on both their medical specialization and partisan affiliation. We find that, even after controlling for other factors, doctors who identify with the Republican Party place a somewhat higher priority on protecting clinical autonomy (and a somewhat lower priority on discouraging clinical interventions with minor or no benefits) than do doctors who identify with the Democratic Party. We cannot say if this partisan split is new or long-standing, but it helps explain why the medical profession has not been a unified voice for efforts to promote evidence-based practices.

Before detailing our survey results, we first provide a brief overview of the role of the U.S. medical profession in the American state, and the challenge this role poses for democratic accountability.

The Dilemma of Professional Self-Regulation

Health care is characterized by uncertainty and asymmetric information. Medical knowledge is specialized and complicated. The typical doctor knows much more than the average patient does about what care he or she needs, and the patient cannot test the "product" before consuming it. As a result of this information asymmetry and the desirability of delegation, society establishes a social institution—the medical profession—based on trust. Professional ethics require doctors to serve as reliable "agents" and put the interests of patients above their own self-interests.[19]

Yet while the social function of the medical profession is to harness expertise on behalf of the public welfare, professional authority is constituted by state power.[20] Governments endow "legitimate" healers—doctors—with cultural status, legal privileges, and the right to prescribe and deliver medical services to patients without supervision. Legitimation occurs through the standardization and subsidization of medical education licensure.[21] As Mark Peterson points out, medical knowledge is power—and this power is applied not only in the clinical work that doctors perform, but in the profession's efforts through lobbying and civil society activities to exert "influence over the entire social structure that defines and regulates the environment in which that work is accomplished."[22] In short, professions are "political entities" that possess "the power to distract, encourage, limit, and inform public recognition of and deliberation over social problems."[23]

John E. Wennberg observes that the acceptance of the agency model as rational from both the patient's and society's point of view rests on strong assumptions. First, the model assumes "that clinical decision making is grounded in medical science; physicians have evidence-based knowledge to diagnose illness accurately and estimate the risks and benefits for the treatments they prescribe."[24] The second assumption is that physicians choose the treatments that individual patients would prefer, if individual patients were to possess the same information as physicians and understand their "true" wants and needs. The third assumption is that professional ethics ensures that doctors will recommend what is best for their patients, even though doctors typically benefit financially from higher utilization of services. A fourth assumption is that "egregious behavior by the few unethical physicians who induce patient demand for self-serving motives is detected and controlled through utilization review and other methods the profession adopts to discipline 'outlier' behavior."[25] The agency model was also assumed to be rational from society's point of view:

> A doctor-patient relationship that works in the way I have just described ensures that the supply of medical resources, including physicians, will not influence demand in a way that is wasteful. . . . Thus, the physician serves as guarantor of the efficient allocation of society's resources: if capacity exceeds that required to produce effective and valued services, capacity in excess will go unused.[26]

Unfortunately, all these assumptions have been shaken by health services research. There is widespread regional variation in the utilization of services and spending in the Medicare program that is unrelated to illness rates.[27] Physician beliefs and behavior are major drivers of this variation. To be sure, most physicians have ethical motivations. Without denying the vast influence of the medical products industry,[28] we strongly agree with Wennberg that most doctors are *not* "cynically rubbing their hands together every time a patient walks in the door, thinking of ways to deliver more care, and thus make more money."[29] Still, most patients delegate decision-making authority to their doctors. Medical education, peer-reviewed research, guideline development, and professional meetings and information sharing are all intended to ensure that patients receive appropriate treatments, but these mechanisms do not always function effectively.

Wennberg develops a typology of three categories of care: effective care, preference-sensitive care, and supply-sensitive care.[30] The category of medicine labeled *effective care*, which Wennberg suggests accounts for no more than 15 percent of total Medicare spending, refers to treatments that are known to work better than alternatives and for which the benefits are greater than the side effects. Delegation does not pose a major risk to the patient because services are backed by reasonably strong medical evidence. The main problem in this category of medicine is *underuse* of necessary care.[31] *Preference-sensitive care* (approximately 25 percent of Medicare spending) consists of services for which evidence does not point to a single best intervention (there are multiple ways of treating a condition, each of which has different outcomes) or evidence is missing altogether. Finally, *supply-sensitive* care, which accounts for roughly 60 percent of Medicare spending, refers to services where the supply of a specific resource (e.g., the number of hospital beds per capita in a given region) has a major influence on utilization rates.

Professional self-regulation should ensure that doctors recommend the best treatments for patients, but it sometimes disappoints. In his important book *Unaccountable*, Marty Makary describes physicians who overlook malpractice by their colleagues and the failure of the medical profession to play a leadership role in curbing rampant medical errors.[32] A key problem concerns the failure of the medical profession to collect and use the information needed to learn from mistakes and improve performance. Makary and his colleagues at Johns Hopkins examined clinical registries that collect data on patient outcomes. Such registries are crucial for comparing the efficacy of treatments and evaluate the quality of care. The study found that 84 percent (98 of 117) of recognized U.S. medical specialties had no national clinical registries, and the registries that did exist were generally of poor quality and lacked the information needed to render them useful for physicians, patients, and policy makers.[33] Of course, the fact that studies like this are increasingly common and that physicians are much more willing to be honest about the performance failures of the medical profession demonstrates how much has changed since the 1950s when there were strong norms against airing the profession's dirty laundry in public.[34] Increasingly, there are leaders who are trying to bring data, transparency, science, and accountability to the medical profession. Yet while significant progress has been made in surfacing the harms from the medical profession's lack of internal accountability mechanisms, financial ties to the medical products industry, and general complacency, a tremendous amount remains to be done.

The Diffuse American Medical Authority Regime

The United States is by no means alone in having doctors who seek to protect their professional authority and clinical autonomy. Yet the broader context in which American doctors practice and organize themselves is distinctive because of the nation's political development, cultural values, and institutional arrangements.[35] While physician services are increasingly financed from public sources as a result of the growth of Medicare, Medicaid, and tax preferences for employer-provided health insurance, public control over providers has "not matched the shift in dollars."[36]

A recent survey of physicians in Canada, Norway, and the United States found that U.S. doctors report much higher perceptions of clinical autonomy than their counterparts in the other two countries (though somewhat lower job satisfaction). Specifically, a much larger proportion of U.S. physicians compared to Canadian or Norwegian physicians strongly agreed with the statement, "I have the freedom to make clinical decisions that meet my patients' needs"(United States, 55 percent; Canada, 10 percent; Norway, 12 percent).[37] While the United States is not an outlier in the use of expensive technologies in every practice area, the overall environment of American medical care broadly permits doctors (many of whom are self-employed) to practice as they see fit. "The policies of both private and public insurers have traditionally offered a more welcoming and cost-unconscious approach to the provision of new healthcare technologies in the United States," observe health economists Alan Garber and Jonathan Skinner. "Almost uniquely among wealthy nations, the United States typically does not consider effectiveness relative to its costs or to the costs of alternative treatments."[38]

History helps explain these cross-national differences. The absence of centralized budgetary or regulatory control of the U.S. medical profession reflects in part the timing of the growth of public health insurance programs. The U.S. medical profession developed well before government efforts to control health care spending. As Deborah Stone observes, "In the United States, professional organization has generally preceded state involvement in health care, though government intervention has often been an impetus to organizational activity of the medical profession."[39]

The story of the U.S. medical profession's rise to sovereignty has been told by Paul Starr in his Pulitzer Prize–winning book *The Social Transformation of American Medicine*. Three points bear emphasis. First, historical forces—not just the rate of scientific progress—explain why the U.S. medical profession's claims to therapeutic authority, social privileges, and economic power were consolidated during the Progressive Era. Whereas the Jacksonian Democrats and Populists of the 1800s viewed expertise with skepticism and resisted the claims of the professions (viewing them as the means to maintain artificial privileges), progressive reformers viewed knowledge as the basis of legitimate power in the modern state. Progressives sought a rationally governed society. They believed that scientific knowledge was complex and inaccessible to the average citizen, and they held up professional authority as a "model of public disinterestedness."[40] In the political domain, Progressives believed that the public leadership of communities of scientific experts could protect citizens from the rough edges of capitalism, enlighten public opinion, and build a consensus for reform.[41] Progressives therefore were supportive of the medical profession's efforts to promote its autonomy.[42] "[O]nce they were institutionalized, standardized programs of [medical] education and [state] licensing [boards]" served as gatekeeping mechanisms, allowing medical societies to contest medical "quackery" and mobilize opposition to competitors like the patent medicine industry.[43] As James A. Morone argues, "Physicians were well constituted to meet the Progressive regulatory ideal of relying on skilled professionals to protect the public from abusive practices."[44]

Second, the growing cultural authority of the U.S. medical profession during the Progressive Era reflected a general increase in the public's confidence in science, but it did not "stem specifically from the development of effective therapeutic agents, which were still few in number."[45] To be sure, nineteenth-century physicians could point to major advances in public health, immunology, and surgery, but in other areas, doctors made recommendations on the basis of little or no evidence. As Starr writes, "cultural authority need not be based on competence. Ambiguity may suffice."[46] This point still resonates; the therapeutic authority of doctors does not appear to have a one-to-one relationship with the quality of medical knowledge in specific specialty areas.

Third, while physicians exercise authority in every health care system, the U.S. medical profession's situation is distinctive because of the weakness of the central American state. In many European nations, national governments and social institutions have a long history of regulating "public health functions such as sanitation, vaccination, and quarantine."[47] This subsequently provided the institutional foundation for centralized oversight over the medical profession's therapeutic decisions. In contrast, medical authority in the United States has traditionally been diffuse. As Daniel Carpenter observes, in Australia, Japan, and Western Europe, licensure, examination and testing, and professional entry processes are regulated at the national level, but in the United States these matters are subnational affairs,[48] much as they are for other professions like lawyers and clinical psychologists. In a comparative historical study of the medical profession in the United States and France through the 1980s, David Wilsford showed that French medical societies are poorly financed, inadequately staffed, and internally divided. The centralized bureaucratic French state was generally able to withstand the pressures of the doctors' groups. By contrast, in the United States centralized state authority was weaker, the financing of medicine was more fragmented, and organized medicine was able to guard its professional autonomy in the name of promoting quality.[49]

In a series of articles, University of Pennsylvania Law School dean Theodore Ruger analyzes the deep historical and constitutional roots of the diffuse authority structure in American medicine. Since the founding of the nation and up to the present, Ruger argues, the main thrust of U.S. medical practices has been "relentlessly centrifugal: therapeutic authority was devolved to and resided in the most granular level of medical interaction."[50] As he writes:

> Central to the individualistic diffusion of medical authority in the United States were three basic devolutions of power generated by a coalescence of constitutional federalism, weak state licensure regimes, and professional eclecticism and resistance to standardization. The first decentralization was a product of constitutional federalism, as regulatory power over medicine was understood to rest with the states, where it largely remains today. To the extent that states regulated medicine at all (and in the nineteenth century, most repealed their licensure laws under popular pressure), they in turn delegated authority to the profession itself in the form of licensure boards. Finally, the medical boards effected a third devolution to individual practitioners through their inability or

unwillingness to actively monitor or standardize the actual practice of medicine.[51]

In short, America's medical authority regime has traditionally delegated most authority over the utilization of medical services to individual physicians and their patients. This approach allows physicians to practice according to their (specialized) training and beliefs, but it also produces troubling results from the perspective of both patient outcomes and system rationality and costs, including wide variations in treatment utilization, and spending and outcomes without apparent logic. To be sure, these problems are not unique to the United States.[52] Compared to its counterparts in other nations, however, the U.S. medical profession is more specialized and fragmented—by one count, there are 37 primary specialties and 92 subspecialties.[53] Doctors in the United States also practice within the context of an overall medical system in which health care is treated as a market good, many doctors still own their own practices, and there are few supply-side constraints to limit overutilization of low-value services, such as controls on high-tech medical capital equipment.

National efforts to regulate health care have built around the constraints posed by traditions of strong professional autonomy. Even when Congress has enacted national legislation to expand insurance coverage, as in the adoption of Medicare over the opposition of organized medicine, there has been pressure to reassure doctors that the government was not a threat to their professional autonomy.[54] The result is that government health insurance programs have largely respected preexisting patterns of therapeutic authority. Despite growing concerns about whether the roughly 18 percent of GDP spent on health care[55] delivers good value for money, federal officials often lack the tools to promote quality, safety, efficiency, or cost control in either Medicare or the health care sector as a whole.[56] The health care sector thus reflects and encapsulates some of the most challenging features of public administration in the United States. As political scientist Terry Moe argues, "American public bureaucracy is not designed to be effective. The bureaucracy arises out of politics, and its design reflects the interests, strategies, and compromises of those who exercise political power."[57] Moe's statement applies with special force to the CMS, which lacks the capacity to routinely defund low-value treatments or even to root out fraud and abuse despite growing concerns about Medicare's cost growth.[58]

Nicholas Bagley, a health law professor at the University of Michigan, summarizes Medicare's administrative pathologies:

Here's the crux of the dilemma. Only physicians have the opportunity, knowledge, and legitimacy to make clinically sensitive judgments about what medical care beneficiaries need and, by extension, what Medicare should finance. And so Congress, in the Medicare statute, put physicians at the center of the program. They judge whether treatments are medically necessary and thus eligible for reimbursement. They must certify the need for institutional care or Medicare pays nothing to hospitals, hospices, or skilled nursing facilities. And they diagnose the medical conditions that establish how much Medicare pays for institutional care. Physicians are Medicare's bureaucrats at the bedside. Taken together, their decisions constitute Medicare policy . . .

However understandable [when Medicare was created in 1965], Congress's design choice has hamstrung subsequent efforts to assert control over the physicians that actually have the administration of the program in hand.[59]

Bagley carefully reviewed the implementation of the four most ambitious efforts to reform Medicare since 1965: peer review organizations, the shift from retrospective to prospective payment, Medicare managed care, and limitations on the coverage of new technology. He finds that while these changes (especially prospective payment) may have slowed the rate of cost escalation, they have done relatively little to make the thousands of private physicians paid by the program—"Medicare's bureaucrats at the bedside"— attentive to government's programmatic health care goals. Further, Bagley argues that while the ACA aimed to reshape the delivery system to reduce costs and improve quality through a transition to "bundled payments" and other changes, "the ACA reforms are inattentive to the structural features of Medicare that have frustrated the development of organized systems of care that have the incentives, bureaucratic wherewithal, and legitimacy to reshape physician practice patterns to accommodate federal priorities."[60]

To be sure, there have been countervailing developments. For example, CMS has sometimes conditioned reimbursement of a new device on the collection of additional evidence about its effectiveness after the device is on the market.[61] Private insurers are increasingly requiring drug companies to supply data on the clinical performance of their new products and using these data when deciding which products to include on formularies that, in turn, shape doctors' treatment decisions. Physicians increasingly are receiving capitated payments or being paid based on outcomes or quality. And key health institutions like Kaiser Permanente are at the vanguard of efforts to rationalize health care delivery. These developments could potentially reconfigure American medicine over time.[62] For now, though, they represent islands of rationality and efficiency in the overall U.S. health care system.

THE FALL OF THE HOUSE OF MEDICINE?

There is no doubt that physicians enjoy less power (and lower job satisfaction) today than their counterparts did during the "golden age" of American medicine during the postwar era.[63] Yet the prevailing view that the professional and clinical autonomy of the U.S. medical profession has crumbled over the past several decades cuts too deeply. Starr persuasively traced the loss of legitimacy and influence after the 1960s to the corporatization of medicine, growing concerns about costs, and the rise of countervailing powers, including insurance companies and social movements questioning all sources of traditional authority.[64] Yet as noted in chapter 3, while public trust in the leaders of medicine has indeed fallen in an *absolute* sense, Americans still believe that doctors have high ethical standards and remain confident in their own physician. Moreover, the public has much more faith in doctors to recommend the "right thing" when it comes to health reform than other groups. The high degree of trust that Americans have in their own doctors colors the way medical societies are perceived. Much of political power is a function of relative trust, and *relative* to the other institutional actors with whom the medical profession competes for influence, doctor groups have maintained a fairly high level of prestige and trust. Medical societies remain powerful vested interests that are often forces for stability who seek to protect their institutions and resist threatening reforms.[65]

Physicians and medical societies in the United States continue to exercise vast influence in policy venues and settings characterized by low visibility and high technical complexity. A canonical example is in the calculation of physician fee schedules under the Medicare program. As Miriam J. Laugesen observes in her important book *Fixing Medical Prices*, the Centers for Medicare and Medicaid Services (CMS) heavily relies on the recommendations of the American Medical Association's Relative Value Scale Update Committee (RUC). Little known to the general public, the RUC has an enormous influence on Medicare financing decisions. Between 1994 and 2010, CMS agreed with 87.4 percent of the committee's recommendations on how much physician time and effort is associated with various physicians' services.[66] There is evidence that the RUC's estimates of the time involved in many procedures are often exaggerated, sometimes by as much as 100 percent, according to a *Washington Post* investigation.[67] To determine how long a procedure takes, the committee relies on surveys of doctors conducted by the medical societies representing specialists and primary care physicians. The doctors who fill out the surveys are told that the reason for the survey is to set their Medicare pay. "What started as an advisory group has taken on a life of its own," said Tom Scully, who administered Medicare under George W. Bush. "The idea that $100 billion in federal spending is based on fixed prices that go through an industry trade association in a process that is not open to the public is pretty wild."[68] The RUC's influence over health policy making is vast; studies show that changes in Medicare's relative value units influence private insurers. When Medicare raises the price of a service by $1, private insurers raise prices by $1.30 on average.[69]

The biggest recent threat to doctors' clinical autonomy occurred with the rise of "managed care" in the 1980s.[70] Directors of managed care insurance plans argued that they, not doctors, were the key to scientific progress and patient welfare.[71] "Armed with treatment protocols and guidelines predicated on the results of clinical trials, outcomes research, quality measures, and patient satisfaction surveys, they have moved to supplant physicians as the primary arbiters of what works and does not work in medical practice."[72] For a time, doctors and patients had to seek permission to use expensive treatments—a textbook definition of explicit rationing.[73] Robert Blendon and his colleagues report that 53 percent of U.S. physicians in 1991 indicated that "external review of clinical decisions for the purpose of controlling health care costs" was a serious problem, compared to 28 percent of Canadian physicians and 43 percent of West German physicians.[74] But managed care restriction generated a furious backlash. "The transition to managed care was rapid and stunning. But the demise was even more rapid and even more stunning. . . . The managed care backlash was typified by the 1997 movie *As Good as It Gets*, in which the Helen Hunt character unleashed a flurry of expletives about managed care, and audiences across the country cheered loudly."[75] Political attacks, along with an outpouring of anti–managed care regulatory initiatives at the state level, succeeded in diluting strong utilization management controls and increasing physicians' clinical autonomy.[76] As David Mechanic observes, while "some managed care strategies are being reintroduced and new ones tried. American doctors and patients want to remain in the driver's seat, and their wishes are likely to affect the range of realistic future options."[77] While the role of doctors in the United States has evolved over time, the main story line is continuity, not change. As medical historian Rosemary A. Stevens wrote in 2001,

Despite the gloom and doom expressed over managed care from the early 1990s to the present, doctors have not lost their normative roles in

American society. They embody a huge reservoir of goodwill, inherited from the past. This is derived in various parts: from long respect of the doctor as healer; from the ideology of medicine as a public service and the doctor as hero; from the huge advances of scientific medicine in the 20th century, continuing through promises for the future; from claims for scientific objectivity; from the symbolic value of medicine as culturally suited to other American values (such as ingenuity, technology, and international superiority); and, not least, from the sheer visibility of national medical organizations, even in the absence of a unified governmental health policy.[78]

National Survey of Physicians on Medical Evidence Issues

Because of these long-standing institutional and cultural features of our national approach to health policy, the future of U.S. health policy will be shaped to a significant extent by the preferences and beliefs of our nation's doctors. It is important to understand how individual physicians think about issues that affect the overall efficiency and performance of the U.S. health care system, such as regional variation in Medicare, the role of medical societies, and professional self-regulation. To explore these issues, we conducted a national survey of 750 U.S. physicians between August 21, 2015, and September 24, 2015.[79] Each survey was accompanied by a letter of introduction and included $20 as a (small) compensation for the physician's time.[80] We received 12 returned envelopes owing to bad addresses and 374 total responses, for a response rate of 50.7 percent (374/738).[81]

We separate the results of our survey of doctors into six subsections. We first discuss doctors' political interest and civic engagement. We then examine doctors' views on how the United States compares to Western European nations when it comes to a variety of health outcomes. Next, we examine doctors' beliefs about the causes of regional variation in Medicare spending. We also report doctors' views of the appropriate role of medical societies in representing physicians' interests and in responding to research challenging the effectiveness of treatments. Last, we discuss the "practice style" of doctors and how it impacts physicians' beliefs about patient care.

PARTICIPATION AND INTEREST IN POLITICS

It is well known that doctors' interest groups such as the AMA and medical societies play an active role in politics, but individual doctors are also influential actors in health care within their social networks and local communities. How engaged are individual physicians in politics?

A study published in the *Journal of General Internal Medicine* that analyzed data from the 1996 and 2002 elections found that physicians vote at rates that are 9 percent lower than the general population and 22 percent lower than lawyers, controlling for socioeconomic variables known to influence voting rates.[82] Yet casting a ballot is not the only or likely the most effective avenue of civic engagement for physicians. Most doctors are much wealthier than the average American and can easily afford to give political donations to candidates and causes they believe in. Bonica, Rosenthal, and Rothman, for example, report that physician campaign contributions increased from $20 million to $189 million between the early 1990s and the 2010s.[83]

In our survey, we asked doctors about their general interest in politics and whether they contact government officials. In terms of political interest, 84 percent of doctors in our sample report following what's going on in government and public affairs at least some of the time (45 percent most of the time; 39 percent some of the time). In comparison, a 2014 Pew report found that 77 percent of the general public reported following what's going on in government and public affairs to the same degree (48 percent most of the time; 29 percent some of the time).[84] Although not a large difference, this suggests that even if doctors do vote at somewhat lower rates than the general population, they are at least as, if not more, attentive to governmental affairs than the general public.

Similarly, our sample of doctors reported having contacted government officials somewhat more than the general public. Thirty-one percent of doctors in our sample reported having initiated direct contact with their members of Congress (either a congressional representative or senator) in the past twelve months.[85] In the same Pew report cited above, 28 percent of the general public reported contacting an "elected official" in the last two years.[86] So, again, doctors appear to be at least, if not more, politically active than the general population. In addition, we also asked our sample of physicians whether they had contacted a White House official, an executive department official, or an official at a regulatory agency. Although fewer doctors reported making such contacts, 14 percent did report contacting an official at a regulatory agency, 5 percent an executive department official, and 2.5 percent a White House official. Although we do not have comparable figures for such contacts among the general population, these findings suggest that a nontrivial number of *individual* doctors, not just interest groups such as the AMA and medical societies, are willing to contact those executive agencies (such as those falling under the purview of the Department of Health and Human Services) involved in rule making that may directly affect their practice/autonomy. In sum, many doctors report being politically engaged. Doctors are geographically dispersed across the country, and it is likely that at some point or another virtually all members of Congress hear from doctors in their districts.

THE UNITED STATES COMPARED TO WESTERN EUROPEAN NATIONS

It is widely believed among health services researchers that U.S. health outcomes are not consistently superior to the health outcomes to those of other rich Western societies, despite our substantially higher level of spending.[87] But what do doctors know about our relative spending levels and what do they think about the relative quality of care? We asked doctors a factual question about whether the level of health care spending in the United States differs from other Western democracies. More than 90 percent of doctors correctly indicated that health care spending as a percentage of GDP is higher in the United States compared to Western European nations, such as France or Germany. Only 7.6 percent of all respondents indicated that the United States was on par with these other nations or spent less as a percentage of GDP. Many doctors expressed concerns about what the United States achieves for its high level of health care spending. A majority of doctors indicated they believe that "the quality of health care" received by the average patient in the United States is "worse" (21 percent) or "the same" (43 percent) as the health care received by the average patient in Western European nations. However, only 36 percent of doctors in our sample stated that the quality of health care in the United States is "better."[88]

REGIONAL VARIATION IN MEDICARE SPENDING AND UTILIZATION

One reason to believe there is wide scope to improve the efficiency and quality of U.S. health care comes from the *Dartmouth Atlas of Health Care*, which documents a more than twofold variation in per capita Medicare spending in different regions of the country.[89] Atul Gawande distilled the lessons from this body of research in a famous 2009 *New Yorker* article, "The Cost Conundrum," describing medical practices in high-spending McAllen, Texas.[90] The essay went viral and became required reading in the Obama White House.[91]

We were interested in gauging whether physicians were aware of the regional variation controversy and what they thought might be responsible for the variation. Before describing the results of the physician survey, we briefly review some of the key findings about the regional variation controversy.

Most of the variation in Medicare spending is due to utilization, meaning the amount of care given to patients. Regional variation in Medicare spending is often said to be "unwarranted" because it does not show a consistent relationship between Medicare patients' use of services on the one hand, and quality or health outcomes on the other.[92] It is important to note that prices do not explain most of the variation in Medicare spending. All providers face the same Medicare reimbursement schedule, adjusted across regions for cost of living, graduate medical education, or low-income subsidies. (As we noted earlier, the situation is quite different in insurance markets under age 65, in which the prices of procedures do vary tremendously across regions. As a result, total per capita regional spending in the under-65 markets is not closely associated with per capita Medicare spending in those markets, even though there is a strong correlation between *utilization* patterns in Medicare and commercial insurance plans.)[93]

If not prices, then what does drive geographic variation in Medicare utilization? Controlling for patients' age, sex, income, race, and health attenuates differences in the amount of services patients receive across areas, but a lot of unexplained variation remains.[94] Additionally, most research suggests that patient preferences for life-prolonging treatments and other services have a relatively small influence on regional variations in Medicare spending.[95] The threat of malpractice is also often mentioned as a cause, but "defensive medicine has yet to be shown to be an explanation for regional variation in spending and utilization."[96]

On the other hand, supply-side factors are clearly a key driver of geographic variation.[97] These include the number of physicians, specialists, and hospitals beds in an area, as well as doctors' beliefs about appropriate practice style.[98] Practice style, which we discuss in more detail at the end of this chapter, can contribute to overtreatment in two ways. First, doctors may use unsupported or discredited treatments, such as the arthroscopic knee surgeries discussed in chapter 2. Here, the physical benefits for all patients who receive the treatments are small or nonexistent. The second and likely much more common situation arises when doctors who have an aggressive practice style use treatments in low-value settings, giving the treatments to patients beyond the appropriate target population based on evidence.[99]

A fascinating recent study found that physician beliefs about treatments (unsupported by clinical evidence) can explain as much as 35 percent of end-of-life Medicare expenditures and 12 percent of Medicare expenditures overall.[100] The authors created vignettes of specific patient scenarios and asked samples of cardiologists and primary care physicians what they would do in each situation; for example, whether to provide intensive care to a heart patient beyond the indications of evidence-based guidelines or attempt to make the patient more comfortable by administering palliative care. Based on these surveys, the authors were able to classify the physicians as either "cowboys" or "comforters" and found that their respective concentrations in a region closely tracked the level of end-of-life spending in that area. The authors also conducted surveys of Medicare enrollees to check if patient preferences were driving the results and determined they were not. The effects of the geographic variation in the practice styles elicited by the vignettes are substantial. The study suggests that physician beliefs about the appropriate care for patients accounts for more than half of the variation in end-of-life spending across areas, as well the frequency with which physicians recommend their patients for routine office visits.

Evidence that regional variation is explained in large measure by physician-specific effects is found in a recent study that followed Medicare enrollees who moved from one part of the country to another. The study concluded that 50–60 percent of the geographic variation in health care utilization is due to place-specific factors, such as doctors' incentives and beliefs, physical and human capital, and hospital market structure. The remainder is due to fixed characteristics of patients that they carry with them when they move, such as preferences and health status. Patient characteristics matter more for outcomes such as emergency room visits than for outcomes such as diagnostic and imaging tests, where the physician is the main decision maker.[101]

Research on regional variation in Medicare received wide media attention during the Obama administration, even showing up in the pages of magazines like the *New Yorker* widely read by educated professionals. How familiar are physicians with the literature on geographic variation, and what factors do they believe cause it? Do physicians' beliefs accurately reflect the state of the academic literature? Although there has been some survey work concerning physician views of and support for CER,[102] the extent to which physicians understand the underlying problems of waste, inefficiency, unwarranted variation, and over- or underutilization that helped justify an increased federal role in CER remains largely unexplored.

First, we asked physicians if they have heard anything about health services research on the regional (or geographic) variation in health care spending within the United States. The typical doctor appears unfamiliar with these important features of medical spending. Just under half of the physicians in our survey (48.5 percent) reported that they had "heard anything about" this research; 51.5 percent said they had not. Moreover, of the doctors who reported that they had heard anything about these studies, less than half reported that they were "very familiar" (4.5 percent) or "somewhat familiar" (40.5 percent) with this research; in other words, given that half the sample stated they had not heard anything about these studies, *doctors who were very or somewhat familiar with this research represent only one-fifth of the entire sample* (80 out of 368 total responses to this measure). And, of course, this is a self-reported measure where we might expect a "social desirability" bias toward overreporting of knowledge.[103]

There were statistically significant differences in knowledge of regional variation across groups. The results of a regression analysis in which we predicted reported familiarity with the studies on regional variation with a series of demographic and other characteristics of the doctors are included in the appendix to this chapter (table A4.1).[104] Reporting a high level of interest in politics ($p<.01$), having had residency training at a VA ($p<.05$), and being in practice longer ($p<.05$) are associated with greater familiarity with these studies.[105]

Next, we provided respondents with some factual information about regional variation in Medicare spending and asked what might be causing this situation. In particular, we investigated what doctors believe are the major factors that explain the observed variation. We asked the following question to all the doctors, regardless of how familiar with the research they reported they were:

> According to a recent Institute of Medicine (IOM) study, there is large and persistent regional variation in health care spending across the United States. We will now ask you some questions about regional variation in the Medicare program. How much do you think each of the following factors contributes to regional variation in Medicare spending?

Doctors indicated to what degree—"none," "little," "some," or "a lot"—each of eight statements contributed to regional variation in Medicare spending (see figure 4.1). All eight factors were thought to contribute "a lot" or at least "some" to regional variation in Medicare spending by at least 65 percent of doctors. However, there were important differences in the factors viewed

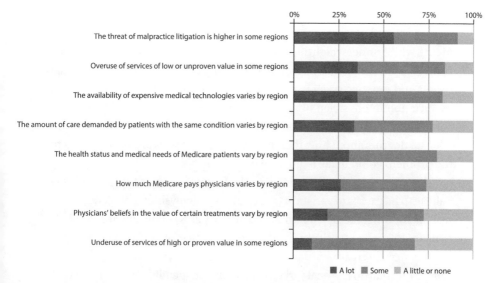

FIGURE 4.1. Doctors' beliefs about what factors contribute to regional variation in Medicare spending. *Note*: Responses to question: "According to a recent Institute of Medicine (IOM) study, there is large and persistent regional variation in health care spending across the United States. We will now ask you some questions about regional variation in the Medicare program. How much do you think each of the following factors contributes to regional variation in Medicare spending?" (*N*=366). *Source*: Fall 2015 survey of physicians.

as most important, and this pattern of emphasis did not always follow the evidence that has accumulated in the health services literature. Many doctors see malpractice suits as the most important driver of variation in the Medicare program. Fifty-five percent of doctors said differences in the threat of malpractice litigation across regions contributed "a lot" to variation with an additional 36 percent saying such threats contribute "some" to explaining regional variation in Medicare spending (leaving only 9 percent saying "a little" or "none"). No other factor was cited by more than half of doctors as contributing "a lot" to variation. In comparison, only 35 percent of doctors said they believe that overuse of services of low or unproven value contribute "a lot" to variation (with 48 percent saying "some" and 16 percent "a little" or "none"). In contrast with recent work focusing on the importance of doctors' beliefs to regional variation in Medicare spending, just 18 percent of doctors said that physicians' beliefs in the value of certain treatments contribute "a lot" to variation (with 54 percent saying "some" and 27 percent saying "a little" or "none."). In sum, doctors' views of the causes of regional variation in Medicare spending are somewhat informed yet off the mark in key respects. Doctors appear to overemphasize systemic factors beyond physician control (for example, the malpractice environment) while underweighting factors that in principle are subject to the control of physicians and their professional organizations (such as physician beliefs and practice styles). To the extent that regional variation is driven by variation in physician practice style and decisions to provide care not based on evidence, a reform movement within the medical profession to educate doctors about how their own clinical decisions are contributing to the problem could make a difference.

There were notable differences in the factors different types of doctors believe to be causes of variation (see regression analysis in table A4.2). Controlling for other factors, doctors who identify as Republicans are *less* likely than doctors who identity as Democrats to say that physician beliefs' in the value of certain treatments and the underuse of services of high or proven value contribute to regional variation in Medicare spending ($p<.05$). A recent study in the Proceedings of the National Academy of Sciences demonstrates that physicians' political worldviews are correlated with their professional decisions on certain politically salient issues.[106] For example, doctors who identify with the Democratic Party are more likely to urge patients against storing firearms in the home, while Republican physicians are more likely to counsel patients on the mental health risks of abortion and to urge patients to cut down on marijuana use. Our survey results show that Democratic and Republican doctors also possess somewhat different understandings of how the medical system works.

Besides partisan differences, we found that medical specialists are *less* likely than primary care doctors to say that differences in the amount of care demanded by patients with the same condition contributes a lot to variation ($p<.05$), whereas surgical specialists are *less* likely than primary care doctors to say that the health status and medical needs of Medicare patients contributes a lot to variation ($p<.05$). Finally, years of practice is positively associated with a belief that how much Medicare pays physicians contributes a lot to variation ($p<.05$).[107]

WHOM DO DOCTORS TRUST?

Suppose one wishes to influence the opinions of doctors or provide evidence that might shape their beliefs. Who should ideally be selected as messenger? Chapter 3 showed that the American public places more trust in doctors compared to other groups, but who do doctors trust to provide accurate,

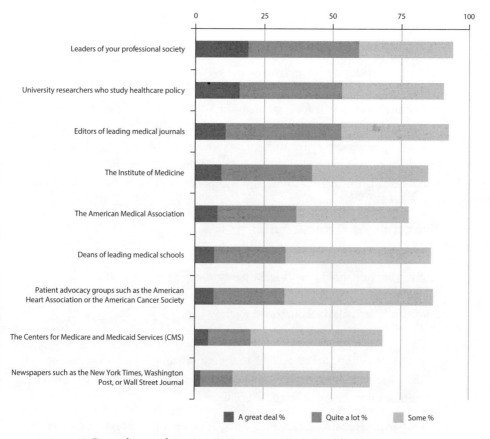

FIGURE 4.2. Doctors' reported trust in various groups. *Note*: Responses to question: "How much would you trust the following groups to provide accurate, factual information about the U.S. health care system?" Unreported percentage is for those who responded "very little." (*N*=373). *Source*: Fall 2015 survey of physicians.

factual information about the U.S. health care system? Do doctors have greater faith in the medical profession or other groups?

The groups we asked about are listed in figure 4.2, where we also report the percentage of respondents who stated they would trust that group "a great deal," "quite a lot," or "some." Doctors reported the highest level of trust in leaders of their own professional society, university researchers, and editors of leading medical journals—a majority of doctors reported either a great deal or quite a lot of trust in these three entities. Doctors expressed the least amount of trust in newspapers and the Centers for Medicare and Medicaid Services (CMS), two entities that less than 25 percent of doctors reported at least "quite a lot" of trust in. In between these most and least trusted entities were several others that received middling levels of trust from doctors. Notably, deans of leading medical schools are not ranked particularly high, and both the American Medical Association and the Institute of Medicine are viewed as less trustworthy than leaders of doctors' own professional societies. The lower level of trust that doctors have in the AMA than in their own societies' leaders is consistent with the declining proportion of physicians who are members of the AMA since the 1950s. The secular decline in AMA membership reflects many factors, including growing allegiance among physicians to specialty groups. In addition, AMA membership took a hit following the organization's endorsement of the ACA.[108]

PRIORITIES OF MEDICAL SOCIETIES

Given that doctors trust their own professional societies more than other actors, what role should they ideally play both in general and with respect to controversies over medical evidence. What do they see as the association's priorities? We first asked doctors the following:

> Medical societies have to set priorities. How important do you think each of the following goals should be to the American College of Cardiology, the American Academy of Orthopedic Surgeons, and other medical societies representing different specialties?

Doctors expressed strong support for five priorities of medical societies (see figure 4.3): "disseminating best practices through guidelines and professional education," "protecting the clinical autonomy of physicians in the society's area of specialization," "finding ways to cut health care costs by discouraging the use of clinical interventions with minor or no benefit to patients," "pointing out where physicians in the society's area of specialization are not following best medical practices," and "advocating for the economic interests of physicians who practice in the medical society's area of specialization." Sixty-five percent or more of doctors thought each of these five goals was at least a *very* important priority for medical societies. The belief of many doctors that advocating for the economic interests of physicians should be a priority of medical societies is notable for the frank admission that medical societies are in a sense trade associations.

Doctors viewed the remaining goal we asked about—"identifying physicians in the society's area of specialization who are not following best medical practices and bringing them to the attention of disciplinary boards"—as a much less important priority. Indeed, less than 20 percent of doctors

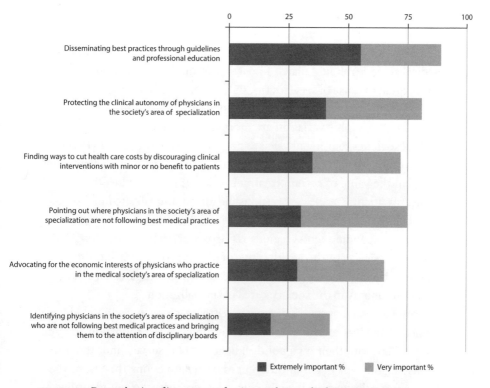

FIGURE 4.3. Doctors' rating of importance of various goals to medical societies. *Note*: Responses to question: "Medical societies have to set priorities. How important do you think each of the following goals should be to the American College of Cardiology, the American Academy of Orthopedic Surgeons, and other medical societies representing different specialties?" Unreported percentage is for those who responded "not that important" or "moderately important." (*N*=373). *Source*: Fall 2015 survey of physicians.

indicated this was an extremely important goal. Thus, although many doctors felt it was important for medical societies to *point out* when best medical practices are not being followed (nearly 75 percent indicated it was at minimum a "very important" goal), far fewer felt medical societies should be in the business of policing their members. This view is perhaps not surprising in light of the failure of peer review organizations in Medicare, which are supposed to sanction providers that abuse Medicare, but in practice have been "paper tigers" and have done little to control costs or improve quality: "Physicians are loath to second-guess their colleagues' work."[109] Coupled with the high level of support doctors had for protecting clinical autonomy, we observe evidence that doctors believe professional societies should protect the interests and autonomy of doctors.

We observe some interesting patterns when we examine the relationship between what a physician believes causes regional variation in Medicare spending (reported in figure 4.1) and his or her view about the role that medical societies should play.[110] In particular, doctors who are more likely to think that overuse of services ($p<.05$), underuse of services ($p<.10$), and availability of expensive medical technology ($p<.05$) in some regions are to blame for geographic variation are more likely to think it is important for medical societies to bring physicians not following best practices to the attention of disciplinary boards. However, respondents who think physicians' beliefs in the value of certain treatments ($p<.05$) and the health status of Medicare patients ($p<.05$) are responsible for variation desire more protection of clinical autonomy. In other words, the more doctors view variation in Medicare spending across regions as the product of the professional judgment of physicians or the health status of patients, the more likely they are to believe it should be a priority for medical societies to safeguard doctor's clinical autonomy in the society's area of specialization.

As noted, recent research demonstrates that Democratic and Republican physicians tend to counsel patients about topics such as abortion and gun safety in line with their own political beliefs.[111] Our survey finds that there are also significant partisan differences on what actions they want their medical societies to prioritize. In particular, doctors who self-identified as Republican rated advocating for economic interests and protecting clinical autonomy as more important priorities for medical societies than doctors who self-identified as Democrats ($p<.05$). In addition, self-identified Republican physicians rated finding ways to cut health care costs by discouraging clinical interventions with minor or no benefit to patients as less important medical society priorities than did Democrats ($p<.05$).[112] Beyond partisan identification, the survey also revealed that doctors whose specialty is primary care rated advocating for economic interests and protecting clinical autonomy as more important than doctors whose specialty is surgical care ($p<.05$). In short, there are important divisions along both partisan and specialization lines about the role that medical societies should play in representing the medical profession's interests in the health care system. (See table A4.4 for details.)

RESPONSE OF MEDICAL SOCIETIES TO RESEARCH CALLING INTO QUESTION THE EFFECTIVENESS OF TREATMENTS

Beyond views about the overall priorities of medical societies, we were especially interested in how doctors think medical societies should respond

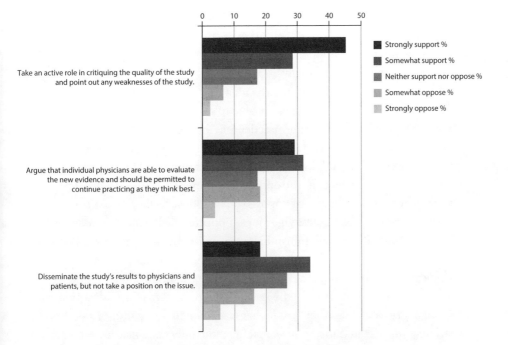

FIGURE 4.4. Doctors' opinions on what medical societies should do when a medical study calls into question a common treatment in practice area. *Note*: Responses to question: "Suppose a leading medical journal publishes a new study (widely covered in the mainstream media) that calls into question a treatment that is commonly used in your practice area. The evidence suggests that the treatment might not be as effective as previously thought. Indicate below the extent to which you would support or oppose each of the following responses by the medical society in your practice area" (*N*=372). *Source*: Fall 2015 survey of physicians.

to new medical evidence about treatment effects. We asked respondents to consider the following scenario:

> Suppose a leading medical journal publishes a new study (widely covered in the mainstream media) that calls into question a treatment that is commonly used in your practice area. The evidence suggests that the treatment might not be as effective as previously thought.

We asked respondents to indicate the extent to which they would support three potential responses by the medical society in their practice area. The pattern of responses indicates doctors want their medical society to push back and defend professional autonomy when treatments are questioned. Figure 4.4 shows that the most preferred response by doctors is for medical societies "to take an active role in critiquing the quality of the study and point out any weaknesses of the study." Almost 75 percent of respondents somewhat or strongly agreed with this posture. An additional 17 percent neither supported nor opposed this response, leaving only 9 percent in opposition (somewhat or strongly).

Many doctors also supported the idea that the medical society should "argue that individual physicians are able to evaluate the new evidence and should be permitted to continue practicing as they think best." Sixty-one percent of physicians supported (somewhat or strongly) the medical society taking this approach. An additional 17 percent neither supported nor opposed this response, leaving 21 percent who opposed it—the vast majority of which (18 of the 21 percent) only somewhat opposed this response by the medical society.

In contrast, there was less vigorous support for having medical societies play a neutral information transmission role without taking a stance. Just a bare majority (52 percent) of doctors (somewhat or strongly) supported the medical society disseminating "the study's results to physicians and patients, but not tak[ing] a position on the issue." Indeed, what makes this response stand apart from the other two is that less than 20 percent of physicians strongly supported this response, making it the only response in which the opposition (somewhat and strong) was greater than those who strongly supported it (21 to 18 percent). This response also had the greatest percentage of physicians who were neutral, at 27 percent.

Although doctors overall want their medical societies to defend clinical autonomy, there are some notable differences among the views of different subgroups of doctors. The results of a regression analysis (reported in table A4.5) indicate that, compared to primary care doctors, doctors with a surgical specialty are more hesitant to support their medical societies taking an active role in critiquing the quality of the study ($p < .01$).[113] Female doctors in our sample were less likely to support the statement that the medical society should disseminate the results but not take a position on the issue compared to their male counterparts ($p < .10$). Republican doctors were more likely than their Democratic counterparts to support the statement that "individual physicians are able to evaluate the new evidence and should be permitted to continue practicing as they think best" ($p < .10$).

PRACTICE STYLES

Finally, we asked doctors to assess their own "practice style." We told respondents that "academic research suggests that physicians practicing in similar organizational settings often exhibit large and persistent 'style' differences in their tendency to prescribe certain treatments and utilize medical resources for similar patients." We asked doctors how confident they were that they could characterize their own practice style compared to the practice styles of other doctors in their area of specialization. Most respondents lacked confidence in their knowledge of their own practice style. Only 31 percent of doctors in our sample said they were "very confident" they could identify their own practice style compared to the practice style of other doctors. An additional 52 percent were "somewhat confident," with 17 percent reporting that they were "a little" (13 percent) or "not at all" (4 percent) confident. These findings suggest there is room for doctors to become more self-aware of their own practice styles—and how they stack up against evidence-based protocols.

Practice styles are important in part because there is growing evidence that tendencies to prescribe certain treatments and utilize certain medical resources or technology are established early on and persist, and that some practice styles can be beneficial or harmful to the welfare of patients with certain conditions.[114] For example, research has documented substantial variation in the practice styles of both cardiologists[115] and obstetricians.[116] Even more central to the concern about overutilization, Lipitz-Snyderman and colleagues find high rates of nonrecommended care in the treatment of cancer patients.[117] These findings "provide strong evidence that some physicians persistently use low-value care."[118]

Our survey results show that physicians are reluctant to be evaluated according to their adherence to simple metrics. We asked the doctors which of the following two statements came closer to their own view:

> It is reasonable to evaluate doctors in terms of their adherence to simple metrics, such as the fraction of their patients who receive influenza immunization or whether patients with coronary artery disease are taking appropriate medications.

Or:

> Decisions about treatment should be tailored to the needs of individual patients, and this type of sensitivity to patient characteristics cannot be captured through adherence to simple rules.

Sixty-nine percent of doctors indicated the second statement came closer to their own view; in other words, less than one-third of doctors felt evaluating doctors in terms of their adherence to metrics was most appropriate. This result is not surprising, but it underscores that medical reformers face an uphill battle to convince doctors that evidence-based metrics can support the diagnostic and treatment capabilities of even skilled physicians. Consistent with the partisan differences concerning the roles of medical societies we report above, compared to Republican physicians, Democratic physicians were more likely to say that evaluating doctors in terms of their adherence to metrics was most appropriate ($p<.05$).

Still, there might be room for medical societies to promote greater self-awareness of practice styles among members. For example, if information about the practice styles of individual physicians were routinely collected, and if these data were used to tease out the influence of practice style on patient outcomes, it might be possible to refine treatment guidelines in order to improve health outcomes.[119] Although altering physician practice styles is difficult, "providing physicians information about how their practice styles compare to their peers" has been shown to change, for the better, physician behaviors.[120] Importantly, a refinement to treatment guidelines need not necessarily imply a reflexive endorsement of reduced use of invasive procedures—in some cases, a careful study might reveal that more aggressive practice styles are superior.[121]

Conclusion

The U.S. medical system has long emphasized the professional and clinical autonomy of physicians. Doctors possess the discretion to prescribe the treatments that patients receive, and their practice styles have a big influence on variation in utilization and spending in Medicare. In addition, doctors, who enjoy a high level of public trust, are heavily involved in health policy making both through their membership in medical societies and in their role as prominent and respected leaders of their local communities. Given that the future of U.S. health policy will be shaped to a significant degree by the preferences of doctors, we surveyed doctors to learn what they think about key medical evidence issues. Our national survey produced several key findings.

First, many doctors do not recognize the important role their own clinical decisions and practice style play in contributing to regional variation in Medicare spending. (The main exceptions are doctors who have been in practice longer, had their residency take place at a VA, or express a high level of interest in politics.) Overall, our survey uncovered little evidence that the leaders of the medical profession have done an adequate job diffusing knowledge about waste and geographic variation to rank-and-file doctors, despite the attention the topic has received from prominent policy makers and researchers.

Second, the survey suggests that many doctors want their medical society to play an "attack dog" role when evidence emerges that treatments in their practice areas may not work as well as previously believed. As the knee surgery case study (chapter 2) showed, leaders of medical societies are often quite aggressive in critiquing the results of even the most rigorous randomized controlled trials.

Finally, while our survey results overall show support for the role of medical societies as guardians of physician discretion and economic interests, our survey uncovered some notable differences in the beliefs of physicians based on their partisan identification. Republican doctors viewed advocating for economic interests and protecting clinical autonomy as more important priorities for medical societies than did Democratic doctors. Republican physicians also viewed discouraging clinical interventions with minor or no benefit to patients as less important than Democratic physicians. As the next two chapters show, partisan polarization and electoral competition has politicized efforts to promote efficiency and quality in U.S. health care. The physician survey findings reported in this chapter raise the possibility that another barrier to the creation of a technocratic consensus on the need for better use of standardized evidence is partisan polarization within the medical profession itself.

5

Zero-Credit Politics

THE GOVERNMENT'S SLUGGISH EFFORT TO PROMOTE EVIDENCE-BASED MEDICINE, 1970s–2008

Imagine a political world in which the value of evidence-based medicine was recognized by policy elites across the political spectrum and had a "taken-for-granted" status, just as it is expected that any nuclear power plant that society chooses to build will reflect accepted engineering safety standards. This world is not so distant from our own. Indeed, despite the increasing politicization of governance, there have been moments in the recent past when the U.S. political system seemed on the verge of developing a bipartisan, technocratic consensus around EBM. A month before the 2008 election, for example, Newt Gingrich (R-GA), John Kerry (D-MA), and Billy Beane (the statistics-loving baseball executive portrayed in the film *Moneyball*) published an op-ed in the *New York Times* entitled "How to Take American Health Care from Worst to First." They pointed out that the United States "spends more than twice as much per capita on health care compared to almost every other country in the world—and with worse health quality than most industrialized nations." A major reason why U.S. health care is so wasteful and low performing, they argued, is that medical practices are not based on clinical evidence of what works best and what does not. "Remarkably, a doctor today can get more data on the starting third baseman on his fantasy baseball team than on the effectiveness of life-and-death medical procedures. . . . To deliver better health care, we should learn from the successful teams that have adopted baseball's new evidence-based methods," they wrote.[1] To be sure, there are dimensions of EBM that could stimulate political polarization, such as legitimate concerns about government interference with doctors' clinical judgment and autonomy. As Sheila Jasanoff, a leading scholar of the role of science in public policy, argues, the "boundaries between science and politics . . . are constructed and maintained through politically inflected 'boundary work'. Put differently, the balance between reliance on science and reliance on politics is itself a product of social accommodation and power plays."[2]

The Gingrich-Kerry-Beane agreement on the need for U.S. health care to become more scientific thus does not demonstrate that the pursuit of better evidence in medicine inevitably "ought" to be a nonpartisan, "good government" issue, but rather points to this potential. The key question we address in this and the following chapter is why a potentially technocratic issue that *could* be handled pragmatically by experts instead becomes politicized.

In brief, our answer is that the politics surrounding efforts to address the medical evidence problem have been "unhealthy." This chapter shows that while the pragmatic case for bringing standardized evidence more systematically to bear on decisions in health care is compelling, federal politicians took only modest actions to support steps to identify and eliminate wasteful, unnecessary services between the 1970s and late 2000s. Moreover, politicians (responding to their electoral incentives) were quick to abandon even these incremental reforms when they sparked opposition from providers and the medical products industry. Then, when the Obama administration surprisingly did focus public attention on the need for more federal investment in research on the comparative effectiveness of treatments—an idea that had support among health care experts associated with both parties— the issue became politicized, as the next chapter shows. Republicans accused the administration of "rationing" and interfering with the doctor-patient relationship. In sum, the government's performance as a problem-solving institution with respect to health care quality and efficiency was doubly disappointing. First, the medical guesswork problem was a low-priority concern, barely registering on the policy agenda; it was an "inside initiative" in which the conversation excluded both politicians and the general public.[3] Later, when the medical evidence problem began to generate the broad attention it deserved, proposed solutions became the object of partisan manipulation and political distortion.

Taken together, the two episodes suggest that systemic failures in the performance of our institutions of collective choice are not automatically self-correcting; they can persist for long periods of time. They also point to the political limits of the Progressive reform model of government as a neutral, problem-solving institution built on professional expertise, scientific management, and enlightened public opinion.[4]

Why the Supply of Political Entrepreneurship May Be Too Low

It is useful to begin by stepping back from the details of the medical evidence problem to ask: Why would government fail to address a major, well-documented problem that is causing the nation to perform below potential year after year? The proximate causes of government failure will of course vary across sectors and over time. Just as each unhappy family is unhappy in its own way (to borrow from Tolstoy), so each story of democratic performance failure is distinctive. The starting point for analysis, however, is that pragmatic problem solving and the promotion of the public interest may quite simply offer meager political returns to reelection-minded politicians.[5]

If, following Joseph Schumpeter, we construe societal problem solving as an unintended by-product of partisan competition and the pursuit of power rather than something that the average politician pursues for its own sake,[6] a tension exists in representative democracy. From the standpoint of social welfare, a new policy should be adopted if the social benefits are greater than the costs, whereas from the standpoint of a politician, a policy should be adopted if the political benefits to the politician are greater than the political costs. Good policies that have large social benefits but small, selective benefits for the politician may not find a political sponsor. Proposing creative, thoughtful solutions to important policy problems may not be the best way for savvy politicians to generate support.

This is so for several reasons. First, the simple act of defining a problem is not straightforward. There may be disagreement over whether some objective societal condition constitutes a "problem" that requires governmental intervention. Is wealth inequality a problem that should be addressed by government action? Is the level of soft drink consumption a social problem? Even if people agree that a problem exists, there will typically be disagreement over what to do about the problem.[7] Is gun control the solution to mass shootings? Is the answer better-trained police forces or better mental health services? These debates are the very stuff of politics. A legislator who genuinely wishes to do good for society, while also doing well for him- or herself, first needs to frame a problem in a way that brings the public along yet also makes sense from the standpoint of instrumental rationality. Finally, to turn an idea into policy, the politician must then "deliberate, bargain, and compromise in a fishbowl setting in a fashion that can swerve both publics and experts toward emergent solutions."[8]

None of this is likely to happen in the absence of political entrepreneurship. Political entrepreneurs are creative actors who invest their time, energy, resources, and political reputations to advocate for an idea or proposal—in order to capture a political reward.[9] They frame issues, create new public demands, build coalitions, and expand the set of issues it is considered legitimate and expected for government to address.[10] To use an economics analogy, political entrepreneurs are "sellers" of problem definitions and proposed solutions who seek to satisfy an unmet social need in exchange for a price, which may take the form of reputational gains or advancement of ideological goals. As legal theorist and federal judge Richard Posner observes, political entrepreneurs can have a large influence on public policy:

> The voting public did not know that it wanted social security, conscription, public education, an independent central bank, an interstate highway system, a Presidency opened to divorced or Catholic persons, the North Atlantic Treaty Organization, or the auctioning of rights to the use of the electromagnetic spectrum before those things were proposed by political entrepreneurs, as distinct from run-of-the-mill politicians.[11]

Taking a step back, the surprising situation of licensed physicians performing procedures and ordering tests not grounded or based on evidence about what works best for patients would seem to be *precisely* the kind of important problem where a healthy dose of political entrepreneurship is warranted. Yet there is no guarantee that the need for political entrepreneurship will generate its own supply. We develop a theory of "zero-credit politics" to explain why this is so. The core idea is not that the supply of political entrepreneurship will *literally* be zero—there will nearly always be some actors who are willing to pursue a cause to make a reputation for themselves or further their personal agenda—but rather that the absence of significant political rewards for tackling an important but thorny problem will lead to a much lower level of entrepreneurship in the policy community than is socially optimal.

THE THEORY OF ZERO-CREDIT POLITICS

The role of political entrepreneurs as agents of policy change has received considerable attention.[12] Despite extensive research on the topic, however, few studies examine the role that political entrepreneurship plays in improving governance and system performance. Many political scientists have casually borrowed a market analogy from economics, but few have followed the logic of the analogy or adapted the theory of entrepreneurship to the special features of democratic politics.[13]

Economists have argued that the activities of private sector entrepreneurs make a vital contribution not only to economic change, but to economic growth and improvements in social welfare.[14] Similarly, political entrepreneurship deserves close attention not only because it provides a channel for innovation and the disruption of existing political equilibria, but also because it can shape the problem-solving capacity of a society. In the short run, a political system's performance depends on the responsiveness of elected officials to extant citizen preferences and needs, but in the long run it depends on the capacity of its leaders and institutions to identify problems, fashion solutions, and adapt to evolving conditions.

Nothing ensures that the supply of problem-focused political entrepreneurship will be adequate from society's standpoint. Political entrepreneurship entails creating a demand among voters for new policy ideas. This task is far more difficult than the routine marketing of proposals already in circulation. This effort to advocate for and propose new policy ideas and solutions might be viewed as making a risky investment. There are two ways the investment can go sour. First, if the public declines to buy the new policy product, the entrepreneur's *own* political reputation may suffer. If a politician pushes a policy idea that conflicts with voters' beliefs or understanding of reality, it is possible that voters will conclude that the politician is a courageous truth teller and change their minds. But, it is also possible (and perhaps more likely) that voters will instead remain skeptical about the proposal and become skeptical about its advocate as well.[15] There are good reasons for voter skepticism. Sometimes politicians are well meaning but out of step with their constituents. Sometimes they really *are* snake oil salesmen. When an uninvited visitor comes knocking with promises to help, it is not absurd to think that the first instinct of many citizens is to slam the door. One thing is certain: the opponents of the policy change can be counted on to pounce if they sense an opportunity to denigrate the proposal and thereby undermine the policy innovator's public standing. And, if the public is initially skeptical, such attacks will have a considerable tailwind.

The second risk arises if the entrepreneur's efforts to build public support for a new policy approach begin to work. In a commercial setting, a risky investment often enjoys legal protections such as patents and trademarks. In a political setting, however, there is nothing to stop an opportunistic opponent who observes the changes in public opinion produced by a rival's hard work from proposing a substantively similar proposal of his or her own. If this effort at political mimicry is successful, the initial, true policy innovator will capture, at best, a small share of the credit for the results of his or her efforts. Worse, the second politician, by hanging back until political conditions become more favorable and observing how opinion unfolds, may generate more support for his or her alternative scheme, a copycat plan tweaked to be better tailored to public opinion. In the ruthlessly competitive world of democratic politics, the political entrepreneur and innovative problem solver could even end up worse off for his or her effort.

We call this dynamic "zero-credit politics," meaning a government intervention or activity that offers no or few "captureable" political returns even though it has large net social benefits.[16] At the extreme, if novel solutions to societal problems are perfectly appropriated, the effect will be to discourage the entrepreneurial investments in the first place.[17]

To be sure, the zero-credit dynamic does not always thwart all efforts at innovative policy reform. One can point to examples where political entrepreneurs were willing to invest their time and energy on behalf of the development and advocacy of proposals, including reforms that served a diffuse public interest.[18] An example is airline deregulation. In the 1970s, the federal government controlled the fares airlines could charge and what routes they could fly. Airline service was generally excellent, but ordinary Americans could not find affordable flights to take them where they wanted to go. Although economists argued on the basis of theory and demonstration studies that the freeing of market forces would be highly beneficial for air passengers, the millions of potential winners from airline deregulation were largely unorganized. In contrast, the major airlines that benefited from anticompetitive regulations were mobilized. Nevertheless, in 1978 Congress passed an airline deregulation bill in the face of strong industry opposition. Key to this reform victory was the entrepreneurial activity of legislators such as Senator Ted Kennedy (D-MA), who saw in airline deregulation the potential to enhance his standing with the burgeoning consumer movement.[19] To be sure, expertise alone did not bring about reform; the forces of good policy and good politics had to be brought into alignment through skillful manipulation of the procedural context in which decisions were made.[20] There is no escape from politics. Yet airline deregulation, together with cases such as the creation of an efficient market trading system to control the sulfur dioxide emissions that cause acid rain, clearly demonstrates that general-interest reform *is* possible in American government, even if it is not an everyday occurrence.[21]

But it is a mistake to infer from these canonical examples that the need for political entrepreneurship to improve system performance will automatically lead actors to supply it. The expected return on political entrepreneurship may simply be too low. While James Q. Wilson emphasized that policy entrepreneurs like Ralph Nader could speak on behalf of the unorganized and serve as an effective agent of change,[22] the incentives to engage in entrepreneurial activity may be much lower when the status quo is dominated not by corporations or labor unions, whom voters may view as motivated by narrow economic interests, but by members of highly esteemed professions, such as doctors, whom voters may view as public regarding.

Empirical Support for the Zero-Credit Politics Model

We offer support for the zero-credit politics model in two ways. At the end of this chapter, we provide a brief historical narrative of the federal government's sluggish efforts to promote EBM between the 1970s and 2008. The narrative shows that relatively few members of Congress sponsored or cosponsored legislation to strengthen the government's role in funding or overseeing comparative effectiveness research to identify what treatments work best. This case study evidence is instructive because lawmakers who did support such proposals were acting as institutional designers. They were not questioning the appropriateness of particular treatments or suggesting that specific medical societies were not behaving responsibly. In most cases, they were merely proposing to create an agency that would conduct research that might someday discredit popular treatments prescribed by doctors. Nevertheless, even tiptoeing into questions about need for greater third-party oversight of doctors' therapeutic authority was evidently seen by members of Congress as a "bad" investment of entrepreneurial energy—presumably because calling attention to the problems of overtreatment and unnecessary spending implicitly challenges the public's trust in doctors as guardians of patient and social welfare. As chapter 6 shows, Congress did eventually vote to increase taxpayer funding of health outcomes and created a new, nongovernmental, nonprofit entity (PCORI) to coordinate the work—but that was only because the proposals "hitched a ride" with two virtually must-pass, omnibus Democratic Party vehicles (the 2009 Recovery Act and the Affordable Care Act). The proposals likely would not have gained traction as stand-alone measures. In sum, the policy history of Congress's role in CER is broadly consistent with the zero-credit politics model.

While a review of past events illuminates what occurred, it tells us less about what could have happened but did not. To appreciate how political forces channel and constrain the incentives for political entrepreneurship, innovation, and pragmatic problem solving, it is also essential to consider what *might* have happened if politicians had been more willing to support evidence-based medicine, even at the cost of challenging doctors. It is important to view the lack of a robust response by elected representatives to the vast gaps in medical evidence as a genuine puzzle that requires an explanation. Imagine a world in which a politician decides to become a political entrepreneur to address medical evidence gaps. Would this politician be punished or rewarded by voters for his or her efforts?

This counterfactual question cannot be answered definitively, but we can illuminate it through survey experiments that employ vignettes about medical evidence controversies. We find that if politicians challenge doctors and medical societies on the appropriateness of treatments, their electoral standing declines, even if the scientific evidence is on the politicians' side. To be sure, politicians are quite reluctant to inject themselves into medical evidence controversies in the real world. The scenarios we describe rarely occur. But that is exactly the point. Challenging doctors is (in the terms of the economist) "off the equilibrium path" behavior. That is, certain kinds of efforts to promote evidence-based policy making, which could produce benefits for society, do not occur because of the political reactions or the punishments they would trigger. In short, in their potential roles as both institutional designers of expert agencies to promote health care quality and efficiency and as "position takers" on specific medical controversies, lawmakers have recognized that even attempting to curb unnecessary treatments and impose new monitoring and accountability mechanisms of the medical profession offers few electoral rewards. The take-away lesson is that the lack of effective political oversight of the use of evidence in the U.S. health care system is the product of powerful incentives. Only by taking such incentives into account can durable and effective reforms occur.

SURVEY ON POLITICAL ENTREPRENEURSHIP

Below we highlight results from a July 2015 web-based survey that we conducted on a nationally representative sample of 1,100 U.S. adults. The survey contained a variety of questions designed to examine the plausibility of the theory of zero-credit politics.

Members of Congress have multiple goals, but they cannot achieve any of them unless they win reelection. That is why most political science theories of legislative behavior start from the premise that legislators want to remain in office.[23] But what specific governing tasks will reelection-seeking lawmakers pursue to win votes? Are some activities more highly valued by the public than others? Can lawmakers reasonably expect to build a base of support among voters on the basis of entrepreneurial problem-solving activities, or would they generate greater electoral rewards by placing their attention elsewhere? To address these questions, we asked respondents to evaluate the performance of a politician based on a list of 18 factors individually.

Specifically, respondents were asked, "Below is a list of factors related to a politician's job performance. Please tell us the extent to which each factor would affect how likely you are to vote for your congressional representative." The response options ranged from "not at all more likely to vote for" to "a great deal more likely to vote for" on a five-point scale. The 18 items we asked about are listed in table 5.1. They range from factors that we did not expect to affect evaluations of politicians all that much (e.g., "spends a lot of time outdoors") to those that were meant to capture activities that in theory directly benefit constituents (e.g., "provides high-quality help to constituents who are running into problems with Social Security") to items that were meant to capture "entrepreneurial activity" related to solving collective problems.

A clear result—unsurprising yet of fundamental importance—is that voters are not clamoring for legislators to devote their time and energy to political entrepreneurship targeted at developing the expertise necessary to address broad societal problems. Only 23 percent of respondents stated that they were much or a great deal more likely to vote for a politician who "is a genuine expert on a policy area that is important to the nation as a whole but is not of special importance to your district," whereas 45 percent were not at all or a little more likely. In contrast, 52 percent were much or a great deal more likely to vote for a politician who "is an expert on the issues of greatest concern to your district," and only 19 percent were not at all or a little more likely.[24]

TABLE 5.1. Activities Related to Public Assessment of a Politician's Job Performance

	More likely to vote for?		
The representative . . .	Not at all / a little (%)	Somewhat (%)	Much more / a great deal more (%)
Generic Political Entrepreneurship and Leadership Roles			
Develops new policy solutions that have not been considered before	23.3	34.2	42.5
Is willing to question conventional wisdom about public policy issues	18.4	30.1	51.5
Has the courage to challenge powerful actors and organizations	19.4	24.2	56.4
Is effective at advancing bills through the legislative process	28.2	30.3	41.5
District Representation			
Is an expert on the issues of greatest concern to your district	18.8	28.9	52.4
Is a genuine expert in a policy area that is important to both the nation and your district	19.5	27.6	53.0
Brings in grants and projects that produce revenue for your district	32.6	32.8	34.6
Provides high-quality help to constituents who are running into problems with Social Security	20.5	27.1	52.4
Takes policy positions that reflect the existing opinions of the majority of the citizens in the district	29.6	30.8	39.6
Has a long history with your district and knows the district very well	29.6	31.8	38.6
Visits your district often	33.5	29.4	37.1
Problem Solving on Behalf of Broad National Interests			
Publicizes national problems that most people were previously unaware of	25.0	33.6	41.4
Is a genuine expert on a policy area that is important to the nation as a whole but is not of special importance to your district	45.0	32.2	22.8
Has average knowledge about the problems of the district, but is a genuine expert on U.S. counterterrorism policy in the Middle East	46.6	30.0	23.4
Other Attributes			
Runs an efficient office and treats the office staff with respect	25.3	27.8	46.8
Has a good sense of humor and is well liked by fellow members of Congress	50.9	30.0	19.1
Has one of the best attendance records at congressional committee hearings	29.3	31.9	38.8
Spends a lot of time outdoors	66.8	22.9	10.3

Note: Question wording (and response options): "Below is a list of factors related to a politician's job performance. Please tell us the extent to which each factor would affect how likely you are to vote for your congressional representative. (Not at all more likely to vote for; A little more likely to vote for; Somewhat more likely to vote for; Much more likely to vote for; A great deal more likely to vote for)."

Source: July 2015 YouGov/Polimetrix survey.

To be sure, it is possible for elected officials to gain public support while engaging in some entrepreneurial activities. We asked respondents to consider two activities relevant to "marketing" new policy products: (1) developing new policy solutions that have not been considered before and (2) questioning conventional wisdom about public policy issues. Both of these factors received high levels of support, as did general leadership traits such as having the courage to challenge powerful actors and organizations and being effective at advancing bills in the legislative process. Yet while these generic political skills may have a bearing on political entrepreneurship focused on problem solving, they can also feed into symbolic activity or legislating on behalf of narrow geographic or group interests. Where entrepreneurship is most needed—and most likely to be undersupplied—is problem solving on behalf of broad, unorganized groups.[25]

Our results suggest that the public is less likely to reward this type of political entrepreneurship, especially when it involves becoming a policy expert and not just publicizing ideas. As an illustrative example, we asked if respondents would be more likely to vote for a legislator who has average knowledge about the problems of the district, but who is a genuine expert on U.S. counterterrorism policy in the Middle East. Just 23 percent of respondents said they would be much more or a great deal more likely to vote for such a lawmaker.

An analysis of the cross section between support for national problem solving and generic political entrepreneurship highlights the limited public receptivity for national problem solving. Of the 617 respondents in our survey who said they would be a great deal or much more likely to vote for a lawmaker who has the courage to challenge powerful actors and organizations, only one in three (32 percent) also said they would be a great deal or much more likely to vote for a representative who is a genuine expert on a policy area that is important to the country as a whole but is not of special importance to their district. Similarly, only 40 percent of the respondents who said they were either a great deal or much more likely to vote for a representative who is effective at advancing bills through the legislative process or developing new policy solutions were also a great deal or much more likely to vote for a representative who is a national policy expert.

PUBLIC SUPPORT FOR LAWMAKERS WHO
STAND UP FOR EVIDENCE-BASED MEDICINE

The survey results discussed above suggest that the safest course for the reelection-minded lawmaker is to focus on district representation, and if the lawmaker does want to develop a policy reputation to focus on the distinctive concerns of his or her constituency rather than broad national challenges. The would-be entrepreneur contemplating devoting his or her scarce time and energy to developing the expertise required not just to publicize but to actually develop and build support for solutions to broad problems knows that it is, at best, a political investment with uncertain returns.

These conclusions were produced by asking respondents about what they value in a representative in a very abstract context. Do we find similar results when respondents are asked about specific legislative actions taken by a representative? What would happen if a lawmaker who understands the problem of overtreatment and unnecessary care stands up for sound science and the promotion of evidence-based medicine? Will he or she be rewarded or punished for such efforts? To address this question, we conducted two survey experiments.

In the first experiment, respondents read a short vignette about a study published in a medical journal that questioned the effectiveness of a procedure to treat heart disease.[26] Respondents (not in the baseline, "study only" condition) were randomly assigned to read about the stances of doctors and/or members of Congress concerning the journal article. After reading the vignette, respondents were first asked to answer a battery of questions concerning use of the procedure, trust in the various entities mentioned in the vignette, and evaluations of a member of Congress (when applicable).

Specifically, all respondents read the following prompt (bolded text was bolded on the screen for respondents):

> A recent study published in a leading, peer-reviewed medical journal shows that a common procedure for heart disease is not effective. **The study concludes that there are better treatments, and the procedure should be used much less often.**

Respondents randomly assigned to the "study only" condition read only this information before answering questions about what they had read. All other respondents were randomly assigned (with equal probability) to one of 10 experimental treatment conditions. We focus on six of those conditions here, each of which is summarized in table 5.2. In short, some respondents read that doctors supported the study's recommendation that "the procedure should be used much less often" whereas others read that doctors opposed the study's recommendation. Similarly, some respondents read that politicians ("Representative X") supported the study's recommendation whereas others read that politicians ("Representative X") opposed the

TABLE 5.2. Summary of Heart Disease Vignette Experimental Conditions

Experimental Condition	Text
STUDY ONLY	A recent study published in a leading, peer-reviewed medical journal shows that a common procedure for heart disease is <u>not</u> effective. **The study concludes that there are better treatments, and the procedure should be used much less often.**
DOCTORS OPPOSE STUDY	["Study only" text plus] Doctors from an association of cardiologists (heart doctors) disagree with the study's findings. They say that they have decades of experience treating patients with heart disease, and the procedure is effective. **The cardiologists say that the study is wrong, and they oppose reducing the use of the procedure. They say reducing use of the procedure would cost many lives.**
DOCTORS SUPPORT STUDY	["Study only" text plus] Doctors from an association of cardiologists (heart doctors) agree with the study's findings. They say this is the first rigorous study of the effectiveness of the procedure for treating patients with heart disease, and the study was well done. **The cardiologists say that the study is right, and they support reducing the use of the procedure. They say reducing the use of the procedure would save many lives.**
MEMBER OF CONGRESS OPPOSES STUDY	["Study only" text plus] A number of politicians disagree with the study's findings. Representative X says that doctors have decades of experience treating patients with heart disease, and the procedure is effective. **Representative X says that the study is wrong, and he opposes reducing the use of the procedure. He says reducing use of the procedure would cost many lives.**
MEMBER OF CONGRESS SUPPORTS STUDY	["Study only" text plus] A number of politicians agree with the study's findings. Representative X says this is the first rigorous study of the effectiveness of the procedure for treating patients with heart disease, and the study was well done. **Representative X says that the study is right, and he supports reducing the use of the procedure. He says reducing use of the procedure would save many lives.**
DOCTORS AND MEMBER OF CONGRESS OPPOSE STUDY	["Study only" text plus "Doctors oppose study" text plus "member of Congress opposes study" text]
DOCTORS OPPOSE STUDY; MEMBER OF CONGRESS SUPPORTS STUDY	["Study only" text plus "Doctors oppose study" text plus "member of Congress supports study" text]

study's recommendation. Importantly, the arguments used were the same, which allows us to measure whether the fact that doctors or politicians are the informational source matters for respondents. In addition, two of the experimental conditions included responses from both doctors and politicians. In one, both doctors and politicians opposed the study's recommendation. In the other, doctors opposed the study's recommendation, but politicians supported it.

The first outcome of interest we present (in figure 5.1) concerns respondent beliefs about whether the procedure should be used more or less often. Specifically, we asked: "Based on the exchange, do you think the procedure should be used: Less often than it is currently used; At the same rate as it is currently used; More often than it is currently used." We scored these responses so that "more often" is given a value of 1, "less often" −1, and "the same" 0. Figure 5.1 presents average responses to this question by experimental condition.

Figure 5.1 shows that, on average, respondents in the Study Only condition agreed with the study's recommendation that the procedure should be used less often—the average response is around −.5. When doctors oppose the study's recommendation, however, this shifts to around −.25. In other words, when respondents learn that physicians oppose the study, support for using the procedure less often declines ($p<.05$ for difference between Study Only and Doctors Oppose Study conditions). The member of Congress (Representative X) making the same argument as doctors has a similar effect on respondents ($p<.05$ for difference between Study Only and Member of Congress Opposes Study conditions); ($p>.10$ for difference between Doctors Oppose Study and Member of Congress Opposes Study conditions). Neither doctors nor politicians supporting the study's recommendation, however, moves opinion about how often the procedure should be used much from where it is in the Study Only condition ($p>.10$ for both comparisons to the Study Only condition, and the comparison of Doctors Support Study and Member of Congress Supports Study conditions). This suggests that although doctors and politicians can both discredit the study (when using the same argument), neither bolster public support for the study's recommendation.

The most interesting comparison is the one between the two conditions in which both doctors and politicians are mentioned. When both doctors and politicians oppose the study's recommendation there is no cumulative effect (i.e., the effect of Doctors Oppose Study and Doctors and Member of Congress Oppose Study are statistically indistinguishable from one another,

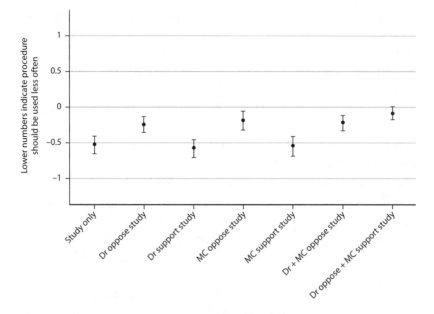

FIGURE 5.1. Effects of elite positions on public support for use of heart disease procedure after study says procedure should be used less often. *Note*: Dots represent means for each experimental condition; whiskers are 95% confidence intervals. In the "Study Only" condition respondents were simply told, "A recent study published in a leading, peer-reviewed medical journal shows that a common procedure for heart disease is <u>not</u> effective. **The study concludes that there are better treatments, and the procedure should be used much less often.**" Other conditions, as displayed in table 5.2, added information for those respondents about whether, for example, doctors opposed ("Dr Oppose Study") or supported ("Dr Support Study") the study's findings. The figure shows that when doctors oppose the study's findings, public support for using the procedure less often declines. *Source*: July 2015 YouGov/Polimetrix survey.

as is Member of Congress Opposes Study and Doctors and Member of Congress Oppose Study). However—and this point is critical—politicians are not able to counteract the opposition of doctors. *When politicians support the study's recommendation to reduce the use of the heart procedure in light of research findings and doctors oppose this recommendation, the average response is no different in this condition compared to when both doctors and politicians oppose the study's recommendation* ($p > .10$ for comparison of Doctors and Member of Congress Oppose Study and Doctors Oppose and Member of Congress Supports Study).

In sum, a politician who takes a stand in support of sound evidence has no independent ability to influence public opinion about the use of the treatment if a doctors' group attacks the recommendation. This would be highly discouraging to any lawmaker contemplating wading into these waters. But

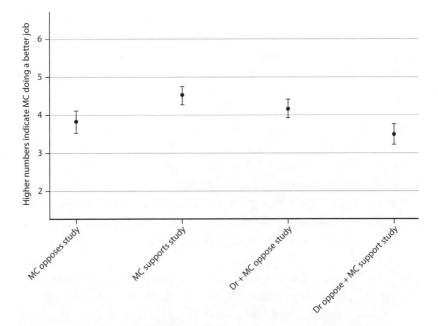

FIGURE 5.2. Effects of elite positions about use of heart disease procedure after study says procedure should be used less often on public approval of job member of Congress is doing. *Note*: Dots represent means for each experimental condition; whiskers are 95% confidence intervals. Question wording: "How likely do you think it is that Representative X is doing a good job as a representative?" Scale ranged from 1 (very unlikely) to 7 (very likely). The figure shows that compared to when the position of doctors is not mentioned, when doctors oppose the study's recommendations the member of Congress's support of the study's recommendations results in views that the member of Congress is doing a worse job. *Source*: July 2015 YouGov/Polimetrix survey.

will the public reward or punish the member for their courage? What are the political returns to supporting or opposing the doctors?

To find out, we also asked respondents who were assigned to a condition that mentioned a politician to evaluate the member of Congress (Representative X). We asked them, "How likely do you think it is that Representative X is doing a good job as a representative?" Responses were recorded on a seven-point scale ranging from "very unlikely" to "very likely." Figure 5.2 presents average responses for the four conditions in which Representative X was mentioned. The primary takeaway from figure 5.2 is that when the member of Congress challenges doctors' opposition to the study's recommendation, the lawmaker receives the most negative evaluation—about 3.5 on the seven-point scale, which falls somewhere between being somewhat unlikely to think the representative is doing a good job and being undecided.

We observe this effect most clearly when we compare the condition in which the legislator supports the study's recommendation without any mention of doctors (second to left dot in figure 5.2) to the one in which the legislator supports the study's recommendation but doctors oppose it (far right dot in figure 5.2). Evaluations of the member of Congress are a full point higher on the seven-point scale when doctors are not mentioned in the vignette compared to when their opposition is described ($p<.05$). Overall, the results of this vignette experiment suggest that politicians face an uphill battle when they face off against doctors in the realm of health care policy, specifically when the use of medical procedures and medical effectiveness is in question.

To see if these findings were robust across contexts, we performed a second survey experiment. Respondents read a short vignette about a recommendation by a task force regarding use of the PSA test. Respondents (not in the baseline, "task force only" condition) were randomly assigned to read about the stances of doctors and/or members of Congress concerning the task force's recommendation. After reading the vignette, respondents were asked to answer a battery of questions concerning use of the procedure, trust in the various entities mentioned in the vignette, and evaluations of the member of Congress (when applicable).

All respondents read the following prompt (bolded text was bolded on the screen for respondents):

> In 2012 a government-appointed, independent panel of national experts in prevention and evidence-based medicine issued a **recommendation that men who have no symptoms of prostate cancer should *not* routinely be given a PSA test, a common test to screen for prostate cancer.** The task force concluded that it is likely "that the service has no benefit or that the harms outweigh the benefits."

Respondents randomly assigned to the "task force only" condition only read this information before answering questions about what they had read. All other respondents were randomly assigned (with equal probability) to one of 11 experimental treatment conditions. We focus on five of those conditions here, each of which is summarized in table 5.3. In this vignette, all respondents read some information about whether politicians (Representative A) supported or opposed the task force's recommendation "that men who have no symptoms of prostate cancer should *not* routinely be given a PSA test." Similar to the design of the previous experiment, when Representative A supported the recommendation of the task force, we also had a condition in which doctors opposed the recommendation. Finally, we had two

TABLE 5.3. Summary of PSA Vignette Experimental Conditions

Experimental Condition	Text
TASK FORCE ONLY	In 2012 a government-appointed, independent panel of national experts in prevention and evidence-based medicine issued a **recommendation that men who have no symptoms of prostate cancer should *not* routinely be given a PSA test, a common test to screen for prostate cancer.** The task force concluded that it is likely "that the service has no benefit or that the harms outweigh the benefits."
REP. A OPPOSES TASK FORCE	["Task force only" text plus] A number of politicians disagree with the task force's recommendations. Representative A says that we should trust doctors to do what is best for their patients, and not base medical practice on the recommendations of so-called experts on a task force. **Representative A says that the task force is wrong. He says that recommending against routine screening would cost many lives.**
REP. A SUPPORTS TASK FORCE	["Task force only" text plus] A number of politicians agree with the task force's recommendations. Representative A says that we should follow the scientific evidence and base medical practice on the task force recommendations. Also, doctors sometimes push for more screening than is medically necessary because they receive money from tests and procedures. **Representative A says that the task force is right. He says that recommending against routine screening is the right decision.**
REP. A SUPPORTS TASK FORCE; DOCTORS OPPOSE	["Task force only" text plus "Rep. A. supports task force" text plus] Doctors from an association of urologists challenge Representative A's support for the task force's recommendations. They say that we should trust doctors to do what is best for their patients, and not base medical practice on the recommendations of so-called experts on a task force. **The urologists say that both the task force and Representative A are wrong. They say that recommending against routine screening would cost many lives.**
REP. A SUPPORTS TASK FORCE; REP. B OPPOSES; DOCTORS SUPPORT	["Task force only" text plus "Rep. A. supports task force" text plus] Representative B challenges Representative A's support for the task force's recommendations. Representative B says that we should trust doctors to do what is best for their patients, and not base medical practice on the recommendations of so-called experts on a task force. **Representative B says that both the task force and Representative A are wrong. Representative B says that recommending against routine screening would cost many lives. Doctors from an association of urologists weighed in to say that Representative B is wrong. They say that Representative A is right and that the task force recommendation against routine screening is the right decision.**
REP. A SUPPORTS TASK FORCE; REP. B OPPOSES; DOCTORS OPPOSE	["Task force only" text plus "Rep. A. supports task force" text plus] Representative B challenges Representative A's support for the task force's recommendations. Representative B says that we should trust doctors to do what is best for their patients, and not base medical practice on the recommendations of so-called experts on a task force. **Representative B says that both the task force and Representative A are wrong. Representative B says that recommending against routine screening would cost many lives. Doctors from an association of urologists weighed in to say that the task force is wrong and Representative A is wrong. They say that Representative B is right that recommending against routine screening would cost many lives.**

conditions in which another lawmaker (Representative B) opposed the task force's recommendation (when Representative A supported it), and doctors either supported (in one condition) or opposed (in a different condition) the recommendation of the task force.

The results of this study are summarized in figures 5.3 and 5.4. As with the heart disease vignette study, the first outcome of interest we present concerns respondent beliefs about use of the procedure (in this case, the PSA test). Specifically, we asked: "Based on the exchange, do you think the screening test should be routinely given to men with no symptoms of prostate cancer?" The response options were, "Yes, screening test should be routinely given to men with no symptoms of prostate cancer"; "No, screening test should *not* be routinely given to men with no symptoms of prostate cancer"; and "I don't know." We scored these responses so that "yes" is given a value of 1, "no" −1, and "don't know" 0. Figure 5.3 presents average responses to this question by experimental condition.

Figure 5.3 shows that, on average, respondents in the Task Force Only condition were uncertain (at 0) about whether the PSA test should be given to men without symptoms. The position of Representative A does move opinion on this issue—when Representative A opposes the task force recommendation, more people think the PSA test should be given to men without symptoms (around .3 on the scale, $p<.05$); when Representative A supports the task force recommendation, more people think the PSA test should *not* be given to men without symptoms (around −.2 on the scale, $p=.18$). However, the next dot over (fourth from the left) shows that Representative A's support of the task force recommendation can be completely counteracted by the opposition of physicians, as the average response in that condition is virtually the same as when Representative A opposed the task force recommendation himself ($p<.05$ for difference between Representative A Supports Task Force and Representative A Supports Task Force and Doctors Oppose Task Force).

The last two entries of figure 5.3 further illustrate the unique power of physicians in this area. In those two conditions, there was a disagreement between politicians. When such disagreements occur, our results suggest that doctors can move opinion. In the face of political disagreement over the task force recommendation, doctors' support of the task force recommendation moves people in the direction of the task force recommendation; doctors' opposition to the task force recommendation, on the other hand, moves people away from the task force recommendation ($p<.05$ for difference between these two conditions).

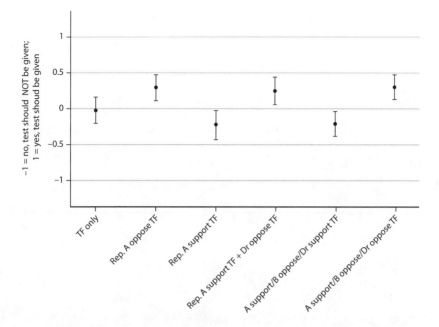

FIGURE 5.3. Effects of elite positions on public support for use of PSA test after task force recommends PSA test should not be given to men without symptoms. *Note*: Dots represent means for each experimental condition; whiskers are 95% confidence intervals. In the "Task Force (TF) Only" condition respondents were told, "In 2012 a government-appointed, independent panel of national experts in prevention and evidence-based medicine issued a **recommendation that men who have no symptoms of prostate cancer should** <u>**not**</u> **routinely be given a PSA test, a common test to screen for prostate cancer**. The task force concluded that it is likely 'that the service has no benefit or that the harms outweigh the benefits.'" Other conditions, as displayed in table 5.3, added information for those respondents about whether, for example, a representative opposed ("Rep. A Oppose TF") or supported ("Rep. A Support TF") the task force's recommendation. The figure shows that compared to the "task force only" condition, when Rep A. supports the task force's recommendation, respondents are somewhat more likely to think the PSA test should not be given to men without symptoms, but not when doctors oppose the task force's recommendation. *Source*: July 2015 YouGov/Polimetrix survey.

We also asked respondents who were assigned to a condition that mentioned a politician to evaluate Representative A. We asked them, "How likely do you think it is that Representative A is doing a good job as a representative?" Responses were recorded on a seven-point scale ranging from "very unlikely" to "very likely." Figure 5.4 presents average responses for the five conditions in which Representative A was mentioned. The primary takeaway from figure 5.4 is that when there is a political disagreement over EBM (last two dots of figure 5.4), evaluations of the member of Congress are more favorable when the lawmaker is on the side of doctors.[27] When

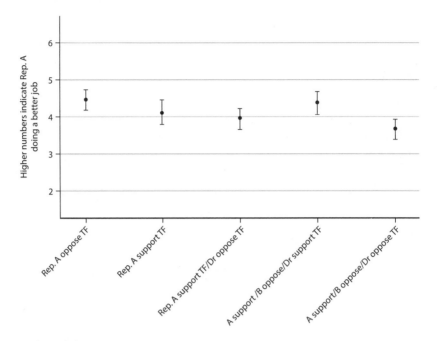

FIGURE 5.4. Effects of elite positions about use of PSA test after task force recommends PSA test should not be given to men without symptoms on public approval of job Rep. A is doing. *Note*: Dots represent means for each experimental condition; whiskers are 95% confidence intervals. Question wording: "How likely do you think it is that Representative A is doing a good job as a representative?" Scale ranged from 1 (very unlikely) to 7 (very likely). Comparing the two dots on the right hand side of the figure suggests that when politicians (Rep. A and Rep. B) are in disagreement over the task force's recommendation, the position of doctors determines whether approval of Rep. A is higher (when doctors agree with Rep. A) or lower (when doctors disagree with Rep. A). *Source*: July 2015 YouGov/Polimetrix survey.

doctors are of the same opinion as Representative A (that is, both support the task force recommendation), Representative A's evaluation is almost 4.5 (somewhere between being undecided and somewhat likely to think the representative is doing a good job). However, when doctors disagree with Representative A and the task force recommendation, Representative A's evaluation falls to just under 3.7 (nearly a full point, difference is statistically significant, $p<.05$). In short, being a policy entrepreneur in this area is likely prudent only when doctors are in agreement with your position.

These survey experiments are simple by design, but they capture a fundamental truth about efforts to tighten oversight of the clinical authority of physicians and medical societies: it is a risky proposition for reelection-minded lawmakers. This, at least in part, helps explain why we have seen relatively little of this activity.

The Government's Sluggish Response to the Medical Evidence Problem, 1970s–2008

The survey experiments described above necessarily abstract from reality. But what has actually happened in Washington? How much effort have lawmakers devoted over the past several decades to tackling the problems of wasteful spending, overtreatment, and bad science in American medicine?

Below, we present a thumbnail history of the federal government's efforts to address the medical evidence gap prior to the Obama administration.[28] Before recounting this history, however, it is useful to ask why government even has a role in funding research on the comparative effectiveness of treatments. Why can't the provision of information about the relative benefits of treatment alternatives be left to the private market? Insurance plans have long conducted some evidence-based technology assessments to inform their coverage decisions[29]—so it is not the case that *no* evidence will be generated without taxpayer money.[30] The reason is that CER is a "public good," which will be undersupplied without government support. As the Congressional Budget Office (CBO) explains:

> The knowledge created by such studies is costly to produce—but once it is produced, can be disseminated at essentially no additional cost, and charging all users for access to that information is not always feasible. As a result, private insurers and other entities conducting research on comparative effectiveness often stand to capture only a portion of the resulting benefits and therefore do not invest as much in such research as they would if they took into account the benefits to all parties. In health plans that do not have exclusive provider networks, some of the benefits probably "spill over" to other health plans using the same doctors, because physicians tend to use a similar approach to care for all of their patients. Even if organizations could keep their findings confidential, so that they captured all of the benefits, some duplication of effort would probably occur. In such a situation, research constitutes a "public good," and economists have long recognized a role for government to increase the supply of such research toward the socially optimal level.[31]

The existence of a market failure does not mean that government will step in to correct it. The perceived costs of more rigorous scrutiny of treatments, tests, and technologies are concentrated on well-organized groups such as device manufacturers and medical specialty societies. This is a classic "diffuse benefits/concentrated costs" situation that Wilson identified as prone to undermining good policy making.[32]

One way to overcome this problem is through "public interest" lobbying. The millions of patients who suffer from cancer, heart disease, and other chronic conditions are dispersed across the nation. Tragically, the patients who are in most desperate need of unbiased information about treatment options are often least able to mobilize politically. "Patient advocacy" groups ostensibly represent the interests of such patients. The number of such organizations has exploded in recent years. Patient advocacy organizations have the capacity to accelerate FDA drug reviews,[33] and they could be an important voice for better use of evidence in medicine. However, research suggests that patient advocacy groups do not act like public interest organizations.[34] They often act much more like nonoccupational trade associations. Many patient groups are underwritten by drug companies.[35] Whether owing to financial or political pressure or organizational maintenance reasons, the patient advocacy community has not prioritized the need to increase the funding of a generic public good like CER. Patient advocacy tends to be disease specific rather than focused on general patient goals or the overall improvement of the health care system.[36]

The theory of zero-credit politics helps account for three observable facts in this history. First, it accounts for the relatively low level of interest in the issue among elected officials, with the important exception of a few lawmakers including Tom Allen (D-ME), Jo Ann Emerson (R-MO), and Max Baucus (D-MT). Second, it helps explain why the most dogged and passionate actors who *have* tried to sell CER have been private citizens (John E. Wennberg), former officials (Gail Wilensky), or political appointees (former Congressional Budget Office and Office of Management and Budget director Peter Orszag), who, compared to elected officials, have not had to worry about pleasing voters and winning elections. Finally, the theory offers insight into why elected officials have often found the payoff from attacking or weakening EBM reforms greater than the payoff from initiating or strengthening them, especially when faced with hostility from doctors and doctors' organizations.

THE RISE AND FALL OF THE NATIONAL CENTER FOR HEALTH CARE TECHNOLOGY

Between the 1970s and mid-2000s, support among politicians for efforts to promote the integration of hard data into clinical decisions was inconsistent.[37]

A few politicians did make entrepreneurial investments of time and energy in the promotion of evidence-based medicine, facilitating the enactment of modest reforms, but most policy makers did not see it as a winning issue. Members of Congress frequently served as allies of industry and medical professionals opposed to reform.

As early as the 1970s, both health services experts and parts of the U.S. health policy community were aware that medical technologies were increasingly diffusing into practice before their effectiveness had been evaluated. Some government officials recognized that the overuse or misuse of expensive technology contributed to the problem of rising health care costs and sought to increase the knowledge base about what interventions work best. A limited (and short-lived) effort to improve the medical evidence base was the National Center for Health Care Technology (NCHCT), which Congress established in 1978 as a small bureau (with a $4 million budget and staff of twenty) inside the Department of Health, Education, and Welfare. Its mission was to generate information about the safety and efficacy of medical technologies and, through its dissemination, to advise the Medicare agency on coverage issues. The act creating the center (PL 95-623) won bipartisan passage in Congress. Hopes were high that the center's work would improve quality and reduce wasteful spending. As the *New York Times* reported, pressing questions, such as what is the best treatment for breast cancer, would no longer be considered "only by individual practitioners, who may have limited access to the facts, or by special-interest professional groups, who may have prejudiced views."[38] The NCHCT managed a program of research grants and was given responsibility for developing standards and norms concerning the use of particular technologies. In addition, the NCHCT provided information on the safety and effectiveness (but *not* cost-effectiveness) of technologies to the Health Care Financing Administration (the precursor agency to the Centers for Medicare and Medicaid Services) for its coverage decisions in the Medicare program. Health and Human Services officials emphasized that the opinions of the NCHCT were only "advisory" and that Medicare did not have to accept them.[39] Between 1978 and 1981, the NCHCT provided Medicare with 75 such evaluations, of which approximately 40 percent were for noncoverage.[40]

But the NCHCT was short-lived. In 1981, the Reagan administration zeroed out the agency's budget, and it ceased operations. (Some of its work was shifted to the National Center for Health Services Research.) Office of Management and Budget director David Stockman viewed NCHCT as an example of excessive government regulation.[41] Yet it would be a mistake to regard sincere ideological opposition as the principal cause of the agency's early demise. Indeed, the conservative Heritage Foundation's book *Mandate for Leadership*, which had a major influence on the Reagan administration's initial budget submissions to Congress, had called for the creation of a research unit to evaluate medical procedures and deny reimbursement under Medicare and Medicaid for procedures that were challenged.[42] While antiregulatory sentiments were clearly a factor in the NCHCT's erosion of support, the most direct cause was the growing opposition of doctors and industry groups. In 1981, the AMA opposed the reauthorization of the agency, arguing that it was a threat to the exercise of individual judgment by physicians:

> The relevant clinical policy analysis and judgments are better made—and are being responsibly made—within the medical profession. Assessing risks and costs, as well as benefits, has been central to the exercise of good medical judgment for decades. The advantage the individual physician has over any national center or advisory council is that he or she is dealing with individuals in need of medical care, not hypothetical cases.[43]

The Health Industry Manufacturer's Association also opposed NCHCT's continuation, fearing that the center would constrain the industry's ability to bring new products to the marketplace.[44]

THE RISE AND FALL OF THE AGENCY FOR HEALTH CARE POLICY AND RESEARCH

While the NCHCT ceased operations in late 1981, the lack of solid, scientific evidence for many common treatments remained a glaring problem. By the mid-1980s, health policy makers in both the legislative and executive branches were becoming increasingly aware of the research on geographical variation in medical practice by Dartmouth professor John E. Wennberg and colleagues. Wennberg's work on Medicare showed that different regions of the United States had marked differences in the use of many health services that could not be explained by age, gender, race, and other population factors, and that high levels of medical services use were not associated with better outcomes such as mortality and functional status.[45] The implication was that a large portion (perhaps as much as 20–30 percent) of health care in the United States may be wasteful.[46] Wennberg himself played an entrepreneurial role in educating elected officials about the practice variation phenomenon through congressional testimony.

Wennberg's research and the need for better information to address unwarranted variation and curb wasteful spending formed an idea that key policy actors judged as plausible, technically feasible, and responsive to the government's needs. The concept entered what political scientist John W. Kingdon calls the "policy stream."[47] When a window of opportunity opened, a proposal to expand the federal government's role in improving the medical evidence base led to the creation of the Agency for Health Care Policy and Research (AHCPR) in 1989. The mission of AHCPR was to carry out and disseminate research on the effectiveness, efficiency, quality, and outcomes of health services. In addition, it was charged with developing clinical practice guidelines. The hope was that better health outcomes research would identify unnecessary or low-value services and help control the growth of Medicare spending. Although the idea of having the federal government establish standards for medical practice had long been anathema to physicians, several medical associations, including the AMA, endorsed the inclusion of practice guidelines in the legislation.[48] Because the law establishing AHCPR was folded into an omnibus budget bill, it never had a separate vote in Congress. The legislative record shows, however, that AHCPR was a bipartisan creation. Key supporters included Congressmen Henry Waxman (D-CA), Bill Gradison (R-Ohio), and Fortney H. (Pete) Stark (D-CA); Senators George Mitchell (D-ME) and David Durenberger (R-MN); and William Roper, Medicare program administrator under President George H. W. Bush.[49] During its first several years of activity, AHCPR sponsored Patient Outcomes Research Teams to study topics such as prostate enlargement and heart attack, and developed 15 clinical practice guidelines. The agency had a low profile, and its work received little attention from politicians. Its budget grew steadily from $115 million in FY 1991 to $159 million in FY 1995.[50]

Although the AHCPR was launched with great enthusiasm, the agency quickly got into political trouble. Both partisan politics and interest group pressures led to the agency's loss of support. In 1994, Republicans gained control of Congress with an agenda (the Contract with America) to reduce federal spending. Even though the AHCPR was created under a Republican administration, with the backing of key GOP lawmakers, the shift in the political environment left the agency vulnerable to budget cuts. (The Office of Technology Assessment [OTA], an even more prominent congressional support agency, also did not survive this period.[51] The OTA's downfall reflected a general lack of congressional support for its research mission, but its health technology assessment work was certainly not without controversy and sparked some medical products industry opposition.) Support for AHCPR among Republicans was further weakened by the perception that it had played an advocacy role in the debate over the Clinton health reform initiative in 1993–94, a perception not helped by the agency's decision to hire several people who had worked on the Clinton plan and Democratic staffers from Capitol Hill.[52]

In addition, the agency set off a firestorm when it released practice guidelines for treating acute lower back pain. The guidelines said that back surgery benefited only 1 in 100 patients and should be avoided, and that doctors should also refrain from using imaging tests, X-rays, and MRIs at the beginning of a back pain episode.[53] The North American Spine Society, the professional group of back surgeons, criticized the study and took their complaints to Congress. Representative Sam Johnson (R-TX) led an attempt to eliminate the AHCPR, arguing that the government should not tell doctors how to practice medicine.[54]

The agency survived the conflict but suffered a sharp reduction in its budget. Moreover, it was stripped of its role as a developer of practice guidelines. Both the continued existence of the agency, which was renamed the Agency for Healthcare Research and Quality (AHRQ), and the narrowing of its mission are significant. That the agency survived at all reflected the fact that it enjoyed residual support among Republican members of the House, such as Bill Thomas (R-CA), John Porter (R-IL), and Speaker Newt Gingrich (R-GA), Senator James Jeffords (R-VT), well-placed committee staffers, and health care expert Gail Wilensky, who had headed the Medicare program under George H. W. Bush. One Republican Hill staffer recalls accompanying his principal to the House Budget Committee and pleading with the legislators not to zero out the budget for the agency: "Are you going nuts?" the staffer recalled saying. "Republicans created this. It is allowing us to figure out what we are spending money on. [Zeroing it out] is just crazy."[55] But the scope of the agency's influence was severely curtailed. No longer would the agency publish guidelines to direct the behavior of clinicians. Instead, its task was reduced to evidence generation, "leaving it to the health care industry to sort what they should be doing."[56] As Harvard School of Medicine professor Jerry Avorn observed, "The linkage between research and policy had been formally renounced, and the nation took one giant step away from bringing science to bear on the systematic assessment of therapeutics."[57]

Efforts to strengthen the role of CER within Medicare during this period also met with political resistance. Under the program's authorizing legislation in 1965, Medicare pays for "reasonable and necessary" services, which was "understood to reflect the prevailing views of physicians, although there were no formal criteria to define this standard at either the local or the national level."[58] In the late 1980s, the Health Care Financing Agency (later the CMS) proposed a requirement that technologies be cost-effective to be covered. The AMA and the Pharmaceutical Research and Manufacturers Association opposed the proposal, and it was withdrawn.[59]

REFORM FORCES IN CONGRESS, 2000–2008

As noted above, to argue that the supply of political entrepreneurship has been below the socially optimal level is not to claim it has been missing entirely. One legislator who did play an important entrepreneurial role was Representative Tom Allen (D-ME). After the failure of the comprehensive Clinton health reform plan in 1994, Allen was searching for more incremental health reforms that could help make health care more affordable and potentially attract bipartisan support. Allen recognized that FDA approval "means less than most people think," that the pharmaceutical industry often buried adverse research results, and that there was no guarantee that expensive drugs worked better than cheaper alternatives.[60] Allen became aware of the drug effectiveness review project started by Oregon governor John Kitzhaber, which sought to integrate drug data into the state Medicaid program, as well as comparative effectiveness initiatives underway in Australia and New Zealand. He became convinced that independent research on the relative effectiveness of drugs would help "reduce system cost and improve quality."[61]

In 2003, Allen and Jo Ann Emerson (R-MO) introduced the Prescription Drug Comparative Effectiveness Act (HR 2356). The bill authorized $50 million for the NIH to conduct research and $25 million for the AHRQ to conduct studies on the comparative effectiveness and cost-effectiveness of prescription drugs. There was a conscious effort not to go as far as drug assessment systems employed in Australia and New Zealand, which used comparative effectiveness information to determine whether particular drugs would be included on a formulary and the price at which the cost of the drug would be reimbursed.[62] The purpose of HR 2356 was simply to generate accurate information on how drugs that treat particular conditions compared to one another and to disseminate this information to patients and providers. Investing time and energy in the development of this issue was not an obvious way to gain political rewards for a new lawmaker. As Allen recollects, "across the country, there was no significant constituency for funding comparative effectiveness research; few even knew what it was."[63]

The bill had eight Republican and seven Democratic cosponsors and was endorsed by consumer groups, the AFL-CIO, the AARP, General Motors, and the American Academy of Family Physicians.[64] Hillary Rodham Clinton introduced similar legislation in the Senate.[65] The Bush administration's support for a Medicare prescription drug bill provided an opening to congressional advocates of CER. Allen and Emerson argued that if the government was going to spend a half a trillion dollars on new drug benefits over the next decade, both doctors and patients should have hard data on what drugs are most effective. It was hoped that this medical evidence base would counterbalance the biased information about drugs that consumers received from television advertising and also help reduce doctor's reliance on pharmaceutical industry marketing in deciding what to prescribe. CER was thus framed as an informational tool that would help doctors push back against the immense influence of drug companies.[66]

During floor debate over the Medicare prescription drug bill, Clinton proposed an amendment authorizing $75 million in research funding. The amendment was defeated 43–52 (Republicans and Independents voted 49–0 against, and Democrats voted 43–3 in favor). Senators Charles Grassley (R-IA) and Mike Enzi (R-WY) spoke against the proposal. Enzi argued that the research would "promote one-size-fits-all medicine," and "end up as a tool for health care rationing by bureaucrats in Washington."[67] Enzi's statement foreshadowed the major criticisms of comparative effectiveness research that opponents would make in 2008–10. Indeed, it is striking how little the anti-CER arguments changed over the decade.[68]

Yet, our interviews with congressional insiders suggest that the GOP opposition to CER at this stage was less sincere than tactical. Passing the prescription drug bill was a top legislative priority for both President Bush and Republicans in Congress, and party leaders wanted to keep the bill "clean" to make it easier to pass.[69] CER funding was an unnecessary diversion at this stage of the process, and even supporters, including Senate Majority Leader Bill Frist (R-TN), a physician by training, voted against the Clinton amendment. Once the passage of the prescription drug bill (the Medicare Modernization Act, MMA) was assured, however, the Republican leadership (most likely Frist, according to our sources) tucked a CER provision into the conference agreement.

As signed into law, Section 1013 of the MMA authorized the AHRQ to spend up to $50 million in 2004 and additional amounts in future years to conduct systematic reviews of existing evidence on the comparative effectiveness of drugs and other treatments. PhRMA opposed the CER program but was unable to block its adoption.[70] The industry was, however, able to get language in the bill prohibiting the AHRQ from using the data to mandate clinical guidelines and stating that the CMS could not use the information to withhold coverage of prescription drugs under Medicare and Medicaid.[71]

Allen and Emerson continued to cosponsor legislation to establish a more ambitious and permanent CER program, and expert support for a major CER initiative grew. In 2006, health economist Wilensky published a widely discussed article in *Health Affairs* calling for a comparative effectiveness center and laying out a range of ideas for how the entity could be organized and financed.[72] Wilensky's article demonstrated that CER was not a partisan idea, but rather a technocratic solution to a national problem. Joseph Antos of the conservative Heritage Foundation was on board:

> We also ought to work on comparative effectiveness research. Information is a public good, and the government is in the best position to collect information. In fact, Medicare collects information on millions of medical treatments and then doesn't use it to better understand what works and what does not. That should be fixed.[73]

The following year, the Congressional Budget Office (CBO), under director Peter Orszag, published a major report on CER.[74] By all accounts, Orszag viewed the Dartmouth Institute's research on regional variation in Medicare as compelling evidence that it should be possible to curb wasteful health care spending by generating better information about the costs and benefits of treatment options. He was known to carry the Dartmouth charts to congressional meetings and to preach "to anyone who would listen about the 'evidence-based' cure for rising medical costs."[75] Under Orszag, the CBO began highlighting the potential for CER to constrain health care costs "without adverse health consequences."[76]

In May 2007, Allen and Emerson introduced a bill authorizing $3 billion for research in AHRQ over five years (HR 2184). Emerson called the bill a "no brainer" that deserved to receive bipartisan support.[77] In June 2007, the Subcommittee on Health of the House Ways and Means Committee, chaired by Stark, held a hearing on CER. Allen, Wilensky, and Orszag advocated for increased government investment in CER. The panel's ranking Republican, Dave Camp of Michigan, likewise expressed the need for a much broader effort on CER. "While we have agencies like the FDA to determine if drugs and devices are safe, we have very little information that compares the actual effectiveness of drug, devices, and medical procedures." Camp and other Republicans did raise concerns about the potential for the Medicare agency to use the information to limit access to certain treatments because they don't work for the "average" patient. However, Allen stressed that the aim of the proposal was not to "drive decisions."[78]

While the Allen-Emerson proposal never made it out of committee, the House folded its language into a larger bill reauthorizing a children's health insurance program that was nearing expiration.[79] The bill, nicknamed "CHAMP" (for Children's Health and Medicare Protection Act) would have created a Center for Comparative Effectiveness under AHRQ. Funding for this center would begin with $300 million from 2008 to 2010 and $375 million per year thereafter. The measure would have created a Comparative Effectiveness Research Trust Fund, fed initially by transfers from the Medicare Trust Funds and over time by a tax on health insurance companies. The CBO projected that the CER provisions contained in CHAMP would reduce total health care spending by half a billion dollars over the 2008–12 period and by about six billion over the 2008–17 period.[80] The projected savings were modest because the CBO assumed that for larger savings the results of studies would "ultimately have to change the behavior of doctors and patients," which, in turn, would require actions by Medicare and private insurers to incorporate comparative effectiveness information in some combination of coverage and payment policies. The CBO thought none of this would be easy.[81] Still, advocates were pleased that the CBO had given CER a "score"—it could save money.[82] But the CHAMP bill did not become law, owing to conflict within Congress, and between Congress and President Bush, over the cost of the children's health program expansion.

DECLINING GOP SUPPORT FOR CER IN CONGRESS

While the incorporation of the Allen-Emerson proposal into the House-passed CHAMP bill might appear to have signaled growing support for CER on the Hill, the proposal would almost certainly not have passed as a stand-alone measure. Indeed, the number of cosponsors of the Allen-Emerson bill *declined* from 15 in 2003 to 7 in 2006 and 5 in 2007. This is not the pattern one expects to see when a clear perception emerges on the Hill that a policy idea's "time has come." By 2007, only one House Republican (Emerson) remained as a cosponsor of the legislation.

The immediate cause of the decline in the number of cosponsors was changes in the composition of Congress. Some of the Republicans who had previously sponsored CER bills retired or lost reelection, and more conservative members who were resistant to any new federal spending initiative replaced them. According to our sources, however, pharmaceutical industry opposition also contributed to the erosion of legislative support. Industry lobbyists had been taken by surprise when CER funding was tucked into the MMA and recognized it needed to become more active on the issue. While PhRMA was unwilling to oppose calls for better information on the comparative effectiveness of drugs, industry leaders wanted to broaden the scope of any CER effort so that the full range of treatments options, not just drugs, were evaluated.[83] They also "wanted CER to focus solely on clinical issues and not at all on cost effectiveness, and resisted any use of so-called quality-adjusted life year (QALY) indices that measure the value of therapies and devices according to expected life years."[84]

———

By late 2008, CER was at a legislative crossroads. The Washington community of health policy experts, including economists associated with both political parties, was solidly behind the idea. The CBO report connected the problem of inadequate research on the effects of treatment options to widely shared concerns about the budget and wasteful and excessive health care spending. In the Senate, Finance Committee chair Max Baucus (D-MT) and Budget Committee chairman Kent Conrad (D-ND) jointly introduced legislation (S 3408) to create a nonprofit entity to direct up to $300 million a year in federal funding for CER. The money would come from general revenues, the Medicare Trust Fund, and fees on private insurance firms.[85]

This constituted progress for CER, yet the effort to win bipartisan support for the idea of better research on medical treatments had stalled on the Hill. Only a handful of members, all of them Democrats, showed a serious interest in the issue by late 2008. There was no major lobbying campaign to raise awareness of the problems of waste and uneven quality in health care, to cultivate an enlightened public opinion, or to explain to ordinary Americans how they would benefit from better research on treatment options. Advocates were playing an inside-the-beltway game, but only a handful of members and policy wonks were participating. The ground was clearly not prepared for legislative action that would bring both parties and the general public along when the Obama administration made investment in CER one of its health reform priorities after the 2008 election. Any remaining chance to build a bipartisan coalition for CER then collapsed entirely when the effort got caught up in the highly charged debates over the economic stimulus measure and Obamacare, as the next chapter shows.

6

Electoral Competition, Polarization, and the Breakdown of Elite-Led Social Learning

Contemporary American politics is characterized by ferocious partisan combat. While bipartisan cooperation has not disappeared entirely from the halls of Congress, many important roll call votes see nearly all Democrats on one side and nearly all Republicans on the other. There are at least two reasons for the high level of partisanship in Washington. The first is sincere ideological disagreement about the role of government. According to quantitative methods for measuring ideological placement, the distance between Democratic and Republican officeholders is much greater today than it was in the 1950s and 1960s, and the two parties have become more internally cohesive.[1] The political center has all but vanished in Congress.[2] Second, partisan conflict also reflects strategic behavior to gain electoral advantage. As political scientist Frances Lee observes, "The period since 1980 stands out as the longest sustained period of competitive balance between the parties since the Civil War. Our politics is distinctive for its narrow and switching national majorities. Nearly every recent election has held out the possibility of a shift in party control of one institution or another."[3]

In this chapter, we argue that elite polarization and a near parity of partisan competition degrades government problem solving in two ways. First, it creates incentives for politicians to transform what plausibly could be consensual "valence" issues, on which nearly all candidates and parties adopt the same stance, into contentious "position" issues, on which candidates and parties take different stances in a zero-sum competition for voter support.[4] Second, elite partisan polarization can stimulate polarization among ordinary voters. Because politically aware members of the public tend to follow the signals of their party leaders, when the parties diverge on an issue, attentive citizens often do so as well, even if the issue has little intrinsic ideological content.[5]

Taken together, these twin dynamics can undercut the processes of elite-led social learning and technocratic problem solving on which social progress to no small extent depends. We show here how these distortions played out in 2009–10, when the Obama administration moved forward with its proposal for a major investment in research on the comparative effectiveness of medical treatments, despite the lack of public buy-in for this reform project.

The Risk of Incomplete Incubation in an Era of Polarization

Writing about the politics of policy innovation, the late political scientist Nelson W. Polsby described a process of "incubation," in which advocates take up an idea, conduct research about its justifications and effects, publicize it, and slowly build acceptance for it among relevant constituencies so that the idea has strong patrons when circumstances permit it to be considered.[6] Incubated ideas often appear in party platforms decades before their formal enactment. The benefits of incubation are considerable. As Hugh Heclo writes, "The very ability to sustain the policy argument over time helps persuade people to the view that there is a real problem that will not go away until something is done. Almost unnoticed, a presumption for policy action can grow."[7]

However, not all innovations are incubated. Sometimes, when the political stars align, new ideas emerge hastily on the public agenda and their supporters find themselves in the right place at the right time.[8] It is perfectly understandable that advocates take advantage of those propitious circumstances to move their ideas forward in the legislative process, but the decision to do so is not without strategic costs.

As described in chapter 5, the incubation process for the idea of building a new CER institute was underway by the time Barack Obama won election in November 2008, but it was clearly incomplete. Policy formation and agenda setting was less the result of a mobilization of public support around the need for a more evidence-based medical system than it was the product of an insider process dominated by experts who enjoyed close access to decision makers.[9] CER was left vulnerable to the baleful influence of partisan forces when proposals to invest tax dollars in research on what works best for patients unexpectedly gained prominence on the president's domestic agenda. While CER funding initiatives did win enactment by being incorporated into two omnibus laws that congressional Democrats viewed as "must pass"—the 2009 economic stimulus measure and the Affordable Care Act—the measures became objects of ideological derision and partisan attack, undermining their technocratic image and political sustainability.

There is a fundamental dilemma at play: Nonpartisan, technocratic solutions to collective problems, grounded in scientific knowledge and neutral expertise, may lack for effective political advocates who can build a broad coalition when the proposals challenge the autonomy of esteemed professional groups, especially when public trust in government is low, as it has been in the United States since the late 1960s. This creates a strong incentive for advocates to employ "under the radar" legislative tactics in the hope that the measures can progress before the opposition can mobilize. Yet embedding these technocratic solutions within broader legislative proposals (like health insurance expansion) before the political ground has been prepared is risky. Opponents may in fact organize and exploit the issue, thus disrupting the elite-led process of social learning and undercutting the consolidation of reform.

CER IN THE 2008 PRESIDENTIAL CAMPAIGN

While bipartisan support for CER was waning on Capitol Hill, both major party nominees made CER a component of their health reform agendas in the 2008 presidential campaign—a signal that, among the small crowd of serious health policy experts who feed ideas to speech writers, medical evidence gulfs were widely regarded as a problem. The Republican nominee, John McCain, who had brought on CER expert Gail Wilensky as one of his health policy advisers, stated, "We must make public more information on treatment options and doctor records, and require transparency regarding medical outcomes, quality of care, costs, and prices. We must also facilitate the development of national standards for measuring and recording treatments and outcomes."[10] In his health care campaign platform, the Democratic nominee, Barack Obama, identified CER as "one of the keys to eliminating waste and missed opportunities" and pledged to

create "an independent institute to guide reviews and research on comparative effectiveness, so that Americans and their doctors will have accurate
and objective information to make the best decisions for their health and
well-being."[11] Several advisers close to Obama were strong CER supporters. Former senator Tom Daschle (D-SD), who would be Obama's initial
nominee to be secretary of the Department of Health and Human Services,
had published a book arguing that the United States needed to create an
independent Federal Health Board that would make coverage decisions
on the basis of scientific evidence.[12] While Daschle was forced to withdraw
his nomination owing to tax trouble, Peter Orszag picked up the mantle in
his new role as Obama's expected OMB director. By all accounts, Orszag
wanted to see CER used as a tool to curb wasteful spending. As he wrote
in an op-ed in the *New York Times*,

> Right now, health care is more evidence-free than you might think. And
> even where evidence-based clinical guidelines exist, research suggests
> that doctors follow them only about half of the time. One estimate sug-
> gests that it takes 17 years on average to incorporate new research findings
> into widespread practice. As a result, any clinical guidelines that exist
> often have limited impact.[13]

Orszag's favorite idea was to create "safe harbors," whereby doctors who
followed evidence-based best practices would be shielded from malpractice
liability.[14] It seemed likely that CER would emerge as a White House priority
regardless of who occupied the Oval Office. Given the fierce environment of
partisan conflict, the real question was whether the issue would then gain
support from lawmakers of the opposition party.

RISING GOP OPPOSITION

Any hope that CER would win the backing of congressional Republicans
after Obama's election victory quickly vanished. There are at least three
explanations for the vociferous GOP opposition to CER during the Obama
years. The first is the general claim that the modern Republican Party simply
does not believe in the use of scientific evidence to guide policy decisions,
or at least believes in science much less than does the Democratic Party. Despite recent arguments about a Republican "war on science,"[15] we are skeptical of such sweeping claims. At times, both parties can be politically opportunistic in the research they support, depending on their evolving electoral
incentives.[16] Further, as previously noted, some prominent Republicans,
including Bill Frist and John McCain, endorsed CER and evidence-based

medicine before 2009. Republican administrations have sought to promote evidence-based health policy making within the constraints of federal law. As Tom Scully, who served as administrator of the Centers for Medicare and Medicaid Services under George W. Bush, stated in 2009:

> I have always been a big fan of comparative effectiveness research if done correctly. . . . There's a lot of fear from some people that it's going to stifle innovation of drugs and devices and other things and I just don't [think] that's correct. . . . I like Senator [Jon] Kyl [who was then voicing strong opposition to the Obama administration's CER agenda], he's a very big free market guy, he's got a lot of doctors in Arizona that are very worried about this. And so, like any member of [C]ongress he tries to please constituents.[17]

Scully went on to say that the attacks of conservative pundits on CER were "just noise" and that since the Republicans are the minority party, "their job is to hurl attacks."[18]

A second argument is that GOP opposition reflected increasingly close ties to the drug and device industry. In European countries where CER and technology assessment are now part of national policy, long before that was the case, drug companies in those countries were sponsoring a lot of research in order to satisfy the growing need to demonstrate "value for money." In their review of CER in Britain, France, Australia, and Germany, Chalkidou and colleagues found that industry had adapted to the evidentiary requirements of coverage and reimbursement systems in Europe.

> CER entities create a more secure environment in which the naturally risk-averse medical technology industry can make its investment choices. The reason is that well-defined and consistent CER is a much more rational and predictable way for payers to make purchasing decisions than for administrators to impose price cuts arbitrarily, to shift costs to individual patients, or to ration needed technologies and services according to ability to pay.[19]

But this adaption may have been as much out of necessity as choice. In the U.S. market, the biggest payer, Medicare, has avoided supply-side technology constraints and price controls on drugs. Many firms wished to keep the U.S. market an outlier in these areas, and hence industrial opposition to CER (seen as a precursor to more far-reaching shifts in policy) in the United States was particularly intense, which then arguably translated into unusually high partisan opposition. Ian Spatz, Merck's former vice president for global health policy, stated that the view of drug companies is that CER is a "slippery slope that leads to NICE—and NICE is seen as pure evil."[20]

A final reason for the GOP's opposition—echoed in Scully's remarks—is that the GOP's turn away from CER during this period was *tactical*, a product of the electoral incentives created by partisan competition and the GOP's desire to block Obama's overall health care agenda and take back Congress. The health experts associated with the Republican Party fully grasped the magnitude of the problem and the need for a government solution—but partisan competition undermined pragmatism.

The Disruption of Elite-Led Social Learning and Problem Solving

As political scientist David R. Mayhew observes, a democratic polity can make public policy in at least three ways.[21] The first two are familiar: distributive politics, in which my district gets a road, your district gets a road, everyone's district gets a road, and partisan politics, in which my party coalition gets what the government has to give and yours pays the taxes. By contrast, "problem solving" entails an "empirically detectable mindset. Some person, or small or large set of persons, needs to frame a state of affairs as exhibiting a 'problem' and to point toward a 'solution.'"[22]

Experts play a key role in the politics of problem solving, in part because the media and politicians often take their cues from policy specialists.[23] Expert communities generate the empirical claims and general perspectives on policy issues that structure the political debate. As political scientist John Zaller has observed, when policy specialists of differing ideological orientations reach a fact-based consensus on the existence of a technical problem, this elite consensus may diffuse out to politicians and then over time to the general public.[24] This broad support in turn makes it easier for coalition leaders to build the legislative majorities necessary to overcome the veto points of the U.S. political system.

However, this idealized social learning process neglects the role of partisanship and electoral competition. When, as is the case today, American politics features intense partisan conflict and the majority party chooses (or is compelled) to "go it alone" on major legislation, the minority party will possess a strong incentive to discredit the empirical claims offered by the other party—even if working from a common set of technical understandings of a problem would be in the national interest. As even sound evidentiary claims are contested owing to partisan conflict, an expert consensus on the seriousness of a given problem may then fail to unify political elites and the public around a course of action. The parties may take opposing stances on the role of government in a particular policy area—even when there is no underlying ideological disagreement between them.[25]

We argue below that this is what happened during 2009–10: CER became an issue "owned"[26] by the Democrats and associated with negative images such as "rationing" and "death panels." A new research agency was established, but the national conversation about the benefits of evidence-based medicine took a giant step backward, at least for a time.[27]

THE RECOVERY ACT DEBATE

The Obama administration's first major push on CER came in the 2009 American Recovery and Reinvestment Act, which included $1.1 billion for CER to be spent by the NIH, AHRQ, and the Office of the Secretary of Health and Human Services.[28] The act also created an advisory board mostly made up of clinicians, the Federal Coordinating Council for Comparative Effectiveness Research, to steer the research effort. As political scientists James G. Gimpel, Frances E. Lee, and Rebecca U. Thorpe argue, the advertised purpose of the $787 billion legislation was to promote economic recovery, but the measure "became a vehicle for a broad array of other policy goals" important to the administration and congressional leaders who "took advantage of an especially wide-open window of opportunity."[29] Among these policy goals was promoting CER.

In the context of the $2 trillion the nation spends each year on health care, $1.1 billion for research on what medical interventions work best is a small investment. Since the idea had been supported by the McCain campaign, one might have expected the Obama administration's CER initiative to have won bipartisan support.[30] But that is not what happened. Republicans used the battle over the Recovery Act as an opportunity to rehearse their arguments against what they knew would be a major drive by the Obama administration to restructure the nation's overall health care system. The Obama administration's health reform agenda—which featured redistribution, tax increases, and an expansion of the welfare state—was bound to be opposed by conservatives on both policy and political grounds. As mentioned earlier, a Republican committee staff member told us that conservatives attacked CER, even though they knew it would advance their long-standing goal to curb wasteful health care spending, because they viewed the battle over national health reform as a "knife fight, and in a knife fight, you don't stop in the middle to tell your opponent, 'Hey, I like your shirt.'"[31] As political scientist Morris Fiorina writes, in an era in which party elites are highly polarized, "[p]olicies are proposed and opposed relatively more on the basis of ideology and the demands of the base and relatively less on the basis of their likelihood of solving problems."[32]

Pharmaceutical and medical device companies viewed the Obama administration's support for a major investment in CER with suspicion, seeing it as the first step toward tighter governmental control over medical service payment decisions. "There was a real fear about the government saying: We know what's best, that drug's too expensive, you can't have it," said former Democratic congressional leader Tony Coehlo.[33] Coehlo, who has epilepsy, was chosen to head the Partnership to Improve Patient Care (PIPC). Funded by pharmaceutical, device, and biotechnology companies, PIPC emerged in 2008 as the medical product industry's watchdog on federal CER efforts.[34] Former Republican congressman Billy Tauzin, president of PhRMA, explained that his industry's mobilization against the CER funding in the Recovery Act was a signal to politicians to be careful about embracing more ambitious policy reforms. "I hope it is a clear warning," Tauzin said. "There are a lot of beehives out there. You don't just go around punching them."[35]

Allegations that Democrats wanted to use studies of treatment effects to reduce wasteful spending were supported by language in a House Appropriations Committee draft report stating:

> By knowing what works best and presenting the information more broadly to patients and health care professionals, those items, procedures, and interventions that are most effective to prevent, control, and treat health conditions will be utilized, while those that are found to be less effective and in some cases, more expensive, will no longer be prescribed.[36]

One could interpret this statement as having no clear implication for overall health care investment, but it was widely read by those hostile to CER as a signal that the Obama administration wanted to use CER as a tool to ration care.[37] Representative Tom Price (R-GA), a physician—who would later be secretary of the Department of Health and Human Services in the Donald Trump administration—sent out an alert through the Republican Study Committee stating that that purpose of the CER measure was to grant Tom Daschle, Obama's nominee for secretary of HHS, "his wish of a permanent government rationing board prescribing care in place of doctors and patients."[38] Former New York lieutenant governor Betsy Mc-Caughey warned on Bloomberg.com that the elderly would be hardest hit, and that the government would use electronic medical records to monitor the behavior of physicians, punishing those that did not comply with the government's clinical practice guidelines.[39] Rush Limbaugh then disseminated the rationing charge on his national radio show.[40] The final version of the stimulus legislation took out the House report language about less effective, more expensive treatments not receiving coverage, and instead referenced the Medicare Modernization Act, which focused on clinical outcomes, not cost.[41] The conference report also stated that "the conferees do not intend for the comparative effectiveness research funding . . . to be used to mandate coverage, reimbursement, or other policies for any public or private payer."[42]

The partisan controversy over the CER language in the stimulus bill greatly raised the issue's public visibility. In 2008, U.S. newspapers and wires ran only 249 articles that mentioned CER and health care or medicine. The following year, the number of such articles increased sixfold to 1,497. Twenty-two percent of the articles published about CER in 2009 mentioned "rationing," the frame that Republcans strategically deployed to tap into the public's long-standing unease with service restricitons and perceived interference with the doctor-patient relationship.[43]

THE AFFORDABLE CARE ACT DEBATE

Despite the controversy over the stimulus act, the Obama administration endorsed an even greater federal role in CER in health reform legislation.[44] By all accounts, President Obama himself believed in CER and the need for stronger evidence about what works. In an interview with the *New York Times*, President Obama explained,

> When Peter Orszag and I talk about the importance of using comparative-effectiveness studies as a way of reining in costs, that's not an attempt to micromanage the doctor-patient relationship. It is an attempt to say to patients, you know what, we've looked at some objective studies out here, people who know about this stuff, concluding that the blue pill, which costs half as much as the red pill, is just as effective, and you might want to go ahead and get the blue one. And if a provider is pushing the red one on you, then you should at least ask some important questions.[45]

While Obama attempted to persuade people that implementing evidence-based medicine is common sense, the controversy over CER continued. Indeed, the backlash over the issue got so harsh that White House chief of staff Rahm Emanuel argued within the White House for abandoning the effort.[46]

Ultimately, the authority and funding for the Patient-Centered Outcomes Research Institute made it into the Affordable Care Act, but not before key concessions were made.

By the summer of 2009, committees in both the House and the Senate were developing CER proposals as part of health reform legislation. The key issues were whether a new agency should be created within or outside government, how it should be funded, and what role it should play in coverage decisions. The House (as well as the Senate Health, Education, Labor, and Pensions Committee, HELP) sought to create a government-based entity within the AHRQ. In contrast, Senator Mike Enzi (R-WY) was an outspoken critic of the HELP bill. He compared the entity to NICE and raised fears that lodging it inside government would lead to rationing.[47]

Whether CER would even remain a feature of health reform legislation was tested during the summer of 2009, when members of Congress returned to their districts for contentious town hall meetings. To an angry, wary, and confused public, CER was of a piece with two other controversial health reform proposals then under consideration: voluntary counseling for Medicare patients about their options for end-of-life care, and the creation of a commission (the Independent Payment Advisory Board) with the mission to achieve savings in Medicare if the program's spending growth was forecast to exceed target levels, but without affecting coverage or cutting benefits. With prompting from opponents, including 2008 GOP vice presidential nominee Sarah Palin and others, these three elements combined in the public mind to give birth to the charge that Obama was seeking to slash Medicare benefits by creating "death panels" for seniors. At one town hall meeting, Senator Charles Grassley (R-IA) stated, "We should not have a government program that determines if you're going to pull the plug on grandma."[48]

After the summer recess, Senate Finance Committee chair Max Baucus (D-MT) proposed the concept of an independent entity, the Patient-Centered Outcomes Research Institute (PCORI). While the institute's name ("patient-centered") and location outside government were intended to allay medical products industry concerns, the proposal remained controversial. Republicans introduced amendments "that would strip out funding for the research institute, eliminate any consideration of cost in the research, and prohibit research results from being used to make coverage decisions or to deny coverage."[49] The Senate Finance Committee sought to strike a balance between addressing the concerns of critics who claimed that the Senate finance bill gave the industry too much influence over the research, and others who remained concerned that the institute would ration care.[50]

In the midst of this controversy over CER, the Obama administration felt compelled to distance itself from new guidelines for breast cancer screening, contained in an awkwardly timed report of the U.S. Preventive Services Task Force. A Pew survey found that 68 percent of people who followed the news about the change in these guidelines very or fairly closely disagreed with the task force's recommendation that most women should not start routine screening until age 50.[51] The Obama administration responded to the public outcry against the change by promising that government insurance programs would continue to cover mammograms for women starting at age 40.[52]

Congressional leaders anticipated a conference committee to resolve differences with the Senate, and some staffers expected that the final version would move closer to the House vision of a less industry-influenced CER-agency located inside government.[53] However, Republicans took control of the upper chamber following Scott Brown's surprising victory to fill the Senate seat vacated by Ted Kennedy's death. To avoid a conference committee and the risk of a filibuster, House Democrats passed the Senate bill, and Baucus's PCORI design prevailed.

As signed into law by President Obama, the ACA established a nongovernmental, "Patient-Centered Outcomes Research Institute."

> The purpose of the Institute is to assist patients, clinicians, purchasers, and policy-makers in making informed health decisions by advancing the quality and relevance of evidence concerning the manner in which diseases, disorders, and other health conditions can effectively and appropriately be prevented, diagnosed, treated, monitored, and managed through research and evidence synthesis . . .[54]

The creation of PCORI was a significant victory in the multidecade effort to improve the evidence base of American medicine, yet the institute's financing, design, and mission reflect legislative compromises designed to protect the entity's independence but also circumscribe its role. To fund PCORI, the ACA created a federal trust fund, fed by annual appropriations, funds transferred from the Medicare trust fund, plus annual $1 fees (rising to $2 in fiscal year 2014) per individual assessed on private health insurance and self-insured plans. Total funding was estimated to reach $650 million annually by 2015. However, PCORI's authorization expires in 2019, leaving the institute only a few years "in which to produce timely, practice-changing results that will build public support for comparative effectiveness research."[55] The legislation also gave the institute less authority than CER entities in other advanced nations. While nothing in the law *prevents* Medicare officials (or private insurers) from using CER research to inform coverage decisions, nothing requires it: PCORI's findings may "not be construed as mandates for practice guidelines, coverage recommendations, payment or policy recommendations."[56] To avoid any resemblance to NICE, PCORI was barred from using a dollars per quality-adjusted life year metric as a threshold for establishing cost-effectiveness.[57]

Ultimately, PhRMA managed to win enough concessions, including representation of three medical products industry seats on PCORI's board of governors, that the trade group came out in support of PCORI. Richard Smith, PhRMA's senior vice president, stated:

> By including the full range of stakeholders in its governance, by defining the scope of research to include the full range of treatment options and the organization, delivery, and management of care, the institute is charting a different, more positive course than agencies in other countries which focus on cost-effectiveness and impose centralized restrictions on access to care.[58]

The CEO of the Advanced Medical Technology Association (AdvaMed) also supported the legislation. He applauded the commitment that PCORI "does not make coverage decisions" and that the studies would not include coverage recommendations or include practice guidelines.[59] The medical profession was not highly visible during this debate. Most medical societies were focused on Medicare reimbursement rates ("the doc fix") and did not provide much input into the shaping of the legislation.[60]

As important as what the ACA accomplishes are the more ambitious changes that it leaves out. The legislation failed to modify Medicare's obligation to cover all "reasonable and necessary" medical services.[61] Peter Orszag's proposal to shield doctors from malpractice suits if they follow evidence-based guidelines made it into the law only as a small pilot program. In sum, while Republican and industry opposition failed to kill CER, the reform project narrowed and lost its pragmatic, technocratic character. No longer a "valence" issue on which Democrats and Republicans could publicly agree (if not necessarily act), CER became a divisive "position" issue on which there were different ideological preferences, based on people's views of the Obama administration's overall domestic agenda.[62] Advocates managed to win support for CER by incorporating language into omnibus bills that congressional Democrats regarded as "must pass" legislation, but the decision-making process reflected (and amplified) partisan conflict and arguably did not lay the foundation for a durable reconfiguration of the use of evidence in the medical system.

Elite Polarization and the Leadership of Public Opinion

As we argued above, elite partisan polarization not only weakens the incentives for pragmatic problem solving in a legislature; it distorts the process by which ordinary citizens learn what and how to think about novel public policy issues.[63] In the U.S. political system, a citizen's political identity (how the citizen thinks of him- or herself) frequently (not always) means a partisan identity.[64] Attentive citizens who follow public affairs typically ask themselves, "What do Democrats (Republicans) like myself think about this issue?" Frequently, the answer is readily apparent: Republicans stand for lower taxes, and Democrats support a more generous safety net, and so on. But when new issues emerge on the agenda, especially those characterized by scientific or technological complexity, the "appropriate" partisan response may not be self-evident. Under these circumstances, partisan identifiers may not initially all share the same views until opinion leaders clarify the "party line." As Levendusky argues, "When elites are polarized, they send voters clearer signals about where they stand on the issues of the day. . . . As voters follow these party cues on multiple issues, they begin to hold more consistent attitudes."[65] This is largely a top-down process, one in which citizens tend to "follow the leader."[66] As Fiorina and Abrams write, "The more visible and active members of a party, especially its elected officials and party activists, sort first and provide cues to voters that party positions are evolving."[67]

Issue publics are not always partisan, but this party-sorting dynamic has clearly shaped the evolution of public attitudes on key topics. Consider opinion on the environment and climate change.[68] Historically, there were only modest partisan differences among the general public in support for environmental protection. Between the 1970s and 1990s, for example, "support for increased spending on environmental protection by self-identified Democrats was typically only around 10 points higher than for self-identified Republicans."[69] But, "[t]he gap began to widen in the late 1990s, likely reflecting voters' tendency to follow cues from party leaders and political pundits."[70] While Richard Nixon had created the Environmental Protection Agency and signed landmark clean air legislation, Ronald Reagan's administration sought to scale back environmental regulations. The polarization of public opinion has been even more pronounced with respect to climate

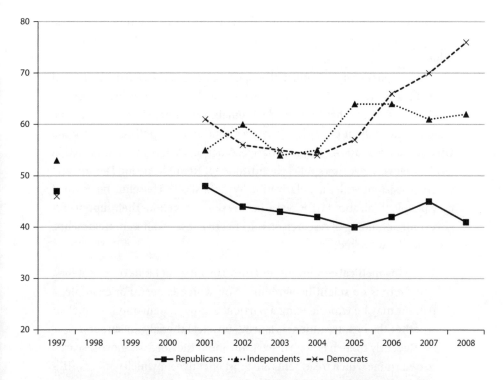

FIGURE 6.1. Percentage of respondents saying the effects of global warming have already begun, by respondent party identification. *Note*: Figure displays the percentage of respondents who said "they have already begun" in response to question "Which of the following statements reflects your view of when the effects of global warming will begin to happen: [rotated: they have already begun to happen; they will start happening within a few years; they will start happening within your lifetime; they will not happen within your lifetime but they will affect future generations; they will never happen]?" From 2001–8, surveys took place in March of each year; 1997 survey was conducted in November. Question was not asked on Gallup surveys 1998–2000. *Source*: Gallup polling data. See Riley E. Dunlap, 2008, "Climate-Change Views: Republican-Democratic Gaps Expand," May 29, http://www.gallup.com/poll/107569/climatechange-views-republicandemocratic-gaps-expand.aspx.

change. According to Gallup polling data, in 1997 nearly identical percentages of Republicans and Democrats said that the effects of global warming were already happening. However, as Republican politicians and pundits began questioning the science behind climate change, while Democratic politicians and environmental activists made belief in climate change a litmus test, a partisan divide among the public began to emerge. As figure 6.1 shows, by 2008, Democrats were 35 percentage points more likely than Republicans (76 percent versus 41 percent) to say the effects of global warming had already begun to occur, with Independents falling in between the two.

This finding of growing partisan (and ideological) polarization on climate change among the public persists in a multivariate analysis that controls for other relevant variables.[71]

What about public opinion with respect to evidence-based medicine and CER? Ideally, we would like to have over-time data to examine whether any partisan differences have changed or remain the same. Unfortunately, the issue was not salient enough to receive attention from pollsters before the Obama administration's major initiative. A national survey we conducted in 2010, however, reveals a split in the attitudes of Republican and Democratic voters consistent with the polarization hypothesis. As a baseline measure of how people think about CER, we asked respondents about their support for government funding of research on the effectiveness of different treatments. Specifically, we asked:

> For many medical conditions, doctors use different kinds of treatments, and there is no scientific agreement on which is best. For example, a patient may be experiencing a particular type of pain and it is unclear whether the best treatment is a drug, physical therapy, or surgery.
>
> Recently there has been discussion about the need for more research to determine which treatments are most effective for which patients. This is sometimes called comparative effectiveness research.
>
> Would you support or oppose government funding of research on the effectiveness of different medical treatments?

Respondents were asked to choose a point on a sliding scale where the far left read "strongly oppose" (scored as 0) and the far right read "strongly support" (scored as 100). The mean rating for the sample was 61.9, suggesting that, on average, people were slightly more supportive of CER than they were in opposition. There were, however, significant differences in support levels across important demographic and political groups. These differences are displayed in table 6.1.[72]

There were important differences among demographic groups. Blacks (68.1) and Hispanics (67.7) were more supportive of government funding of CER than whites (60.0), respondents with a college degree or higher level of education were more supportive (65.3) than those with a high school education or less (59.9), and respondents aged 18–37 were more supportive (66.3) than those aged 65 and over (55.8).[73] There was not a statistically significant difference between men and women or across income groups.

The most important factor in explaining support for CER, however, was partisanship. Although evidence-based medicine might seem to be a technocratic issue that should generate bipartisan support, consistent with our discussion in the previous sections concerning elite polarization, there were substantial differences between Democrats and Republicans in the mass public. Democratic Party identifiers were more supportive of government funding of CER (70.9) than Independents (59.8), who, in turn, were more supportive than Republicans (50.7). Significantly, these partisan differences hold only for respondents who reported voting in the 2008 election. Among those who voted in 2008, support for government funding of CER was 72.0, 59.1, and 49.8 among Democrats, Independents, and Republicans, respectively. Among those who did not vote, however, there was not a large or statistically significant difference in support across Democrats (63.9), Independents (61.4), and Republicans (59.8). During the debate over the stimulus bill and President Obama's health reform proposal, evidence-based medicine evolved from a technocratic issue into a partisan issue. The two parties took opposing stances on the federal government's role in CER, which may have led to the significant partisan split among the most attentive (voting) citizens.

We conducted a follow-up survey in 2014 to see if these partisan differences persisted.[74] We asked the same question we did in 2010, but with one wrinkle. Although the first two paragraphs of the question were identical to the question we asked in 2010, half of the respondents in 2014 were randomly assigned to receive some text that made an explicit link between CER and Obamacare. Specifically, respondents assigned to this Obamacare "treatment" condition received the following text:

> Obamacare (the Affordable Care Act) includes increased funding for comparative effectiveness research. Do you support or oppose government funding of research on the effectiveness of different medical treatments?

The other half of the respondents simply received the following, "control" condition text:

> Do you support or oppose government funding of research on the effectiveness of different medical treatments?

This design allows us to address two important questions. First, did overall public opinion on CER shift between 2010 and 2014? Second, does making an explicit partisan link to Obamacare exacerbate partisan differences on this issue?

As in 2010, respondents were asked to choose a point on a (0–100) sliding scale where the far left (0) indicated strong opposition and the

TABLE 6.1. Americans' Support for Government Funding of Comparative Effectiveness Research, 2010

		Support for CER[a]	p-value[b]
Overall		61.9	N/A
Voted in 2008	No	61.9	>.10
	Yes	61.9	
Party ID	Dem	70.9	<.01
	Rep	50.7	
	Ind	59.8	
Party ID (Voted in 2008)	Dem	72.0	<.01
	Rep	49.8	
	Ind	59.1	
Party ID (Did Not Vote in 2008)	Dem	63.9	>.10
	Rep	59.8	
	Ind	61.4	
Age	18–37	66.3	<.01
	38–51	60.2	
	52–64	61.0	
	65+	55.8	
Education	High school or less	59.9	<.01
	Some college	62.3	
	4-year college degree or higher	65.3	
Race	White	60.0	<.01
	Black	68.1	
	Hispanic	67.7	
Income	Less than $30,000 per year	61.9	>.10
	$30,000–60,000 per year	61.8	
	More than $60,000 per year	63.3	
Gender	Male	61.4	>.10
	Female	62.5	

Note: N=2,017. [a]Responses range from strongly oppose (0) to strongly support (100) CER and are weighted sample means. [b]p-values are from tests of whether support varied across groups. *Source*: May 21–24, 2010, YouGov/Polimetrix survey. A version of this table was originally published by Project HOPE/*Health Affairs* as exhibit 1 in Alan S. Gerber, Eric M. Patashnik, David Doherty, and Conor M. Dowling. 2010. "The Public Wants Information, Not Board Mandates, from Comparative Effectiveness Research." *Health Affairs* (Millwood) 29 (10): 1872–81. The published article is archived and available online at www.healthaffairs.org.

far right (100) indicated strong support. The mean rating for the sample was 60.2 (very close to the mean rating in 2010 of 61.9), suggesting that the American public overall remained moderately supportive of CER in fall 2014. Moreover, among the public as a whole, there was no significant difference between the two question wordings. The average rating for respondents who received the Obamacare language was 60.0, and it was 60.4

TABLE 6.2. Americans' Support for Government Funding of Comparative Effectiveness Research, by Respondent Party Identification and Obamacare Cue, 2014

	Obamacare Cue			No Obamacare Cue		
	All Respondents	Voted in 2012	Did Not Vote in 2012	All Respondents	Voted in 2012	Did Not Vote in 2012
Democrats	72.9 (1.73)	74.0 (2.02)	70.0 (3.44)	66.7 (1.74)	69.2 (1.79)	63.5 (4.38)
Independents	60.1 (2.76)	56.3 (4.46)	62.5 (3.52)	54.7 (2.54)	49.9 (4.64)	57.3 (2.83)
Republicans	45.0 (2.38)	41.6 (2.47)	60.0 (6.92)	53.7 (2.01)	53.6 (2.27)	53.7 (4.09)

Note: $N=802$. Cell entries are weighted means with standard errors in parentheses. Higher numbers represent more support for CER on 0–100 scale. For the entire sample, overall mean rating is 60.2, and for the Obamacare Cue and No Obamacare Cue conditions it is 60.0 and 60.4, respectively. Obamacare Cue: "Obamacare (the Affordable Care Act) includes increased funding for comparative effectiveness research. Do you support or oppose government funding of research on the effectiveness of different medical treatments?" No Obamacare Cue: "Do you support or oppose government funding of research on the effectiveness of different medical treatments?" "Independents" include any respondent that did not identify with one of the two major parties, including those who responded "not sure." *Source*: Alan S. Gerber, Cooperative Congressional Election Study, 2014. Yale University Content. [Computer File] Release: February 2015. New Haven, CT. [producer] http://cces.gov.harvard.edu.

for those that received the standard (control) language in which Obamacare was not mentioned.

There were, however, large and statistically significant differences in support levels across partisan groups, differences that were exacerbated by the Obamacare language. We display these differences in table 6.2. Focusing initially on respondents who did not receive the Obamacare language, and are therefore most comparable to the sample of our 2010 survey, support for government funding of CER was 66.7, 54.7, and 53.7 among Democrats, Independents, and Republicans, respectively. This 13-point gap between Democrats and Republicans is smaller than the 20-point gap we observed in 2010, but still quite substantial. As was the case in 2010, these differences are larger among voters. However, the difference is not as stark as it was in 2010. Specifically, there is a 16-point gap in 2014 between Democrats and Republicans among voters (69.2 v. 53.6) and a 10-point gap among nonvoters (63.5 v. 53.7). Thus, it appears that polarization of opinion on CER may have followed a diffusion process—from party elites and opinion leaders in 2009 to voters by 2010 to party identifiers among the general public by 2014.[75]

When explicit reference is made to Obamacare, partisan differences become even sharper. As table 6.2 shows, Democrats and Republicans move in opposite directions when CER is explicitly linked to Obama's health reform law. Democrats become more supportive of CER, whereas Republicans become less supportive. The average rating among Democrats is 72.9 (up from

66.7 in the "control" condition, a 9 percent increase).[76] Among Republicans, the average rating is 45.0 (down from 53.7 in the "control" condition, a 16 percent decrease).[77] In short, a 13-point gap between Democrats and Republicans in terms of their support for CER when no reference to Obamacare is made more than doubles to a gap of nearly 28 points when Obamacare is referenced. This simple partisan cue experiment thus illustrates the extent to which public opinion on even technocratic issues like CER can become highly polarized when the issues are deliberated in partisan debates by policy elites.

Summary

The Obama administration's political strategy to hitch a technocratic reform to two partisan, omnibus bills (the Economic Recovery Act and the Affordable Care Act) was both reasonable and understandable. In an area characterized by legislative stalemate and gridlock, any savvy president will look for "moving trains" on which to place agenda items. Yet there was a cost to this strategy too. While it is not easy to isolate technocratic, "good government" ideas from partisan contests over welfare state expansion and the politics of redistribution, the failure to do so can cause these solutions to become the "property" of one party and the electorally charged object of political derision for the other. The result can be to undercut efforts to cultivate an enlightened public opinion and potentially weaken the measure's long-term impact and political sustainability. The story of how CER morphed into a symbol of rationing and government interference with the doctor-patient relationship offers a cautionary lesson about the limits of elite-led problem solving in an era of intense partisan competition and heightened polarization.

Conclusion

POSTENACTMENT COALITION BUILDING (AND OTHER STRATEGIES FOR SUSTAINING REFORM IN A POLARIZED AGE)

While public investment in CER increased significantly during the Obama years, it is unclear whether this policy achievement will lead to durable improvements in the efficiency, quality, and cost-effectiveness of U.S. health care.[1] There were ample grounds for skepticism even before Donald Trump's surprising victory in the 2016 presidential election created new uncertainty over the future of U.S. health policy making. While PCORI expects to spend over three billion dollars over its first decade of operation, it faces a sunset date of September 2019. Enacted as part of an omnibus bill (the ACA) that passed without a single Republican vote, PCORI may not command the bipartisan support on Capitol Hill necessary to win reauthorization, even if the ACA survives repeal. The entity had only a few short years to prove the value of its work and develop an esteemed reputation that would lead members of Congress to conclude that supporting CER is in their electoral interests, and there is little evidence PCORI has done so. Indeed, even sympathetic observers, such as health economists who are strong advocates for CER, believe that while the agency has sometimes produced good work, some of its grants have funded low-priority research that has generated little insight into the most pressing health care questions.[2]

What makes the failure of PCORI to generate wide esteem and growing support for the broader evidence-based medicine project all the more unfortunate is that PCORI's leadership has been at pains to avoid antagonizing stakeholders. They have used their administrative discretion, not to push the envelope, but to stay well inside it. For example, while the ACA permits research that considers costs,[3] PCORI's executive director has publicly stated, "You can take it to the bank that PCORI will never do a cost-effectiveness analysis."[4] Yet this conflict-avoidance strategy plainly did not cure the "unhealthy politics" that surrounds efforts to bolster the scientific foundation and efficiency of American medicine.

From the outset, PCORI's architects recognized that consolidating political support for an expanded federal role in CER would be a daunting challenge. Memories of Congress's attacks on the Agency for Health Care Policy and Research back in the early 1990s after it had issued a report questioning the benefits of back surgery were still fresh.[5] PCORI's designers were painfully aware that any new CER entity could be similarly vulnerable. As Gail Wilensky wrote in a 2006 essay laying out the major design options for building a federal comparative effectiveness institute, "The center's findings might anger various stakeholders affected by the findings, who, in turn, could use the political process to threaten the continued existence of the agency that produces the 'threatening' material."[6] It was hoped that PCORI's design as an "independent, nonprofit, nongovernmental organization," funded out of an earmarked trust fund, would afford the agency some measure of political insulation. In view of the politicization of health policy and the massive economic stakes in debates over coverage and reimbursement decisions, however, *any* organization like PCORI will inevitably encounter political risk.

To be sure, it remains possible that technological changes, including the growing use of Electronic Medical Records and computer-assisted clinical decision support tools in hospitals and doctor offices, may help close information gaps and integrate evidence into treatment decisions in the decades ahead. However, early attempts to use these techniques and mechanisms to promote evidence-based decision making have "had poor adoption rates and hence little influence on the clinical environment."[7] In addition, without government support, there will probably still be an undersupply of research on the comparative effectiveness of treatment alternatives.

Ultimately, if the EBM project is to realize its aspirational goal to improve the quality and efficiency of U.S. medical care, it is necessary but insufficient for research agencies like PCORI to endure. In the long run, patterns of medical governance must change. There will need to be stronger mechanisms in place to promote the uptake of evidence in clinical decision making. There is no shortage of plausible reform ideas, including options that would aim to change the behavior of physicians through financial incentives (e.g., value-based payments, changes in malpractice rules to create a safe harbor for evidence-based decision making) or nonfinancial educational strategies (e.g., the "academic detailing" approach to continuing medical education, in which noncommercial, evidence-based information about drugs is provided to doctors) as well as options that would aim to empower patients (e.g., through shared decision making).[8] Strategies to reduce the delivery of low-value care will require sensitivity to the public anxieties and concerns about rationing and interference with the doctor-patient relationship identified in our public opinion surveys. As Mark Schlesinger and Rachel Grob observe, building robust public support for measures to reduce low-value care may require "shifting the focus from particular tests and treatments to emphasize, instead, the potential for better communication and more personalized attention if clinicians spend more time talking and less time testing."[9]

No matter what approaches are tried, it will be critical for advocates to evaluate the effectiveness of particular strategies through randomized controlled trials or other rigorous methods. One notable randomized controlled trial found that a multifaceted package of educational interventions aimed at making the care of back pain more evidence-based produced a significant, but relatively small (9 percent) reduction in the rate of low-back surgery although it is unclear if these effects endured beyond the 30-month study period.[10] The evaluation of the long-term impact of interventions to promote the uptake of evidence and curb overtreatment and unwarranted variation should be a priority of the research community.

Government also has a vital role to play. PCORI (or whatever entity succeeds it) must develop a reputation among key stakeholders for competence, relevance, and impact that causes policy makers to conclude that supporting EBM is in their own political interest. Improving the effectiveness, quality, and affordability of medicine in the United States will thus require *more* politics, not less.[11]

Rather than relying on procedural independence and conflict avoidance as the keys to consolidating and deepening support for EBM, we argue here that a more promising approach is to recognize that any worthy reform project must seek to curb the use of low-value treatments and therefore must seek to change how the health care system works. History suggests that the most resilient domestic policy reforms do not leave a light footprint;

instead, they reconfigure the political dynamic.[12] Accordingly, the task is less to insulate a CER entity from politics, although obviously researchers must be shielded from improper interference. *Rather, the aim is to build a robust base of support so that future policy makers will possess an incentive to sustain and deepen the project over time.*

How can countervailing pressures to improve the quality and efficiency of the U.S. health care sector be unleashed? In this concluding chapter, we draw on lessons from the literature on U.S. state building to develop strategies to load the dice in favor of the political sustainability and success of the EBM project, including postenactment coalition building, agency reputation building, and lateral network building and strategic partnerships. As a preface to this discussion, we briefly review the challenges of political sustainability that face any new agency or policy.

Why the Political Sustainability of Agencies and Policies Cannot Be Taken for Granted

Given how difficult it is to revise an existing law, it might seem that the durability of an agency or program is assured once Congress establishes it. In his 1976 book *Are Government Organizations Immortal?*, political scientist Herbert Kaufman argued that "government activities tend to go on indefinitely."[13] More recent empirical research shows, however, that policy constructions—including agencies, statutes, and programs—are regularly subject to modification and even elimination. According to one study, a federal program has a 1 percent chance of death *every year* in its first 10 years of life, after which the probability of termination slowly begins to decline.[14] New policies are trial and error affairs; they do not always pan out. New policies can be killed. An example is the Medicare Catastrophic Coverage Act of 1988, which Congress terminated when seniors soured on the measure.

What is true of policies and programs is also true of bureaucracies. In 1972, Congress established the Office of Technology Assessment (OTA) to give members expert advice on a wide range of scientific issues, including the use of medical technologies. When Republicans were searching for agencies to cut to reduce the budget deficit during the mid-1990s, the OTA found itself on the chopping block. Not only did the OTA lack for powerful defenders, but some of its health technology assessment reports had antagonized organized medicine and the drug and device industries.[15]

In sum, the process of consolidating support for a new policy or agency— especially ones with general-interest purposes—can be more challenging than winning their enactment in the first place.[16] A crucial issue is political sustainability: whether a public policy or bureau possesses the capacity to maintain its integrity and use its core principles to guide its course amid inevitable political pressure for change.[17] Many factors clearly shape whether a new construction will "take." Here we focus on four: *the level of support it has at enactment, institutional design, the generation of self-reinforcing policy feedback, and the creative destructiveness of market forces.* We first briefly describe these factors and then evaluate how the Obama administration's CER project stacks up.

Commitment at enactment. Some new policies or agencies enjoy overwhelming support at inception; others pass narrowly in the teeth of intense opposition. There is risk in building "minimum winning coalitions." Political scientists Forrest Maltzman and Charles Shipan have shown that the greater the roll call opposition when a law is passed, the more likely the law is to be amended by a future Congress.[18] A key question is whether *partisanship* exacerbates the problem of divisive enactment. There are good reasons to believe it might. As David Mayhew argues, a cross party opposition to a policy might fade, but "[a] party that loses on a congressional issue and stays angry may have an incentive to keep the conflict going."[19]

Political institutions. Policies (and agencies) become more durable, all else being equal, when they destroy the structural bases of support of their opponents, shift decision-making control to venues in which intended beneficiaries are advantaged, and significantly alter governing capacities, such as by enlarging administrative staffs who possess the technical expertise to implement policies in an effective manner.

Policy feedback. Public policies are not merely the products of politics, but also causes. Policies shape the material resources, civic engagement, and incentives of voters and interest groups and, in so doing, affect governing possibilities going forward.[20] Policies may generate increasing returns and path dependence, raising the cost of subsequent policy change. Constituency groups may adapt to existing policies, "get stuck in their adaptations," and then engage in politics to protect their adaptations.[21] For example, the AMA opposed Medicare's creation in 1965, yet once the program was up and running, physicians began aligning their practice plans to Medicare's coverage policies and fee schedules. Over time, Medicare's enormous resource flows even began to shape decisions about what areas of medicine doctors choose to specialize in.[22] Policy feedbacks may also influence the behavior of interest groups. When Social Security was created in 1935, for example, the American Association of Retired Persons did not exist. Rather than senior mass-membership groups pushing for the enactment of Social Security, Social Security's growth transformed seniors into the most active and best organized participatory age group in the country, providing them resources and enhancing their sense of political efficacy.[23] Finally, durable policy reforms also recast institutions and upset existing power monopolies; they establish new norms and expectations; they eliminate or reduce the organizational cohesion of coalitions opposed to reform; and most importantly they create new vested interests and stimulate investments whose value is tied to the reforms being maintained. When reforms accomplish these things, officeholders find it impossible or unattractive to reverse course.[24]

Yet the generation of self-reinforcing policy feedback is not automatic; many public policies have negative or nonexistent feedback effects, increasing their vulnerability to downstream erosion.[25] Feedback effects may be weak when policies offer broadly dispersed benefits to the public as a whole.[26] The low per capita stakes give ordinary citizens little incentive to mobilize if the reform is challenged by groups who would profit from the measure's unraveling.

The Tax Reform Act of 1986 illustrates how general-interest reforms can fail to remake politics. A landmark reform, the TRA closed many special interest tax loopholes over the opposition of the oil industry, realtors, and other formidable clientele groups. The act had bipartisan support in Congress and the strong backing of President Ronald Reagan. Nevertheless, no interest group emerged to defend the reform against the (inevitable) postenactment efforts of politicians and lobbyists to reverse course and reclaim the tax code as a vehicle for particularistic favor provision. The per capita benefits of base broadening were too meager to activate civic participation. As a result of this imbalance of political forces, the reform crumbled. Congress began creating new tax breaks almost as soon as the ink on the 1986 law was dry, and many of the achievements of the law have been lost.[27] In sum, even if reformers manage to triumph during the initial enactment battle, *they haven't really won.* Concentrated groups—such as firms or professional societies—who feel threatened by a reform are unlikely to throw in the towel just because a vote or two in Congress did not go their way; indeed, they likely will continue to enjoy organizational advantages, allowing them to reassert their influence during the postenactment phase. A reform statute is only words on paper; the real struggle to reconfigure politics has only just begun.[28]

Creative destructiveness of market forces. It is rarely the case that a reform victory will cause every politician who voted against the reform to lose in the next election; they may well return to fight another day. Although political losers can hang around as long as their constituents are willing to tolerate their losing positions, the market actors who lose market share in a postreform environment sometimes disappear. The surviving firms are the ones who adapt their business models to the new policy context.

Airline deregulation illustrates this dynamic. Beginning in the 1930s, air carriers and their unions benefited from a highly inefficient regulatory system that determined rates and routes and blocked new entry into the market. In 1978, a reform coalition, animated by public concerns about price inflation, was able to overcome the intense opposition of these groups and enact sweeping reform. Over time, the new market system drove some legacy carriers into bankruptcy. New discount carriers appeared, and business actors were compelled to invest heavily in route systems, schedule tools, and other forms of organization compatible with the new market environment. Supporting industries and suppliers (e.g., aircraft equipment suppliers, hotels, rental cars, restaurants, and corporate office parks) began to grow up around the new system. Each had a vested interest in the reform's maintenance. To be sure, there were still groups that would have preferred a heavier government role in the airline sector. However, the emergence of new carriers postreform greatly lowered the political and economic cohesion of the airline industry. While each airline would like to receive government protections, the airlines increasingly check and balance each other, since more rent for one would reduce the profit of the others. In sum, the politics of the airline sector has been thoroughly reconfigured, making it all but impossible for policy makers to reverse course.[29]

Is the Obama Administration's CER Project Sustainable?

Based on this political sustainability recipe, the Obama administration's CER project appears to lack key ingredients. First, the recovery act and the ACA both passed on narrow, party-line votes. The GOP has continued to tar CER as "rationing" and "cookie-cutter medicine."[30] In contrast to the growing willingness of the GOP to acquiesce to Medicare payments to physicians for counseling patients about their end-of-life care options[31]—another policy that was caught up in the "death panels" debate—many Republicans have continued to criticize PCORI (and the Independent Payment Advisory Board)[32] as examples of government overreach.

Second, and importantly, PCORI failed to generate new supportive interests or alter coalitional alignments. Ann C. Keller, Robin Flagg, Justin

Keller, and Suhasini Ravi at UC Berkeley School of Public Health performed an insightful study of PCORI's political strengths and vulnerabilities. Based on elite interviews, content analysis of public comments, congressional hearings, and media and Internet content about PCORI (including trade association press), the authors found that PCORI's leadership has successfully mobilized patient advocacy groups and researchers in support of the agency's mission. However, patient advocacy groups and researchers have tended to mobilize *within* rather than across disease categories, limiting their organizational cohesion and impact in broader debates over the future of CER and EBM. Few new supporters of CER have emerged.[33] Moreover, the organizational bases of support of the reform's skeptics were not destroyed; there remained plenty of opposition to PCORI from medical industry groups and members of Congress. The authors found that legislators who discussed PCORI during congressional hearings were far more likely to view the entity as having a negative regulatory impact than a positive, market-correcting one. In particular, lawmakers expressed concerns that PCORI was harming taxpayers, that the agency was not truly independent from HHS, that CER would impose a regulatory burden on the drug and device industry, and that PCORI would ration care.[34]

Third, the Obama administration's investment in CER has not brought about shifts in institutional arrangements. The project's major structural innovation was PCORI's establishment as an independent, nongovernmental entity, rather than as an office within HHS. But this design has not shielded PCORI from criticism. At the same time, efforts to require Medicare administrators to use clinical and cost-effectiveness information in coverage decisions were "rebuffed not only by the legislative staffs but by the White House healthcare policy people."[35] In sum, the establishment of PCORI did not bring about durable shifts in wider patterns of medical governance. The creation of PCORI failed to rearrange surrounding institutional authority, as it impinged only lightly on existing federal health programs and bureaucratic activities.[36]

When new policy frameworks stick, they do more than resist the pressure of actors opposed to the shifts. They induce private firms to alter their business models to comply with the new rules of the game; firms unable to do so are more likely to go broke or merge with firms more able to comply, making the new policy regime self-reinforcing.[37]

It is unclear whether the new emphasis on CER is stimulating hard-to-reverse financial investments in the medical products industry. To the extent that pharmaceutical firms and device manufacturers believe that their future profitability will *hinge* on the capacity to demonstrate that their products are superior to alternatives on comparative clinical and/or cost-effectiveness grounds, they should be investing heavily in the development and marketing of such products. As one health industry analyst writes,

> Pharmaceutical manufacturers must recognize that the drugs in the laboratory today are those that will be commercialized in 2020. They will very likely be launched into a market that demands evidence of economic and clinical value as the price of entry. Guidelines based on cost effectiveness developed by payers or providers will increasingly determine market access. Consideration of economic and clinical value must be integrated into the entire product development and commercialization process . . .[38]

However, this analyst goes on to report that the changes he recommends are "not happening quickly enough."[39] Why not? On the one hand, "private payers in the US are aggressively moving to utilize CER in their decisions regarding pricing and reimbursement."[40] For example, a large health care insurer, WellPoint, has "released its own standardized CER guidelines for use in its evaluations of drug coverage."[41] Another large insurer, United Healthcare, has suggested that CER will foster the broader use of copay structures that discourage patients from seeking higher-cost treatments that offer no real benefit over use of lower-cost drugs.[42] On the other hand, the supply of CER studies remains small, and the traditional regulatory procedures for approving new products have not been revised to make a demonstration of superior clinical or cost-effectiveness a priority. For example,

> the Food Drug and Cosmetic Act of 1938, as amended in 1962 and subsequently, does not require assessment of comparative effectiveness, and the legislative history in 1962 made it very clear that there was no relative effectiveness requirement. A new drug does not have to be better than, or even as good as, existing treatment.[43]

For a variety of reasons, including methodological concerns and turf-protection, the FDA's senior drug review officials have expressed a measure of "skepticism of CER in recent years."[44] While some movement toward greater use of CER can be seen in the decisions of both Medicaid and private insurance company administrators, Medicare's coverage and payment policies remain largely unchanged.

For now, it appears that drug companies and the medical device industry do not regard a focus on comparative effectiveness as a central reality around which to base major investment decisions. There is little reason to believe that the evolving industrial organization of the medical products industry, or the vested interests of individual firms, will serve as the guarantor of the overall EBM project's future impact and sustainability.[45]

Toward More and Better Medical Politics

In "The Political Transformation of American Medicine," Peter Swenson shows that between roughly 1870 and 1910, American medicine experienced a progressive phase in which professionals and lay activists joined forces to improve the quality, economy, and equality of health care. Their major goals were three: (1) reforming the drug industry and the marketing of its products; (2) creating a cabinet-level national health department; and (3) improving the quality of the nation's medical schools. The reformers' victories were only partial, and they made important enemies—including parts of the medical profession. Ultimately, the progressive medical reform movement got too far ahead of the rank and file, especially on issues like compulsory national health insurance. Their achievements generated a backlash that helped give rise to the medical establishment's turn toward organizational conservatism and self-protection during the 1920s. But the turn of the century was nonetheless an era of progress in medical education, hospitals, and other areas.

A key lesson from this earlier period is that improving the quality, economy, and rationality of medical care requires reformers to embrace politics.[46] Progress cannot be made without the leadership and buy-in of the medical profession, but it also cannot be made without building support among policy makers, activists, and educated voters.

Given the context of contemporary American politics, what can be done to promote medical progress and the political sustainability of CER and the overall EBM project? We offer three ideas for consolidating and deepening support—postenactment coalition building, building a reputation for competence and efficacy, and lateral network building and strategic partnerships.

POSTENACTMENT COALITION BUILDING AMONG ELECTED OFFICIALS

The first step is to recognize that the task of building support for a new line of policy making does not end when a policy is enacted; it has only just begun.

One of the ways that policies can unravel after enactment is if bureaucracies charged with implementing them shirk or otherwise fail to serve the goals of the policy's designers. An influential line of argument developed by McNollgast—the nom de plume of social scientists Mathew McCubbins, Roger Noll, and Barry Weingast[47]—suggests a solution to this problem: leaders who won the enactment battle can "stack the deck" to establish a context that endures long after the enacting coalition has frayed, ensuring that the coalitions that generated the program's adoption will also hold sway during the postenactment phase. Deck stacking can be accomplished structurally by insulating agencies from executive control and procedurally by crafting administrative rules (i.e., rules concerning what interest groups can intervene in agency decision making). These strategies can work. For example, research shows that bureaus given agency status are more durable than are bureaus subject to direct presidential control.[48]

Yet there are limits to deck stacking as a strategy for sustaining policies over time. First, the deck-stacking perspective overstates the ability of "winners" to impose their preferences on "losers," who often have the opportunity to embed some of their goals into policy designs as well. For example, opponents of efforts to use CER as a tool for cost control won language in the ACA constraining how PCORI could use QALYs in its decision making. As Terry Moe has argued, it is not only a program's strongest supporters who can seek to embed their structural preferences into agency design, but the organization's skeptics as well.[49]

Second, deck stacking is more effective as a strategy for preventing undesired policy outcomes than it is as a strategy for ensuring good government performance. As Daniel P. Carpenter agues, "designing constraints is easier than designing capacities."[50] It is one thing to prevent an agency from taking actions that an enacting coalition would have opposed, quite another to ensure that an agency has the ability to solve problems and benefit from its expertise. History suggests that the greater risk is not that a CER agency will make decisions that its original designers would not have supported, but that it will lack the capacity to catalyze reform of medical governance.

Third, the deck-stacking hypothesis is static. It fails to recognize that contexts and coalitions mutate over time, and that design-stage choices can be nullified by decisions made during the implementation phase. As William N. Eskridge and John Ferejohn argue, the deck-stacking model treats the preferences of actors as exogenous, but such preferences are also "a product of deliberation and feedback, not anterior to it."[51] From the standpoint of political sustainability, the issue is not only whether the goals of the original enacting coalition will persist, but also whether a policy causes new supportive coalitions to emerge during the postenactment phase.

But perhaps the most important limitation of the deck-stacking perspective is that it assumes the enacting coalition provided an adequate base of support. The seminal articles by McNollgast on structural politics were written during the 1980s and early 1990s. This was an era in which Democrats had a seemingly permanent majority in Congress. Many laws had bipartisan support, at least on final passage. What members of Congress feared is that their legislative creations would be undermined after enactment by presidents and bureaucrats, who often responded to different constituencies and incentives.[52] So the key challenge was to lock in the political bargain and prevent its downstream erosion.[53]

By contrast, as we have seen, lawmaking today takes place in a highly competitive, polarized environment in which bills often pass by narrow, temporary partisan majorities. The two parties compete at relative parity, meaning that a shift in party control could be only two years away.[54] These changes can have significant effects on the politics of policy development. According to a careful statistical study of more than 2,000 federal domestic programs established between 1971 and 2003, changes in the partisan composition of Congresses have a strong influence on program durability. Program life spans are shortened when the Congress that inherits a program is different in partisan terms from the Congress that created it.[55] The political sustainability challenge today is less to preserve a policy accomplishment from being undone than it is to generate a bipartisan base of support among officeholders in the first place. Only by broadening the enacting coalition can a policy be sustained in an era of polarization and electoral uncertainty. Long-range thinking remains crucial, but some of the entrenchment strategies employed in the past may no longer be quite so effective.

What can be done? Although there are no silver bullets, we suggest several ideas. First, high-level appointments to public interest purpose agencies like PCORI should be made with an eye not only to technical competence, integrity, and experience—which obviously remain important—but to the imperatives of postenactment coalition building. Strategic leaders should aim to appoint well-qualified officials who can broaden, rather than merely preserve, the agency's base of support and signal that the policies the officials will be responsible for carrying out have broad public purposes, not merely partisan goals. Richard Kronick, the distinguished former head of the highly valuable yet politically vulnerable health services research agency AHRQ, demonstrates the limits of a conventional appointment strategy. Kronick was an extraordinary well qualified expert with a stellar reputation. Yet Kronick had worked in HHS on implementation of the ACA and before that was a health policy maker in Massachusetts. As one author notes,

> That background did not bode well for bonding with the GOP majority in the House, and today Republicans control the Senate, too. Republican opposition to 'Obamacare' has often been frenzied, fanatical and unfair, but the job of an agency head, particularly at an embattled one, is to get along with those who control your budget.[56]

In 2015, House Republicans threatened to zero out AHRQ's budget.[57] In the end, the agency survived with a moderate size (about 8 percent) budget cut—but not without having to wage an exhausting campaign to avoid termination.

To be sure, presidents have long appointed a handful of cabinet officials from the other party. This personnel strategy is often used to burnish a president's reputation as "president of the whole country" rather than designed to widen support for important yet contested policy goals. Typically, presidents appoint officials from the other party to agencies that are already above the partisan fray. For example, George W. Bush appointed Democratic congressman Norman Mineta to be secretary of transportation, and Barack Obama appointed Republicans Ray LaHood and Robert Gates to be his secretary of transportation and secretary of defense, respectively. But politicians support transportation projects primarily for constituent or geographical representation reasons, and defense policy (while not uncontroversial) does not directly implicate partisan debates over the role of government in the economy.

In today's environment, in which general-interest reform projects like EBM can become politicized, it would be worth considering more strategic use of cross aisle appointments to build support among opponents. To be sure, there are limits to what even the most brilliant appointment can accomplish. The forces that generate partisan conflict over policies are rooted in both electoral incentives and fundamental value conflicts. Nonetheless, leaders make a difference.

With the benefit of hindsight, it might have been a more prudent strategy to appoint someone who would have signaled a broadening of the political base, someone like Gail Wilensky, to be the inaugural PCORI director. (We hasten to add that we do not know if Wilensky was considered or if she would have accepted if asked; furthermore, it should be noted the power to appoint the executive director belonged to the board of governors of PCORI rather than to the president or Congress.) In offering this idea, we do not intend to denigrate the person who was appointed to this role, Joe Selby, who had an ideal background if the sole requirements for the job were technical expertise, integrity, and experience. (Selby is a family physician, clinical epidemiologist, and health services researcher who was with Kaiser Permanente for three decades.) But his appointment did little to change the political image of PCORI or forge linkages to Republicans or conservative think tanks. Our claim is not that the appointment of a prominent Washington health policy veteran like Wilensky would have completely insulated PCORI from attack, merely that it would have signaled that the entity's mission draws support from health experts on both sides of the partisan aisle. Strategic appointments like this might help distance the EBM project from continuing debates over the ACA and give Republican officeholders the space to reconsider their positions on CER over time.

BUILDING A REPUTATION FOR
COMPETENCE AND EFFICACY

No public organization can be effective if it lacks the capacity to chart its own course and pursue its core mission without constant harping or second-guessing by politicians. Americans, however, have traditionally viewed bureaucratic power with skepticism, fearful that unelected administrators will shirk, trample on the liberties of citizens, or pursue illegitimate goals unsanctioned by their democratically elected principals. Hence, federal agencies are often subjected to tightly drawn rules and procedural constraints designed to keep agencies on a short leash.[58]

Some federal agencies, however, have managed to gain significant power and the capacity to leverage their authority to exercise vast influence not only over the activities of government, but on private sector actors as well. Key to gaining this organizational power is reputation. When a bureaucracy cultivates a reputation for effectively providing unique services and promoting the public welfare, it can gain the admiration of the general public and the respect of elite audiences, such as scientific and professional organizations. It then becomes costly for politicians to ignore or resist the agencies' ideas, further increasing the agencies' autonomy. The most powerful agencies exert their influence less by imposing their will on recalcitrant actors than by defining the "basic terms of debate, essential concepts of thought, learning and activity."[59]

In *Reputation and Power*, Daniel Carpenter illustrates this argument through a detailed historical study of the Food and Drug Administration.[60]

While the FDA has had a smaller budget than many other federal agencies, it nonetheless became one of the most powerful regulatory agencies in the world during the late twentieth century.[61] The FDA exercises gatekeeping authority over the U.S. pharmaceutical marketplace. It has the power to limit advertising and product claims, to determine what cures are available or unavailable to patients, and to define the very scientific concepts used by experts in the medical field. To be sure, the FDA's power has limits. Under pressure from doctors' groups, the FDA has largely steered clear of the regulation of medical practice. It has not cracked down on "off-label" usage of drugs and has generally eschewed comparative efficacy judgments, which threaten the authority of the medical profession over standards of care.

Despite these limitations, the FDA's perceived performance during the 1950s and 1960s offers vital lessons for EBM advocates who would like a CER entity that builds reputation among both the public and elites for promoting sound science, protecting patients against the risks of overtreatment, and policing the medical profession when it fails to police itself. During the postwar era, the FDA developed increasingly rigorous scientific standards for evaluating the effectiveness of drugs—standards that went well beyond its original statutory mandate to test drugs only for safety. What permitted the FDA to build its capacity was its growing reputation as a competent and vigilant agency, symbolized by its decision to reject the drug thalidomide (which was intended to prevent morning sickness in pregnant women) in 1962. When it was discovered that thalidomide (which was available in Europe) caused severe birth defects, the agency's image as an essential guardian of public welfare was further enhanced. The episode received extensive media coverage and made a celebrity out of Frances Kelsey (the FDA regulator who stood her ground despite pressure from both industry and some actors within the agency to approve the drug), giving advocates an opportunity to ratify the FDA's expanded regulatory powers though the Kefauver-Harris Amendment. As political scientist Steven Teles observes, while critics have chipped away at the FDA's image in recent years, the agency's "powerful reputation gave it a great deal of insulation when an antiregulatory chill took hold in the 1980s."[62]

PCORI has so far failed to develop a reputation for doing important work. In January 2014, the Center for American Progress, a liberal think tank closely tied to the Obama administration, issued a harsh assessment of PCORI's early record.[63] The report pointed out that most of the studies funded by PCORI were broad and focused on methodology, education initiatives, and communication tools, rather than on questions directly relevant to clinical practice. During the time frame of the study, PCORI failed to issue a *single* CER study of medical devices, launched only a few CER studies of drugs, and produced few studies that focused on the priority areas identified by the Institute of Medicine.[64] PCORI's work did accelerate over the ensuing years. In 2016, the Center for American Progress issued a revised evaluation. It found that PCORI had made some progress, allocating 58 percent of its grant funding to CER.[65] The agency commissioned new studies to address a range of important topics, including the "use of radiation therapy for breast cancer, effective treatments for bipolar disorder, and lifestyle interventions versus drug therapy for diabetic patients."[66]

Yet PCORI continued to fund some projects that experts viewed to be as not of central clinical significance (such as a study of hoarding behavior)[67] and remained virtually unknown to the general public. There has been almost no mainstream media coverage of PCORI's work. Even more damaging, key stakeholders did not perceive CER as advancing rapidly. In a 2015 survey of 122 medical sector players—insurers/health plans, government officials, employers, researchers/thought leaders, business coalitions and associations, 81 percent of respondents said that over the past year, CER had "no effect" on health care decision making or led to a "slight" improvement," while 19 percent said it had led to a "moderate" or "substantial" improvement.[68] Wilensky's assessment is particularly damning: "PCORI seems to have become almost invisible. Maybe they think that's the best way to stay under the political radar screen," she said, adding that the institute has yet to "offer much value."[69]

PCORI's leadership faced many challenges. They had to get a new organization up and running, establish procedures for awarding grants, set priorities, and disseminate hundreds of millions of dollars in research support. The "patient-centered" aspect of PCORI's mission—added at the behest of the medical products industry—required PCORI to spend considerable time developing methods to include patients in the research process and educating researchers about the need to incorporate patient concerns into their studies.[70] Yet the most critical task facing PCORI's leaders was not technical, but political: demonstrating its value to members of Congress before its funding expires in 2019. While PCORI developed a strategic plan focused on "funding and conducting highly relevant research that is likely to change practice and improve patient outcomes,"[71] the agency never found an effective strategy for burnishing its reputation and winning reauthorization. In 2012, Dr. Harold Sox (who was later hired as a senior adviser to PCORI) implored the agency to implement "a strategy to make the largest possible impact before its day of reckoning."[72] The agency emphasized that it is "funding studies to answer questions about common, serious conditions like cardiovascular disease, cancer, and mental illness, which affect millions of Americans."[73] That is as it should be, but we offer three more specific suggestions.

First, it should be recognized that the biggest single threat to the political sustainability of CER is its association with "rationing." To overcome this association, PCORI (or future CER entities) should actively seek to distinguish the EBM project—which at its core is about better science, better information, and higher quality care—from service denial. One way to do this is to support and publicize research on the comparative effectiveness of worthy treatments that are being *underused*. Headlines associating the agency with research demonstrating the need for *more* medicine will help build the agency's reputation as a scientific body, rather than a cost-cutting board.

The United States can here learn from the U.K. experience. When the National Institute for Health and Care Excellence, which makes recommendations for covering medical interventions and treatments on the basis of cost-effectiveness analysis, was established in 1999, one of the main rationales was to end the "postcode" lottery in which the availability of services and treatments under the National Health Services depended on where a British citizen happened to live. (In the U.K. single-payer system, such geographical variation is considered to be a problem on *equity* grounds, not just efficiency grounds.) NICE's conclusions (including the denial of some cancer drugs available in the United States) generated controversy in the U.K., but it helped that NICE was created during a period when the U.K. was seeking to increase access to medical services and that following NICE's guidance usually meant spending *more*, rather than less.[74]

Another thought is that strategic leaders should link CER not only to geographic variation, but also to the investigation of the heterogeneity of treatment effects across groups, such as children, women, and the elderly. This approach could quell the refrain that CER creates insights only about population averages and does not help guide MDs in treating specific patients. If PCORI publicized findings that helped target specific groups, it could blunt this criticism.

Finally, PCORI needs to put "points on the board" to make the benefits of evidence-based medicine far more salient to ordinary Americans. That means studying treatments that affect millions of Americans and producing research that is relevant and helpful to physicians, that is understandable to patients and policy makers, and that warrants extensive (and favorable) media coverage.

LATERAL NETWORK BUILDING, FEDERATED
DESIGN, AND STRATEGIC PARTNERSHIPS

Because public administration is inescapably political, all public agencies require advocates. One of the most common mistakes made by institutional designers is to believe that the only political support that matters resides "inside the beltway." In America's fragmented governance system, however, the support that counts most is often locally rooted.[75]

Consider the Veterans Administration. Despite recent scandals, a deserved reputation for bureaucratic sluggishness and incompetence in some quarters, and calls for organizational reform, the VA has survived over many decades and even expanded its clientele base in recent years. Key to the VA's durability has been its federated design. The VA has a Washington-based bureaucracy, but it also entered into strategic partnerships with powerful private organizations, including academic medical centers at prestigious universities. The VA thus has a major presence in a large number of congressional districts around the country. These lateral network ties and public-private partnerships give the VA a geographic and distributive foundation. In addition, they allow the VA to "borrow" the reputation of other revered institutions.[76] A broadly analogous story of networked capacity building can be told about the success of the Department of Agriculture in bringing policy expertise to bear on its decisions during the New Deal through its close ties to state land-grant colleges and experiment stations.[77]

PCORI does not perform medical studies in-house; it distributes grants to researchers across the country. But the entity's visibility in local communities—and before local elite audiences—is much weaker than it could be. Imagine how much more robust the agency might be if instead of one Washington-based organization, Congress had created a dozen (smaller) comparative effectiveness institutes around the country, based at academic medical centers or major research hospitals. Perhaps a Center for Comparative Effectiveness and Cardiology could have been established at the University of Alabama, a Center for Comparative Effectiveness for Breast Cancer at Duke, and so forth. Each time each locally rooted center issued a study, a press conference would be held, attended by the state's congressional delegation.

Most importantly, the entity should develop close ties to leading doctors and local medical societies in communities around the nation, who could work with national organizations such as "Choosing Wisely" and consumer groups to help patients understand evidence-based medicine, the meaning of research findings for patient decision making, the significance of regional variation, and the problems of over- and underutilization. While the American medical profession clearly must lead at the national level as well, our physician survey results (chapter 4) suggest that rank-and-file doctors have strong views about the role of their medical societies. Until most doctors become well-informed about the waste and inefficiency of U.S. health care and politically engaged on these issues, little is likely to change. Indeed, physicians often appear to take the opposing stance and rally against efforts to promote the efficient use of health care dollars. For example, a recent proposal to test new payment models for Medicare Part B drugs, which would have reduced incentives for doctors to prescribe expensive drugs that generate higher reimbursement instead of cheaper drugs that are just as effective, generated intense opposition from medical societies.[78] Yet, local doctors enjoy the individual trust of their patients and could be an important counterweight to national policy makers who oppose EBM reform initiatives.[79]

Finally, PCORI could develop strategic partnerships with payers and providers participating in accountable care organizations (ACOs) around the country to implement PCORI's findings into their clinical management decisions. By collaborating with ACOs, PCORI can

> ensure that a subset of clinical decision makers will translate their recommendations to clinical practice. PCORI can then follow this subset of recruited ACOs, track the clinical outcomes before and after they begin following their recommendations, and compare outcomes with nonparticipating ACOs and providers.[80]

To be sure, a decentralized strategy is not without risks. There are more opportunities for agency heads to lose control over managing controversies, as in the recent case of VA hospitals.[81] In the American federated system, however, there are huge advantages to locally rooted policy.

———

The progressive desire to root out waste, inefficiency, and bad science in the U.S. health care system is well-founded, but the project needs deeper grounding in America's local communities and political culture, greater bipartisan support, and much stronger and more visible public leadership from the medical profession. We have shown that powerful political forces will need to be harnessed to improve the quality, rationality, and efficiency of American medicine. The work will be difficult, but the first step is to recognize that this is primarily a *political* challenge, not a technocratic one. Forging new linkages between expertise, power, and democratic accountability is vital to the durable reform of medical governance—and crucial to American government's performance as an effective problem-solving institution in the twenty-first century.

APPENDIX TO CHAPTER 3

The results of the survey experiment discussed in this chapter suggest that medical associations have the ability to influence public opinion on health care cost control, but the question remains whether the support or opposition of physician groups would be less (or more) effective when the endorsement or opposition cue explicitly references CER.[1] We carried out a second survey experiment to address this question. Respondents were told,

> Some people have suggested that we allow the government and insurance companies to refuse payment for treatments or procedures if their effectiveness has not been demonstrated by rigorous scientific evidence. Suppose you learned that [group cue conditions] and [political cue conditions]. What about you? Would you support this policy?[2]

The five political cue conditions were almost identical to those used in the experiment reported in the chapter, but with slightly different phrasing that fit the vignette better: (a) "congressional Democrats support this policy but congressional Republicans oppose this policy," (b) "congressional Republicans support this policy but congressional Democrats oppose this policy," (c) "both congressional Democrats and Republicans support this policy," (d) "a bipartisan commission supports this policy," or (e) no political group cue was given. These five conditions were randomly assigned with equal probability independently of the group cue treatments.

The group cue treatments, however, were different. We randomly assigned respondents to one of four groups—"leading doctors," "leading patient advocacy groups," "high-level government administrators," or "top drug companies"—or to receive no group cue. The support or opposition of the group for those assigned to one of the four groups was also randomly assigned, such that there were nine total group cue conditions.[3] As in the first experiment, some respondents were presented with a single cue (e.g., the endorsement of leading doctors) while others were presented with both a political cue and a group cue.[4]

For each of the 45 experimental conditions, table A3.1 reports the average (weighted mean) for the outcome measure. The table also reports the average for each political cue condition, collapsing group cue conditions (in row 10), and the average for each group condition, collapsing political cue conditions (both including the "no political cue" cases [in column F] and not including those cases [in column G]). We focus on three results.

First, the support of doctors increases public support for the CER health care cost-control proposal. Focusing on column G, we find that respondents who received the leading doctors support cue (row 2) had a higher level of support for the proposal (mean=47.8) than respondents who received the leading doctors oppose cue (row 3, mean=42.1). This net difference (of 5.7 units) is statistically significant (p=.09, two-tailed) and is consistent with the results of the first experiment.[5] Taken together, the results from both experiments provide evidence that public support of a proposal to use CER to help control health care spending is likely to be significantly influenced by the support of physicians.

Second, the influence of doctors is distinctive in that only their support boosts public acceptance of the CER cost-control proposal. The support of other groups either has no effect or else diminishes public support for the proposal (in comparison to opposition from the group). Surprisingly perhaps, the position of patient advocacy groups has no effect on public opinion about the proposal (p=.90 and .80 for the difference between patient advocacy groups oppose [row 4] and patient advocacy groups support [row 5] in columns G and F, respectively). Two groups—top drug companies and high-level government administrators—have so little standing with the public when it comes to CER and cost control that their *opposition* (not their endorsement) boosts respondents' support for the proposal. In column G, the −4.7 unit difference between support and opposition of high-level government administrators is statistically significant (p=.09), as is the −5.6 unit difference between the support and opposition of top drug companies (p=.04).[6] In short, of the (nonpolitical) group cues we tested, only the *support* of leading doctors increases public support of a CER proposal to help control health care spending. The support of other groups was either inconsequential or counterproductive (compared to the same group's opposition).

Third, as in the first experiment, we find only small differences across political cue conditions. Collapsing the group cue conditions (row 10 of table A3.1), we find that in the absence of a political cue, average support for the CER proposal is 42.4 (column A). The largest difference from this baseline condition is obtained when Democrats support the proposal but

Republicans oppose it (mean=45.6), a statistically significant (p=.09) 3.1 unit difference. When the bipartisan commission cue is given, average support is approximately 44.8 (column C), a 2.4 unit difference from the no political cue condition that is not statistically significant (p=.24).[7] Thus, we again find that the support of a bipartisan commission does not significantly increase public support for a proposal to help reduce health care spending—in this case, one specifically linked to CER. Moreover, as with the previous experiment, the effect of support from a bipartisan commission does not vary across respondents with differing partisan identities, including those who identify as Independent (p>.10 for all pairwise comparisons). Finally, collapsing across group cue conditions (row 10), there are no statistically significant differences between the four political cue treatment conditions (p>.10 for all six pairwise comparisons).

TABLE A3.1. Results of Group and Political Cues Experiment

	A No Political Cue (N=728)	B Democrats Support (N=739)	C Bipartisan Commission Supports (N=709)	D Both Parties Support (N=708)	E Republicans Support (N=674)	F All Political Conditions, with "No Political Cue" (N=3558)	G All Political Conditions, without "No Political Cue" (N=2830)
1 No Group Cue (N=759)	38.60 (1.85)	44.04 (1.79)	47.11 (1.86)	46.37 (1.91)	43.36 (1.72)	43.70 (0.82)	45.10 (0.91)
2 Doctors Support (N=362)	49.65 (3.69)	40.16 (2.88)	54.32 (3.41)	46.96 (3.08)	48.49 (2.19)	48.07 (1.39)	47.75 (1.49)
3 Doctors Opposition (N=354)	44.35 (2.61)	43.67 (2.59)	36.04 (2.94)	41.11 (3.03)	48.05 (3.62)	42.70 (1.32)	42.08 (1.53)
4 Patient Adv. Groups Support (N=317)	43.15 (2.64)	43.69 (2.68)	42.00 (2.58)	45.36 (2.99)	41.31 (3.23)	43.16 (1.25)	43.16 (1.42)
5 Patient Adv. Groups Opposition (N=358)	44.60 (2.45)	51.19 (2.76)	37.23 (3.03)	44.79 (2.52)	40.61 (2.58)	43.74 (1.21)	43.50 (1.39)
6 Gov't Admin. Support (N=361)	39.68 (2.66)	47.00 (3.29)	44.18 (3.03)	42.25 (2.63)	37.40 (3.41)	42.41 (1.34)	43.20 (1.55)
7 Gov't Admin. Opposition (N=364)	42.90 (3.65)	50.79 (2.38)	43.98 (2.23)	44.98 (2.44)	52.47 (2.94)	46.98 (1.23)	47.92 (1.26)
8 Drug Comp. Support (N=330)	47.86 (3.95)	42.97 (2.74)	42.66 (2.94)	40.21 (2.37)	39.49 (2.63)	42.51 (1.31)	41.39 (1.35)

9 Drug Comp. Opposition (N=353)	35.80 (3.16)	47.96 (3.20)	51.01 (2.49)	46.35 (2.66)	40.91 (3.02)	45.26 (1.31)	46.99 (1.41)
10 All Group Conditions (N=3,558)	42.44 (0.94)	45.57 (0.88)	44.80 (0.90)	44.37 (0.86)	43.77 (0.90)	N/A	N/A

Notes: Cell entries are weighted means with standard errors in parentheses. Total *N*=3,558.

Complete question wording: "A variety of public policies have been proposed to help reduce the amount we spend on health care. Some people have suggested that we allow the government and insurance companies to refuse payment for treatments or procedures if their effectiveness has not been demonstrated by rigorous scientific evidence. Suppose you learned that [10 Group Treatment Conditions: none / leading doctors support this policy / leading doctors oppose this policy / nationally recognized patient advocacy groups support this policy / nationally recognized patient advocacy groups oppose this policy / the high-level government administrators who run Medicare and Medicaid suppo:t this policy / the high-level government administrators who run Medicare and Medicaid oppose this policy / top drug companies support this policy / top drug companies oppose this policy] [IF Group Treatment <> none and Political Treatment<> none then "and"] [Five Political Treatment Conditions: none / congressional Democrats support this policy / congressional Democrats oppose this policy / both congressional Democrats and Republicans support this policy / a bipartisan commission supports this policy]. What about you? Would you support this policy? (Selecting the midpoint of the scale would mean that you neither support nor oppose this policy.) Outcome measure ranges from 0 ("strongly oppose") to 100 ("strongly support").

Source: November 9–22, 2011, YouGov/Polimetrix survey. A version of this table was originally published as table 3 in Alan S. Gerber, Eric M. Patashnik, David Doherty, and Conor M. Dowling. 2014. "Doctor Knows Best: Physician Endorsements, Public Opinion, and the Politics of Comparative Effectiveness Research." *Journal of Health Politics, Policy and Law* 39 (1): 171–208. Copyright 2014, Duke University Press. All rights reserved. Republished by permission of the publisher. www.dukeupress.edu.

TABLE A3.2. Results of AMA and Political Cues Experiment, by Respondent Party Identification

	A	B	C	D	E	F	G
	No Political Cue	Democrats Support	Bipartisan Commission Supports	Both Parties Support	Republicans Support	All Political Conditions, with "No Political Cue"	All Political Conditions, without "No Political Cue"
Republicans	(N=57)	(N=87)	(N=89)	(N=83)	(N=78)	(N=394)	(N=337)
1 No AMA Cue (N=132)	N/A	-0.71 (0.20)	0.43 (0.18)	0.09 (0.17)	1.13 (0.17)	0.20 (0.11)	0.20 (0.11)
2 AMA Support (N=134)	0.20 (0.18)	-0.58 (0.21)	0.24 (0.18)	0.44 (0.21)	0.83 (0.19)	0.24 (0.09)	0.25 (0.11)
3 AMA Opposition (N=128)	-0.21 (0.15)	-0.71 (0.24)	-0.34 (0.22)	-0.36 (0.22)	0.87 (0.24)	-0.17 (0.11)	-0.16 (0.13)
4 All AMA Conditions (N=394)	0.03 (0.12)	-0.67 (0.12)	0.14 (0.12)	0.07 (0.12)	0.95 (0.11)	N/A	N/A
Democrats	(N=78)	(N=105)	(N=123)	(N=106)	(N=106)	(N=518)	(N=440)
1 No AMA Cue (N=162)	N/A	0.85 (0.15)	0.29 (0.14)	0.38 (0.12)	-0.89 (0.14)	0.12 (0.08)	0.12 (0.08)
2 AMA Support (N=182)	0.43 (0.13)	0.71 (0.18)	0.54 (0.15)	0.50 (0.15)	-0.15 (0.19)	0.41 (0.07)	0.41 (0.09)
3 AMA Opposition (N=174)	0.20 (0.16)	0.59 (0.17)	-0.08 (0.17)	-0.22 (0.16)	-0.57 (0.24)	-0.01 (0.09)	-0.05 (0.10)
4 All AMA Conditions (N=518)	0.35 (0.10)	0.71 (0.10)	0.25 (0.09)	0.22 (0.09)	-0.57 (0.11)	N/A	N/A

Independents	(N=68)	(N=107)	(N=106)	(N=105)	(N=114)	(N=500)	(N=432)
1 No AMA Cue (N=150)	N/A	−0.10 (0.14)	−0.05 (0.17)	0.01 (0.15)	−0.40 (0.19)	−0.13 (0.08)	−0.13 (0.08)
2 AMA Support (N=161)	0.01 (0.11)	0.50 (0.21)	−0.01 (0.14)	0.07 (0.17)	0.51 (0.13)	0.19 (0.07)	0.24 (0.08)
3 AMA Opposition (N=189)	−0.15 (0.15)	−0.42 (0.17)	−0.16 (0.18)	−0.30 (0.20)	0.25 (0.14)	−0.14 (0.08)	−0.14 (0.09)
4 All AMA Conditions (N=500)	−0.06 (0.09)	−0.07 (0.10)	−0.06 (0.09)	−0.10 (0.10)	0.14 (0.09)	N/A	N/A

Notes: Cell entries are weighted means with standard errors in parentheses. Total N=1,412. See notes to table 3.3 for question wording.

Source: February 17–23, 2011, YouGov/Polimetrix survey. A version of this table was originally published as table 2 in Alan S. Gerber, Eric M. Patashnik, David Doherty, and Conor M. Dowling. 2014. "Doctor Knows Best: Physician Endorsements, Public Opinion, and the Politics of Comparative Effectiveness Research." *Journal of Health Politics, Policy and Law* 39 (1): 171–208. Copyright 2014, Duke University Press. All rights reserved. Republished by permission of the publisher. www.dukeupress.edu.

APPENDIX TO CHAPTER 4

TABLE A4.1. Doctors' Reported Knowledge of Regional Variation in Health Care Spending Studies

	Familiarity with studies about geographic variation in health care spending (0–4)
Female (1=yes)	−0.029 [0.164]
Region=West	−0.109 [0.187]
Region=Northeast	−0.073 [0.200]
Region=Midwest	−0.019 [0.212]
Political interest (0=hardly at all; 3=most of the time)	0.337 [0.084]**
Respondent PID (−3=Str. Dem; 0=Ind.; 3=Str. Rep.)	−0.01 [0.039]
Years in practice	0.014 [0.007]*
Residency take place at VA? (1=yes)	0.321 [0.147]*
Practice affiliated w/academic med center (1=yes)	0.241 [0.166]
Respondent specialty=Medical specialty	−0.187 [0.181]
Respondent specialty=Surgical care	0.103 [0.187]
Income source=Salary plus bonus	0.146 [0.202]
Income source=Billing only	0.112 [0.211]
Income source=Other (including shift work or wages)	0.673 [0.315]*

	Familiarity with studies about geographic variation in health care spending (0–4)
Practice Type=Office based (specialty group)	0.216 [0.378]
Practice Type=Hospital based	0.216 [0.180]
Practice Type=Other (including group or staff model HMO)	0.242 [0.211]
Constant	−0.355 [0.321]
Observations	324
R-squared	0.109
Mean of Dependent Variable	1.174

Note: OLS regression coefficients with robust standard errors in brackets. Dependent variable: 0=have not heard anything about studies; 1=not at all familiar; 2=only a bit familiar; 3=somewhat familiar; 4=very familiar. Omitted reference categories: Region=South; Respondent specialty=Primary Care; Income Source=Salary; Practice Type=Office based (solo or two-person). * significant at 5%; ** significant at 1%
Source: Fall 2015 survey of physicians.

TABLE A4.2. Doctors' Reported Reasons for Regional Variation in Health Care Spending

	Overuse of services of low or unproven value (1=a lot)	Health status and medical needs of Medicare patients (1=a lot)	Physicians' beliefs in the value of certain treatments (1=a lot)
Female (1=yes)	−0.026	0.029	0.027
	[0.064]	[0.062]	[0.051]
Region=West	0.081	−0.068	0.007
	[0.075]	[0.072]	[0.054]
Region=Northeast	−0.019	−0.136	0.08
	[0.071]	[0.073]	[0.064]
Region=Midwest	0.091	−0.165	0.052
	[0.081]	[0.074]*	[0.064]
Political interest (0=hardly at all;	0.015	0.049	0.049
3=most of the time)	[0.033]	[0.033]	[0.026]
Respondent PID (−3=Str. Dem;	−0.012	−0.001	−0.031
0=Ind.; 3=Str. Rep.)	[0.014]	[0.014]	[0.013]*
Years in practice	0	−0.003	0
	[0.003]	[0.003]	[0.002]
Residency take place at VA? (1=yes)	0.039	−0.06	−0.029
	[0.054]	[0.053]	[0.044]
Practice affiliated w/academic med	0.023	−0.04	−0.031
center (1=yes)	[0.064]	[0.059]	[0.049]
Respondent specialty=Medical specialty	0	−0.024	−0.061
	[0.068]	[0.069]	[0.053]
Respondent specialty=Surgical care	0.107	−0.139	−0.01
	[0.072]	[0.069]*	[0.059]
Income source=Salary plus bonus	−0.015	0.129	−0.025
	[0.071]	[0.069]	[0.061]
Income source=Billing only	0.097	0.052	−0.013
	[0.078]	[0.073]	[0.065]
Income source=Other (including shift	0.03	0.115	−0.064
work or wages)	[0.128]	[0.118]	[0.082]
Practice Type=Office based (specialty	0.201	0.046	0.042
group)	[0.136]	[0.115]	[0.108]
Practice Type=Hospital based	0.014	0.047	0.02
	[0.071]	[0.067]	[0.051]
Practice Type=Other (including group	0.039	0.019	0.096
or staff model HMO)	[0.079]	[0.078]	[0.064]
Constant	0.173	0.341	0.074
	[0.123]	[0.134]*	[0.117]
Observations	322	324	324
R-squared	0.045	0.067	0.061
Mean of Dependent Variable	0.355	0.314	0.185

Note: OLS regression coefficients with robust standard errors in brackets. Dependent variable: 1=item contributes "a lot"; 0=all other responses. Results are statistically and substantively similar when estimated using logistic regression. Omitted reference categories: Region=South; Respondent specialty=Primary Care; Income Source=Salary; Practice Type=Office based (solo or two-person).* significant at 5%; ** significant at 1%

Source: Fall 2015 survey of physicians.

How much Medicare pays physicians (1=a lot)	Amount of care demanded by patients with the same condition (1=a lot)	Availability of expensive medical technologies (1=a lot)	Threat of malpractice litigation is higher (1=a lot)	Underuse of services of high or proven value (1=a lot)
0.02	0.012	0.113	−0.044	0.035
[0.058]	[0.060]	[0.067]	[0.068]	[0.039]
0.1	0.038	0.013	−0.023	0.022
[0.067]	[0.070]	[0.071]	[0.076]	[0.040]
0.1	0.169	0.09	0.092	0.064
[0.068]	[0.075]*	[0.076]	[0.078]	[0.050]
0.079	0.011	0.029	−0.036	0.054
[0.073]	[0.076]	[0.077]	[0.084]	[0.051]
0	0.058	0.078	0.015	−0.033
[0.033]	[0.034]	[0.032]*	[0.037]	[0.022]
−0.02	0.019	0.017	0.021	−0.02
[0.014]	[0.015]	[0.015]	[0.016]	[0.010]*
0.006	−0.002	−0.004	−0.001	0
[0.003]*	[0.003]	[0.003]	[0.003]	[0.002]
−0.004	0.034	0.057	−0.021	−0.036
[0.049]	[0.053]	[0.054]	[0.057]	[0.034]
−0.03	−0.044	−0.015	0.045	−0.008
[0.055]	[0.060]	[0.060]	[0.064]	[0.038]
−0.094	−0.135	−0.005	−0.031	−0.02
[0.064]	[0.067]*	[0.068]	[0.073]	[0.041]
−0.062	−0.039	0.092	0.02	−0.009
[0.066]	[0.071]	[0.070]	[0.074]	[0.046]
−0.014	−0.061	0.004	−0.035	0.001
[0.067]	[0.075]	[0.075]	[0.079]	[0.057]
−0.045	0.011	0.1	−0.049	−0.13
[0.072]	[0.079]	[0.079]	[0.082]	[0.053]*
0.069	−0.043	−0.123	0.084	−0.098
[0.117]	[0.120]	[0.105]	[0.129]	[0.064]
−0.021	0.107	−0.003	0.167	0.025
[0.123]	[0.137]	[0.127]	[0.133]	[0.114]
−0.091	−0.082	−0.017	0.007	−0.069
[0.065]	[0.069]	[0.071]	[0.074]	[0.046]
−0.009	0.075	0.029	0.055	−0.093
[0.077]	[0.080]	[0.080]	[0.083]	[0.051]
0.201	0.263	0.108	0.521	0.263
[0.122]	[0.135]	[0.141]	[0.145]**	[0.104]*
320	324	323	324	321
0.049	0.066	0.064	0.032	0.087
0.26	0.336	0.356	0.551	0.108

TABLE A4.3. Beliefs about the Causes of Regional Variation in Medicare Spending Predicts Doctors' Beliefs about the Importance of Various Goals to Medical Societies

	Protecting clinical autonomy (1=not that important; 4=extremely important)	Identifying physicians not following best practices and bringing to board (1=not that important; 4=extremely important)
Overuse of services of low or unproven value	0.028	0.198
(1=none; 4=a lot)	[0.076]	[0.084]*
Health status and medical needs of Medicare	0.144	0.036
patients (1=none; 4=a lot)	[0.060]*	[0.082]
Physicians' beliefs in the value of certain	0.151	−0.072
treatments (1=none; 4=a lot)	[0.066]*	[0.091]
How much Medicare pays physicians	0.083	0.124
(1=none; 4=a lot)	[0.068]	[0.071]
Amount of care demanded by patients with the	0.007	−0.041
same condition (1=none; 4=a lot)	[0.079]	[0.095]
Availability of expensive medical technologies	−0.073	0.207
(1=none; 4=a lot)	[0.074]	[0.087]*
Threat of malpractice litigation is higher	0.106	0.026
(1=none; 4=a lot)	[0.084]	[0.085]
Underuse of services of high or proven value	0	0.163
(1=none; 4=a lot)	[0.084]	[0.092]
Female (1=yes)	0.118	−0.054
	[0.112]	[0.133]
Region=West	−0.128	−0.021
	[0.119]	[0.156]
Region=Northeast	−0.16	−0.053
	[0.113]	[0.167]
Region=Midwest	−0.236	0.022
	[0.140]	[0.159]
Political interest (0=hardly at all;	0.107	−0.026
3=most of the time)	[0.062]	[0.080]
Respondent PID (−3=Str. Dem; 0=Ind.;	0.087	0.018
3=Str. Rep.)	[0.027]**	[0.032]
Years in practice	−0.014	−0.005
	[0.005]**	[0.006]
Residency take place at VA? (1=yes)	−0.005	−0.109
	[0.093]	[0.116]
Practice affiliated w/academic med center	−0.107	0.024
(1=yes)	[0.107]	[0.124]
Respondent specialty=Medical specialty	−0.048	0.253
	[0.112]	[0.147]
Respondent specialty=Surgical care	−0.24	−0.088
	[0.120]*	[0.163]

	Protecting clinical autonomy (1=not that important; 4=extremely important)	Identifying physicians not following best practices and bringing to board (1=not that important; 4=extremely important)
Income source=Salary plus bonus	−0.063	0.099
	[0.123]	[0.160]
Income source=Billing only	−0.005	−0.096
	[0.125]	[0.171]
Income source=Other (including shift work or wages)	−0.116	−0.092
	[0.232]	[0.254]
Practice Type=Office based (specialty group)	0.026	−0.343
	[0.206]	[0.321]
Practice Type=Hospital based	−0.015	−0.031
	[0.116]	[0.151]
Practice Type=Other (including group or staff model HMO)	−0.181	−0.006
	[0.141]	[0.164]
Constant	2.16	0.628
	[0.455]**	[0.579]
Observations	315	312
R-squared	0.165	0.127
Mean	3.177	2.397

Note: OLS regression coefficients with robust standard errors in brackets. Dependent variable: 1=not that important; 2=moderately important; 3=very important; 4=extremely important goal. Omitted reference categories: Region=South; Respondent specialty=Primary Care; Income Source=Salary; Practice Type=Office based (solo or two-person). * significant at 5%; ** significant at 1%

Source: Fall 2015 survey of physicians.

TABLE A4.4. Doctors' Beliefs about the Importance of Various Goals to Medical Societies

	Advocating for economic interests (1=very/extremely important)	Protecting clinical autonomy (1=very/extremely important)
Female (1=yes)	−0.064	0.041
	[0.065]	[0.049]
Region=West	0.039	−0.059
	[0.071]	[0.057]
Region=Northeast	−0.051	−0.064
	[0.072]	[0.054]
Region=Midwest	0.03	−0.099
	[0.079]	[0.064]
Political interest (0=hardly at all; 3=most of the time)	0.011	0.017
	[0.034]	[0.026]
Respondent PID (−3=Str. Dem; 0=Ind.; 3=Str. Rep.)	0.032	0.04
	[0.015]*	[0.013]**
Years in practice	−0.006	−0.004
	[0.003]*	[0.002]
Residency take place at VA? (1=yes)	−0.001	−0.059
	[0.054]	[0.045]
Practice affiliated w/academic med center (1=yes)	−0.078	−0.037
	[0.060]	[0.054]
Respondent specialty=Medical specialty	−0.056	0.015
	[0.065]	[0.050]
Respondent specialty=Surgical care	−0.156	−0.121
	[0.069]*	[0.058]*
Income source=Salary plus bonus	0.092	−0.1
	[0.076]	[0.060]
Income source=Billing only	0.095	−0.032
	[0.081]	[0.062]
Income source=Other (including shift work or wages)	0.062	−0.093
	[0.120]	[0.104]
Practice Type=Office based (specialty group)	0.008	0.1
	[0.137]	[0.083]
Practice Type=Hospital based	−0.079	−0.014
	[0.069]	[0.056]
Practice Type=Other (including group or staff model HMO)	−0.071	−0.119
	[0.080]	[0.067]
Constant	0.824	1.047
	[0.138]**	[0.110]**
Observations	329	329
R-squared	0.083	0.104
Mean of Dependent Variable	0.654	0.81

Note: OLS regression coefficients with robust standard errors in brackets. Dependent variable: 1=very/extremely important goal; 0=not that/moderately important goal. Results are statistically and substantively similar when estimated using logistic regression. Omitted reference categories: Region=South; Respondent specialty=Primary Care; Income Source=Salary; Practice Type=Office based (solo or two-person). * significant at 5%; ** significant at 1%
Source: Fall 2015 survey of physicians.

Pointing out where physicians not following best practices (1=very/extremely important)	Disseminating best practices (1=very/extremely important)	Finding ways to cut costs by discouraging clinical interventions with minor or no benefit (1=very/extremely important)	Identifying physicians not following best practices and bringing to board (1=very/extremely important)
−0.029	0.027	0.06	0.013
[0.057]	[0.039]	[0.057]	[0.065]
−0.026	0.012	−0.117	−0.037
[0.068]	[0.044]	[0.067]	[0.075]
−0.073	−0.021	−0.198	−0.014
[0.071]	[0.050]	[0.071]**	[0.080]
0.026	−0.037	−0.053	0.005
[0.070]	[0.052]	[0.070]	[0.082]
−0.013	−0.001	0.026	−0.005
[0.031]	[0.022]	[0.032]	[0.037]
−0.027	−0.008	−0.03	0.002
[0.014]	[0.011]	[0.013]*	[0.016]
−0.002	−0.003	−0.002	−0.001
[0.002]	[0.002]	[0.003]	[0.003]
−0.029	−0.013	−0.073	−0.073
[0.050]	[0.036]	[0.050]	[0.056]
−0.012	−0.038	0.051	0.001
[0.057]	[0.042]	[0.057]	[0.063]
0.101	−0.027	0.113	0.139
[0.062]	[0.041]	[0.064]	[0.072]
0.016	−0.064	−0.006	−0.005
[0.068]	[0.044]	[0.067]	[0.072]
0.033	−0.073	0.006	0.081
[0.066]	[0.039]	[0.066]	[0.077]
−0.118	−0.095	0.028	0.03
[0.074]	[0.043]*	[0.071]	[0.080]
−0.115	−0.092	−0.082	−0.021
[0.117]	[0.078]	[0.116]	[0.128]
−0.097	0.067	−0.01	−0.085
[0.124]	[0.067]	[0.117]	[0.140]
−0.048	0.043	0	−0.009
[0.066]	[0.048]	[0.064]	[0.073]
−0.003	0.014	0.036	0.002
[0.074]	[0.055]	[0.071]	[0.081]
0.863	1.043	0.74	0.408
[0.129]**	[0.077]**	[0.123]**	[0.146]**
328	329	328	326
0.053	0.041	0.076	0.03
0.747	0.893	0.72	0.424

TABLE A4.5. What Should Medical Societies Do When a Medical Journal Publishes a Study That Calls into Question a Treatment?

	Individual physicians do not need to adhere (1=Support)	Disseminate results, but don't take position (1=Support)	Take an active role in critiquing (1=Support)
Female (1=yes)	−0.093	−0.121	−0.004
	[0.065]	[0.066]	[0.058]
Region=West	0.081	0.014	−0.026
	[0.075]	[0.075]	[0.065]
Region=Northeast	0.076	0.058	−0.04
	[0.077]	[0.077]	[0.069]
Region=Midwest	0.081	−0.046	0.065
	[0.079]	[0.083]	[0.070]
Political interest (0=hardly at all;	−0.016	−0.012	0.05
3=most of the time)	[0.034]	[0.035]	[0.032]
Respondent PID (−3=Str. Dem;	0.026	−0.005	−0.018
0=Ind.; 3=Str. Rep.)	[0.015]	[0.016]	[0.013]
Years in practice	−0.002	0.004	0.002
	[0.003]	[0.003]	[0.003]
Residency take place at VA?	−0.038	0.009	−0.065
(1=yes)	[0.055]	[0.057]	[0.050]
Practice affiliated w/academic	−0.06	−0.002	−0.031
med center (1=yes)	[0.061]	[0.064]	[0.057]
Respondent specialty=Medical	−0.054	−0.091	−0.094
specialty	[0.069]	[0.072]	[0.061]
Respondent specialty=	−0.058	−0.006	−0.191
Surgical care	[0.070]	[0.075]	[0.064]**
Income source=Salary plus	−0.069	0.043	0.074
bonus	[0.073]	[0.077]	[0.069]
Income source=Billing only	−0.032	0.013	−0.005
	[0.076]	[0.081]	[0.075]
Income source=Other (including	−0.023	0.198	−0.01
shift work or wages)	[0.115]	[0.121]	[0.121]
Practice Type=Office based	−0.17	−0.103	0.094
(specialty group)	[0.143]	[0.135]	[0.098]
Practice Type=Hospital based	−0.096	−0.087	−0.011
	[0.069]	[0.073]	[0.064]
Practice Type=Other (including	−0.093	0.007	−0.109
group or staff model HMO)	[0.076]	[0.079]	[0.075]
Constant	0.859	0.529	0.731
	[0.132]**	[0.140]**	[0.132]**
Observations	328	329	327
R-squared	0.051	0.047	0.072
Mean of Dependent Variable	0.615	0.516	0.738

Note: OLS regression coefficients with robust standard errors in brackets. Dependent variable: 1=support (somewhat or strongly); 0=oppose (somewhat or strongly) or neither oppose nor support. Results are statistically and substantively similar when estimated using logistic regression. Omitted reference categories: Region=South; Respondent specialty=Primary Care; Income Source=Salary; Practice Type=Office based (solo or two-person). * significant at 5%; ** significant at 1%
Source: Fall 2015 survey of physicians.

NOTES

Notes to Introduction

1. See Kolata 2002a; also see Moseley, O'Malley, et al. 2002; Ashton and Wray 2013.
2. Felson and Buckwalter 2002; Gerber and Patashnik 2006; David T. Felson, personal communication, September 27, 2004.
3. Gerber and Patashnik 2006.
4. Quoted in Kolata 2002b.
5. IOM 2007.
6. Ashton and Wray 2013, 3.
7. Brownlee 2008.
8. Ashton and Wray 2013.
9. J. Wennberg and A. M. Gittelsohn 1973; J. E. Wennberg 2010.
10. Balas 1998; Morris, Wooding, and Grant 2011.
11. Carey 2006.
12. Some more precise definitions are in order. Comparative Effectiveness Research (CER): "The direct comparison of two or more existing healthcare interventions to determine which interventions work best for which patients and which interventions pose the greatest benefits and harms. The core question of CER is which treatment works best, for whom, and under what circumstances." Patient-Centered Outcomes Research (PCOR): "Research that helps people and their caregivers communicate and make informed healthcare decisions, while allowing their voices to be heard in assessing the value of healthcare options. This research answers patient-centered questions." See http://www.pcori.org/funding-opportunities/how-apply/glossary. Cost-effectiveness analysis, which is used by the National Institute for Health and Care Excellence (NICE) in the United Kingdom: "An economic analysis that compares the relative costs and outcomes of two or more courses of action (or nonaction)." The PCORI is not permitted to develop or employ dollars per quality-adjusted life year (or similar) measures as a threshold to establish what type of health care is cost-effective or recommended. For background, see "Health Policy Brief: Comparative Effectiveness Research" 2010.
13. PCORI website: http://www.pcori.org/about-us.
14. www.pcori.org/sites/default/files/PCORI_Authorizing_Legislation.pdf
15. See Fairbrother et al. 2014.
16. Gray, Gusmano, and Collins 2003; J. Avorn 2009; Gerber and Patashnik 2010.
17. Buchbinder et al. 2009; Kallmes et al. 2009.
18. McGlynn, Asch, et al. 2003.
19. Aaron and Ginsburg 2009; Berwick and Hackbarth 2012; D. Cutler 2013; D. M. Cutler 2014a; Laugesen and Glied 2011.
20. J. Wennberg and A. M. Gittelsohn 1973.
21. J. E. Wennberg 2010.

22. Skinner et al. 2009.

23. Chandra, Finkelstein, Sacarny, and Syverson 2016.

24. Cooper et al. 2015.

25. Cooper et al. 2015.

26. Cooper et al. 2015.

27. Skinner, Goodman, and Fisher 2015.

28. Sackett, Rosenberg, Gray, et al. 1996, 71; see also Ashton and Wray 2013, chapter 5.

29. M. Rodwin 2001, 439.

30. IOM 2011; see http://nationalacademies.org/hmd/Reports/2011/Learning-What -Works-Infrastructure-Required-for-Comparative-Effectiveness-Research.aspx. The difference between the United States and other countries in their approach to EBM reflects, "at least in part, different approaches to health care financing" (Fairbrother et al. 2014, 1). While health care in Europe, Australia, and Canada is, generally speaking, organized and financed centrally, the United States has a complex mix of public and private payers. But there are also many points of similarity between the U.S. health care financing system and those of other advanced nations, including the use of fee-for-service and prospective payment systems and expert concerns about unwarranted variation, quality, and costs. The weakness of countervailing pressure to address the bad science and waste endemic to U.S. medical care requires careful explanation, especially with respect to the Medicare program.

31. De Vries and Lemmens 2006.

32. On the benefits and limits of standardization in medicine, see Timmermans and Berg 2003.

33. Tanenbaum 2012.

34. We thank David Mechanic for helpful insights on these points.

35. Schlesinger and Gray 2016.

36. We thank Mark Schlesinger for this formulation.

37. Gawande 2015, 42.

38. Sirovich, Woloshin, and Schwartz 2011.

39. McGlynn, Asch, et al. 2003; Welch 2015.

40. Blumenthal and Squires 2014.

41. Wilson 1973.

42. Skowronek, Engel, and Ackerman 2016.

43. See Baumgartner and Jones 1993.

44. For detailed information on the medical product industry's campaign contributions and lobbying activities, see: http://www.opensecrets.org/industries/indus.php?cycle=2014&ind=H04.

45. Jerry Avorn and Kesselheim 2015; Jerry Avorn and Kesselheim 2017.

46. Mazer and Curfman 2017; see also Jerry Avorn and Kesselheim 2015.

47. Mechanic 2006.

48. "Health Policy Brief: Reducing Waste in Health Care" 2012.

49. Callahan 2009, 7.

50. See, e.g., T. R. Marmor 2000; M. Peterson 2001.

51. For a similar approach, see Terry Moe's recent essay on the need to study the power of vested interests (2015).

52. Starr 1982; T. R. Marmor 2000; M. Peterson 2001; Laugesen 2016.

53. Cruess and Cruess 2004.

54. On the role of expertise, values, and institutions in health care, see Weimer 2010.

55. Starr 1982; M. Peterson 2001; but see Laugesen 2016.

56. Feldstein 2011; Mechanic 2004b; Robinson 2001.

57. Hall 2003.

58. Ferguson, Dubinsky, and Kirsch 1993.

59. Laugesen and Rice 2003; Laugesen 2009.

60. Arrow 1963.

61. Parsons 1939.

62. Dzur 2008, 56.

63. Dzur 2008, 65; Freidson 1970.

64. Freidson 1970; Starr 1982; M. Peterson 2001.

65. Cruess and Cruess 2004.

66. ABIM 2005, 2.

67. T. R. Marmor 2000.

68. M. Peterson 2001, 1156; see also L. R. Jacobs 1993.

69. Susan Bartlett Foote 2002; Bagley, Chandra, and Frakt 2015.

70. On path dependence, see Pierson 2000.

71. Bagley 2013, 533.

72. Oberlander 2016.

73. Mayes and Berenson 2006.

74. Goldhill 2013.

75. Chambers, Chenoweth, Thorat, and Neumann 2015.

76. See Orren and Skowronek 2004; but see also Frakt 2015a.

77. Swenson n.d.

78. M. Peterson 2001.

79. Mechanic 2004a, 1419.

80. Knox 2012.

81. AAOS 2013a.

82. Rosenberg et al. 2015.

83. Gray, Gusmano, and Collins 2003.

84. Roman and Asch 2014; Ubel 2015.

85. Blumenthal 2014.

86. Tilburt et al. 2013.

87. M. Peterson 2001.

88. Wilson 1973; Sheingate 2003; Posner 2003; Volden and Wiseman 2014.

89. Gerber and Patashnik 2006.

90. Stokes 1963.

91. Lee 2009.

92. J. Avorn 2009.

93. Moe 2015.

94. E.g., Delli Carpini and Keeter 1996.

95. E.g., Zaller 1992.

96. Skowronek, Engel, and Ackerman 2016.

97. Belkin 1997; Morone and Belkin 1995.

98. Stone 2011.

Notes to Chapter 1

1. McGlynn, Meltzer, and Hacker 2008, 88.

2. McGlynn 2004; Fuchs and Milstein 2011.

3. Chandra, Holmes, and Skinner 2013, 261.

4. See Chandra, Holmes, and Skinner 2013.

5. Squires 2011.

6. Fuchs 1974; Skinner et al. 2009.

7. See A. M. Garber and Skinner 2008.

8. Aaron and Ginsburg 2009, 1262.

9. D. M. Cutler 2014a.

10. D. M. Cutler 2014a, 21.

11. A. M. Garber and Skinner 2008.

12. IOM 2013, 102; see also Skinner 2011. For a thoughtful critique of the literature on waste and inefficiency in the U.S. healthcare system, see Glied and Sacarny 2017.

13. IOM 2013, 103.

14. D. M. Cutler 2014a.

15. Berwick and Hackbarth 2012.

16. "Health Policy Brief: Reducing Waste in Health Care" 2012.

17. Berwick and Hackbarth 2012.

18. Kolata 2017.

19. As quoted in Kliff 2013.

20. As quoted in Kliff 2013; see also Sirovich and Welch 2004.

21. Kliff 2013.

22. J. Miller 2014.

23. Quoted in J. Miller 2014.

24. Welch, Schwartz, and Woloshin 2011.

25. Gawande 2015.

26. Brownlee 2008.

27. Quoted in Brown 2011.

28. D. Epstein 2017.

29. D. Carpenter 2010.

30. Olson 2014.

31. Ashton and Wray 2013.

32. Ruger 2012b, 252.

33. CBO 2007a, 4 (note 3).

34. Jerry Avorn 2005.

35. We thank Mark Schlesinger for this point.

36. Jerry Avorn and Kesselheim 2015.

37. Ashton and Wray 2013, 28.

38. Chalkidou et al. 2009, 364.

39. For example, there are stark differences between the United States and European countries in how evidence shapes drug coverage decisions. A 2013 *Health Affairs* study found that European authorities "systematically assess most newly approved cancer drugs and use a variety of methods of comparative effectiveness research to arrive at recommendations on prescribing and reimbursement. . . . In contrast, drug reimbursement decisions in the US Medicare program appear less based on evidence" (J. Cohen, Malins, and Shahpurwala 2013, 767–68). For a proposal to reform U.S. drug pricing using the German reference price model, see Bahr and Huelskoetter 2014.

40. Bagley, Chandra, and Frakt 2015, 8.

41. There is some evidence that CMS is scrutinizing evidence more tightly for national coverage decisions under Medicare (Chambers, Chenoweth, Cangelosi, et al. 2015), but the vast majority of coverage decisions continue to be made by local contractors hired by CMS. These contractors have limited capacity and incentive to restrict coverage of low-value technologies. It remains to be seen what posture CMS will adopt for coverage determinations under the Medicare reforms that may be signed by President Donald Trump.

42. Tunis, Berenson, Phurrough, and Mohr 2011, 3.

43. CBO 2007b, 32.

44. Pearson and Bach 2010.

45. Pear 1991.

46. Susan Bartlett Foote 2002.

47. Susan Bartlett Foote 2002; Chandra, Jena, and Skinner 2011.

48. Neumann 2006.

49. Neumann 2006.

50. Neumann 2006.

51. IOM 2007.

52. CBO 2007b, 11.

53. Deyo 2014.

54. Mello and Brennan 2001.

55. Skinner 2011.

56. Fisher, Bell, et al. 2010.

57. Finkelstein, Gentzkow, and Williams 2016.

58. Westfall et al. 2007.

59. McGlynn, Asch, et al. 2003.

60. Skinner 2006.

61. For a synopsis by a leading figure in the field, see J. E. Wennberg 2010.

62. Brown 2011; Rosenthal 2014.

63. Welch et al. 2011.

64. Deyo and Patrick 2005.

65. Brownlee 2008.

66. Abramson 2008.

67. Clifton 2009.

68. Callahan 2009.

69. Chandra, Jena, and Skinner 2011, 30.

70. The application of scientific research on what works best for patients for every possible treatment option would move the country to point B. The nation would be spending *more* on medical care, but all possible health-related gains would be exhausted. Economists recommend point C over point B because the marginal gains in population health that would be realized by moving to the peak of the production frontier would not be worth it from a cost-effectiveness standpoint— too much consumption of nonhealth goods (e.g., education, clothing, housing, consumer goods, etc.) would have to be sacrificed to reach the peak (Chandra, Jena, and Skinner 2011).

71. Chandra, Jena, and Skinner 2011, 32; Perlroth, Goldman, and Garber 2010.

72. Ashton and Wray 2013, 77.

73. Department of Justice 2012.

74. Makary 2012.

75. Chandra, Jena, and Skinner 2011.

76. Groopman 2010.

77. See Chandra, Jena, and Skinner 2011.

78. Garber and Tunis 2009, 1926.

79. Wilson 1989.

80. Derthick and Quirk 1985; Patashnik 2008.

81. P. Peterson and West 2003.

82. Patashnik 2008.

83. Chalkidou et al. 2009; Stabile et al. 2013; Bevan and Brown 2014; Sorenson et al. 2014.

84. Stabile et al. 2013, 648.

85. Sorenson et al. 2014.

86. T. Marmor, Oberlander, and White 2009; Chalkidou et al. 2009.

87. Sorenson 2015, 205.

88. Sorenson 2015.

89. Steinbrook 2008.

90. McKee 2016.

91. We thank Michael Gusmano for helpful conversations on these issues.

92. On the limited responsiveness of American government to low-income Americans, see Gilens 2012.

Notes to Chapter 2

1. Timbie et al. 2012.

2. Timbie et al. 2012.

3. Jennings 1986.

4. Moseley, O'Malley, et al. 2002, 81; Katz, Brownlee, and Jones 2014.

5. Moseley, O'Malley, et al. 2002.

6. Arrow 1963.

7. Sihvonen et al. 2013.

8. Sihvonen et al. 2013.

9. Belluck 2013, A16.

10. Rosenberg et al. 2015.

11. Felson and Buckwalter 2002.

12. Burman, Finkelstein, and Mayer 1934; Yang and Nisonson 1995.

13. Hanssen et al. 2000.

14. Sprague 1981.

15. Use of subjective measures that are based on remembering something like "pain" levels many months earlier are unlikely to be as accurate as those that ask individuals to reflect on their present state or to engage in more immediate recall. A number of the subsequent studies employed a prospective design and so obtained measures of pain and functionality prior to the operations to compare postoperative measures to.

16. For a comprehensive list of clinical studies published up to 2003, along with a brief description of their designs and main results, see appendix B of CMS 2003.

17. Yang and Nisonson 1995; also see Moseley, O'Malley, et al. 2002.

18. Kalunian et al. 2000; Ravaud et al. 1999; Dawes et al. 1987.

19. Moseley, O'Malley, et al. 2002.

20. Yang and Nisonson 1995.

21. Bernstein and Quach 2003; also see Moseley, O'Malley, et al. 2002.

22. Hanssen et al. 2000, 1769–70.

23. Quoted in McGinty et al. 1992, 1573.

24. Ashton and Wray 2013, chapter 4; Harris 2016; Langreth 2003. We wish to emphasize that our claim is not that orthopedic surgery is generally ineffective. For example, convincing evidence supports major joint replacement operations, such as total knee replacement and hip replacement. These operations improve quality of life and may also be cost saving, because they replace the frequent doctor visits and drug expense associated with chronic care, reduce costs by eliminating falls, and permit the patient to resume more normal activity including employment (David T. Felson, personal communication, October 27, 2004).

25. Buchbinder et al. 2009.

26. Wulff, Miller, and Pearson 2011.

27. Deyo, Nachemson, and Mirza 2004. There have been no studies that we are aware of to determine if spinal fusion works better than placebo.

28. Bunker, Hinkley, and McDermott 1978, 937.

29. Spodick 1975, 35–36.

30. In 1959 the *New England Journal of Medicine* published the results of a sham surgery trial that found that a procedure known as internal mammary artery ligation worked no better than a placebo (L. Cobb et al. 1959). A more recent placebo-controlled trial of implantation of embryonic neurons in patients with Parkinson's disease found a very strong placebo effect, though those who received the real procedure did experience slightly greater improvement along certain dimensions (McCrae et al. 2004). On the case for sham surgery studies, see Carroll 2014.

31. The strong taboo against the use of placebo controls in the evaluation of surgeries raises an intriguing ethical question: If fake operations make people feel better, should surgeons perform them? We are skeptical. If patients were told that their operations did not involve real medical interventions, they would likely experience a much smaller placebo benefit. Moreover, because all medical interventions likely produce some placebo benefits, the knowledge that placebos were now an accepted course of personal medical therapy might lead to worse patient outcomes in general. Keeping patients in the dark about the use of placebos (outside of control arms in clinical trials) would only create more problems. Such deceptions would inhibit open communication between physicians and their patients and erode trust in the health care system. It would also damage the medical research enterprise, discouraging the identification of procedures with true medical benefits.

32. F. Miller 2014, 159; as Baruch Brody, the ethicist who participated in the Moseley study, points out, this ethical conclusion "is not based upon a commitment to a utilitarian philosophy that allows for the mistreatment of subjects if it is sufficiently socially or scientifically valuable." Risks still must be sufficiently minimized, and special steps must be taken to ensure that prospective participants in the trial really understand the nature of the placebo control group. See Baruch A. Brody, "Criteria for Legitimate Placebo Controlled Surgical Trials" (www.bcm.edu /pa/knee-drbrody.htm [October 25, 2004]).

33. AMA cited in F. Miller 2004; also see Tenery, et al. 2002.

34. Spodick 1975, 36.

35. Moseley, O'Malley, et al. 2002, 82.

36. Quoted in Burling 2002, A1.

37. At the time of the trial, the Houston VA (unlike many other VA hospitals around the nation) did not routinely cover the procedure for patients with knee arthritis because an excess of patient demand relative to the supply of available surgical suites forced local hospital officials to set priorities, and other surgical procedures were considered more important. The only way Houston area veterans could receive the procedure from the VA for this condition was by entering the trial (Nelda P. Wray, personal communication, October 5, 2004).

38. Felson and Buckwalter 2002.

39. Okie 2002; Kowalczk 2002.

40. Bandolier (http://www.bandolier.org.uk/booth/Arthritis/arthrokn.html).

41. The authors believe that the placebo effect was responsible for the improvement in part because most of the patients in the study had fairly stable symptoms at the time they entered the trial. They did not have acutely worsened symptoms that would be expected to naturally regress to the mean (J. Bruce Moseley, personal communication, December 7, 2004).

42. The study was conducted at a VA hospital, and therefore most subjects were men, but OA of the knee affects women more than men. There is, however, no medical reason to think surgery response varies according to sex, and critics did not press this argument very hard.

43. Moseley and Wray classified "popping," "clicking," "locking," and "giving way" as mechanical symptoms for purposes of their subgroup analysis (J. Bruce Moseley, personal communication, April 10, 2006). David T. Felson states that orthopedic surgeons generally regard locking and giving way as mechanical indications for arthroscopic surgery, but not popping and

clicking (David T. Felson, personal communication, March 15, 2006). We are unaware of any systematic data on surgeons' actual clinical decisions or behavior in this area.

44. As it turned out, however, some patients with a torn meniscus inadvertently entered the study. (Such patients often had false-negative magnetic resonance imaging findings.) For ethical reasons, an unstable meniscal tear found among patients in the lavage and debridement arms was treated. Although the number of such patients was too small for firm conclusion, they did not appear to do substantially better than patients in the placebo arm. The authors believed this required further study, but that, until clear evidence emerged, arthroscopy should continue to be performed on those with conditions like a bucket-handle tear (J. Bruce Moseley, personal communication, November 1, 2004).

45. David T. Felson, personal communication, September 27, 2004.

46. "Arthroscopic Surgery for Osteoarthritis of the Knee" (multiple letters) 2002; also see Wray et al. 2003.

47. Dervin et al. 2003.

48. There is a general consensus that the procedure is appropriate for patients with an unstable meniscal tear, though Moseley and Wray believed more research is needed on this question (J. Bruce Moseley, personal communication, November 1, 2004).

49. Felson and Buckwalter 2002.

50. David T. Felson, personal communication, September 27, 2004; also see Felson 2010.

51. Quoted in Burling 2002, A1; see also Jackson 2002.

52. Nelda P. Wray, personal communication, October 8, 2004.

53. Felson and Buckwalter 2002.

54. Quoted in Kolata 2002b.

55. Bagley 2013.

56. Kolata 2002c.

57. Shamiram Feinglass, personal communication, October 22, 2004.

58. The report (AAOS 2002), was endorsed by the American Academy of Orthopaedic Surgeons, the American Academy of Hip and Knee Surgeons, the Arthroscopy Association of North America, the American Orthopaedic Society of Sports Medicine, and the Knee Society.

59. CMS 2003.

60. See, for example, AETNA 2003; CIGNA 2004.

61. Shamiram Feinglass, personal communication, October 22, 2004.

62. Sung 2003.

63. Sung 2003.

64. Moseley and Wray's results may have been strong enough that CMS would have been justified in denying coverage of debridement for patients with OA, with an exception for those patients with anatomic abnormalities, such as one that produces locking of the joint, preventing a complete extension of the knee. Ideally, CMS coverage decisions should be based on strong medical evidence, yet CMS acknowledged that the clinical evidence for benefits to subgroups came from case series studies that the agency considered to be methodologically deficient. In light of the agency's own concerns about the existing level of evidence data, one reasonable approach would have been for CMS to have made no coverage changes regarding debridement for the time being but to have announced that it would stop paying for the procedure after some time period (say, three years) unless more rigorous evidence was presented to demonstrate the procedure's benefits. This would have created a powerful economic incentive for defenders of the procedure to replicate Moseley and Wray's study.

65. CMS has taken some steps to address this information problem. In November 2004, CMS chief administrator, Dr. Mark McClellan, who is both an internist and an economist, announced that the agency would make payments for certain new expensive treatments, such as implantable defibrillators for heart patients, conditional on agreement by companies and other

actors to pay for studies on whether these new methods are effective on the Medicare population. But this "coverage with evidence development" initiative has struggled owing to poor study designs and insufficient funding and statutory authority. See Neumann and Chambers 2013.

66. Pearson and Bach 2010. Pearson and Bach propose a new Medicare payment model in which CMS would pay more for services demonstrated by research to provide superior clinical benefits compared to alternatives. New services without such evidence would be reimbursed under standard Medicare rates for a limited time but then be reevaluated as evidence emerged.

67. Kirkley et al. 2008.

68. Katz, Brownlee, and Jones 2014.

69. David T. Felson, personal communication, September 27, 2004; also see Felson 2010.

70. S. Kim et al. 2011.

71. D. Howard et al. 2012.

72. Quoted in Kolata 2008.

73. AAOS 2013b.

74. Englund et al. 2008.

75. Englund et al. 2008.

76. Sihvonen et al. 2013.

77. Katz, Brownlee, and Jones 2014, 152.

78. Järvinen, Sihvonen, and Englund 2014, 216 (citing Moseley, O'Malley, et al. 2002, Herrlin, Hållander, et al. 2007, Kirkley et al. 2008, and S. Kim et al. 2011). In 2015, the *British Medical Journal*, a leading medical journal, published a meta-analysis and systematic review of the benefits and harms of arthroscopic surgery for the degenerative knee. It found no significant benefit on physical function, and some studies finding significant harms. Yet the procedures remain in use. The authors concluded: "Available evidence supports the reversal of a common medical practice. However, disinvestment of commonly used procedures remains a challenge, and use of arthroscopy seems to be undiminished, in analogy with use of vertebroplasty following the publication of trials showing absence of benefit of this procedure. Surgeon confirmation bias in combination with financial aspects and administrative policies may be factors more powerful than evidence in driving practice patterns" (Thorlund et al. 2015, 7).

79. Sihvonen et al. 2013.

80. Sihvonen et al. 2013.

81. Katz, Brownlee, and Jones 2014.

82. Katz, Brophy, et al. 2013.

83. Sihvonen et al. 2013; Belluck 2013.

84. As described by Järvinen, Sihvonen, and Malmivaara 2014. Two other studies showed that APM and exercise therapy were not superior to exercise alone in the treatment of degenerative meniscal tears in patients with varying degrees of knee OA (Herrlin, Wange, et al. 2013; Yim et al. 2013).

85. Quoted in Emery 2013.

86. Bhatia 2014.

87. Sihvonen et al. 2013, table 1.

88. Elattrache et al. 2014, 542.

89. Quoted in Emery 2013.

Notes to Chapter 3

1. Unless otherwise noted, all results are from surveys we conducted. The first survey was conducted November 5–December 31, 2009 ($N=1,100$); the second May 21–24, 2010 ($N=2,200$); the third July 30–31, 2010 ($N=2,000$); the fourth February 17–23, 2011 ($N=1,500$); the fifth November 9–22, 2011 ($N=3,600$).

2. The surveys were conducted by YouGov/Polimetrix, an international Internet-based survey research firm based in the United Kingdom. For each survey, YouGov/Polimetrix interviews more respondents than are required (from their panel of over 1.5 million participants) and then uses a combination of sampling and matching techniques to approximate a nationally representative sample. The surveys were contracted by the researchers, and approved by the institutional review board at Yale University.

3. All the analysis presented below uses the analytical weights provided with each data set. Although we cannot rule out the possibility of bias in this sampling method, it is reassuring that the nationally representative survey samples (i.e., the weighted data) produce responses similar to other surveys on baseline questions about insurance coverage and health status: in the May 2010 and February 2011 surveys, for example, 20 and 23 percent report being uninsured, and 72 and 76 percent report their health as "good" or better.

4. As Mark Peterson writes, "Based on the same claims to science and knowledge that medicine has used to invite our dyadic trust in physicians at the individual level, the medical profession has long sought, and often obtained, broad-based social trust in its leadership of health care policy making by local, state, and federal governments" (2001, 1146).

5. M. Peterson 2001.

6. For a review of agency models in political science, see Moe 1984.

7. Maynard and Bloor 2003; see also Arrow 1963.

8. Lupia and McCubbins 1998.

9. Mechanic 1998b; 2004a.

10. Blendon, Hyams, and Benson 1993; L. R. Jacobs and Shapiro 1994.

11. Buhr and Blendon 2011, 21.

12. See Hetherington 2005.

13. Buhr and Blendon 2011.

14. Buhr and Blendon 2011.

15. Cited in Buhr and Blendon 2011, 22.

16. Blendon, Hyams, and Benson 1993; L. R. Jacobs and Shapiro 1994; Krause 1996; M. Peterson 1993; 2001; Schlesinger 2002.

17. Gallup 2009; Rasmussen Reports 2010.

18. All the differences in the public's assessment of doctors compared to other professions are statistically significant at $p<.05$, two-tailed, with the exception of the differences between doctors and school teachers on the "interested in helping people" ($p=.26$) and "can be trusted" ($p=.25$) items.

19. See Schlesinger 2002.

20. Lillis 2010.

21. Wulff, Miller, and Pearson 2011.

22. Frakt 2015b, A27.

23. Currie, MacLeod, and Van Parys 2016.

24. Carman et al. 2010.

25. On average, we found that people were 5.2 percentage points more likely to find the arguments in favor of treatment guidelines to be somewhat or very convincing when the block of arguments against was presented first. The order of the blocks did not affect evaluations of the arguments against treatment guidelines.

26. Deyo and Patrick 2005; Hadler 2008.

27. Carman et al. 2010.

28. Men were substantially more likely than women to state that more than half of their own care (59.8 percent versus 41.3 percent) and more than half of the care received by others (53.3 percent versus 33.7 percent) is backed by evidence. This suggests that women were more skeptical than men about the evidence basis of medicine.

29. Zaller 1992.

30. Additional analysis revealed that this stylized debate had more of an effect on certain groups. Overall (across all conditions), the mean change in support among Republicans was −9.0; among Independents it was −7.2; and among Democrats the average change was only −5.2. Because Democrats began more supportive of CER than Republicans, exposure to the stylized debate led to greater partisan polarization of opinion regarding comparative effectiveness research. We also found that those with a college degree or more were, on average, less responsive to the debate (−5.6) than individuals with a high school diploma or less (−8.0). We did not find any differences across age groups or between voters and nonvoters.

31. Full argument wording: [*doctors want it*] "Many doctors' groups and medical associations are calling for comparative effectiveness research because the research will give doctors the information they need to identify the best treatments for their patients." [*scare tactic (one-size-fits-all)*] "The argument that this research will lead to one-size fits-all medicine is just a scare tactic. Doctors will be free to treat patients in the way they think is best." [*works best for most*] "It is unrealistic to expect doctors to view every patient as completely unique. Instead it is important to provide doctors with scientific evidence about what works best for most patients with a given medical condition." [*can incorporate group differences*] "Medical studies can be designed not only to identify which treatments work best for the average patient, but also which work best for patients with different medical conditions and backgrounds."

32. The mean persuasiveness ratings for the *scare tactic* and *works best for most* arguments were statistically indistinguishable from 50 (*p*-values=.522 and .216, respectively). We also tested the effectiveness of three rebuttals to the "ration care" argument. An argument that "there is so much waste in the health care system that we can reduce costs without harming patients" was most effective (mean score of 57.2). The other two arguments were statistically indistinguishable from 50: "In a time of budget deficits, difficult choices must be made to get health care costs under control. Every patient cannot get every possible treatment. Comparative effectiveness research will make sure that limited resources are allocated in the fairest and most effective way" (mean score of 51.8); "The rationing argument is just a scare tactic because Congress can prohibit research findings from being used to deny patients access to effective treatments" (mean score of 50.9).

33. Druckman, Hennessy, et al. 2010; Eagly and Chaiken 1993; Lupia 1994.

34. Like other work on public opinion concerning health care politics and policy (e.g., Gollust and Lynch 2011), we adopt Druckman, Hennessy, et al.'s definition of a "cue": Information "that enable[s] individuals to make simplified evaluations without analyzing extensive information" (2010, 137).

35. The full question wording stated, "A variety of public policies have been proposed to help reduce the amount we spend on health care. Suppose you learned that a proposal was [American Medical Association cue conditions] and [political cue conditions]. Would this make you more or less likely to support the proposal?"

36. The effects of the AMA cues are very similar for Republicans (a .41 unit difference between AMA support and opposition), Democrats (.46 unit difference), and Independents (.38 unit difference). The differences across partisan groups are statistically insignificant (*p*>.10 for all pairwise comparisons). This suggests that public support of a proposal to help reduce health care spending is likely to be significantly and similarly (across party lines) influenced by the position of the AMA—Republicans, Democrats, and Independents are no more or less likely to respond to the position of the AMA.

37. Twenty percent of the people who received the bipartisan commission supports cue said they were (somewhat or much) less likely to support the proposal, while 17 percent of the people who received no political cue did so; 31 percent of the people who received the bipartisan commission supports cue said they were (somewhat or much) more likely to support the proposal, while 27 percent of the people who received no political cue said the same.

38. The effect of support from a bipartisan commission does not vary across respondents with differing partisan identities, including those who identify as Independent ($p>.10$ for all pairwise comparisons). In fact, none of the political cue treatment conditions significantly affected Independents relative to the no political cue condition.

39. This finding is consistent with prior work on the effect of partisan cues (e.g., Kam 2005; Popkin 1994; Rahn 1993).

40. Moreover, in additional analysis, we found evidence of "cue substitution"—respondents giving particular weight to the cues they see as most informative (e.g., Schaffner, Streb, and Wright 2001; Ansolabehere et al. 2006). Respondents who identified as Republicans or Democrats (rather than as Independents) relied particularly heavily on cues from the AMA when no directional party cue was provided (i.e., in the Bipartisan Commission Supports, Both Parties Support, and No Political Cue conditions). In the absence of a directional party cue, the effect of an AMA endorsement—rather than AMA opposition—was .566 ($p<.01$) among partisan respondents. However, when a directional party cue (i.e., the Republicans Support or Democrats Support conditions) *was* given to partisan respondents, the effect of the AMA position was substantially smaller and not statistically significant (estimated effect=.171; $p=.305$). In other words, partisans relied on cues from their party when available; but when cues from their own party were not available, partisans were influenced by information about the AMA's position. As we would expect, there was less evidence of cue substitution among self-identified Independents. When a directional partisan cue was given to Independents, the estimated effect of an AMA endorsement was somewhat larger (estimated effect=.548) than it was when no directional partisan cue was given (estimated effect=.234). However, this difference in effect size falls short of conventional levels of statistical significance ($p=.135$). This analysis was conducted by estimating a regression model predicting support for the proposal with indicators for each of five treatment conditions (1) Directional Party Cue, AMA Supports; (2) Directional Party Cue, No AMA Cue; (3) No Directional Party Cue, AMA Supports; (4) No Directional Party Cue, No AMA Cue; (5) No Directional Party Cue, AMA Opposes. The model also included an indicator set to 1 for respondents who identified as either Democrats or Republicans and 0 otherwise. Finally, the model included interactions between this "partisan indicator" and each of the treatment indicators.

41. Some limitations should be kept in mind. The magnitude of the effect sizes we identify in the survey experiments are modest (e.g., the estimated effect of receiving "leading doctors support" rather than "leading doctors oppose" was approximately 6 points on a 100-point scale [0.25 standard deviations]). This is particularly important to note given that these experiments present respondents with a highly simplified representation of the world and, thus, may overstate the size of the effects that would occur outside of the experimental context (Barabas and Jerit 2010). Thus, although this stripped-down framework demonstrates that physician and medical association endorsements are potentially important to public support of health policy proposals, we cannot assume that such endorsements would result in similar effects when other information is available to citizens. We believe the public's high level of confidence in doctors and medical associations is robust to alternative models, but further experimentation that embeds more detailed and complex information about the health care system may provide a more complete picture of the types of information people encounter in the real world and the potential effects that doctors and medical associations can have on public opinion.

Notes to Chapter 4

1. USPSTF 2008.
2. Harris 2011.
3. Welch, Schwartz, and Woloshin 2011, 58.
4. Parker-Pope 2012a.

5. Ablin 2010, A27.

6. USPSTF 2012.

7. Quoted in Jaslow 2013.

8. Quoted in Marshall 2012.

9. Quoted in Jaslow 2012.

10. Pollack 2013.

11. The change in recommendation was "based in part on additional evidence that increased the USPSTF's certainty about the reductions in risk of dying of prostate cancer and risk of metastatic disease." USPSTF 2017.

12. Drazer, Huo, and Eggener 2015. See also Jemal et al. 2015; Sammon et al. 2015.

13. Drazer, Huo, and Eggener 2015.

14. D. H. Howard, Tangka, Guy, et al. 2013.

15. Quoted in Azvolinsky 2015.

16. In October 2015, the American Cancer Society announced that it was recommending that women at average risk of developing breast cancer begin getting annual mammograms at age 45, rather than 40 (the previous recommendation), and that at age 55 women transition to screening every two years. The group also recommended that women no longer receive physical breast exams where doctors feel around for bumps (Grady 2015). Yet the recommendations did not sit well with many doctors. In the *New York Times*, a trio of prominent radiologists and breast surgeons wrote that they "profoundly disagree" with the new guidelines, and that they would continue to recommend that women receive annual screening mammograms starting at age 40 (Drossman, Port, and Sonnenblick 2015). The main message that critics prompt the public to hear is that recommendations "will be used 'to prevent me or someone I care about from getting something that I believe is important for my health and well-being'" (quoted in Ashton and Wray 2013, 246).

17. M. Kim, Blendon, and Benson 2001.

18. Ubel and Asch 2015; Bach 2012.

19. Arrow 1963.

20. D. Carpenter 2012, 298; M. Peterson 2001.

21. Abbott 1988; Freidson 1988; Starr 1982.

22. M. Peterson 2003, 273.

23. Dzur 2002, 178.

24. J. E. Wennberg 2010, 24.

25. J. E. Wennberg 2010, 24.

26. J. E. Wennberg 2010, 24.

27. Regional variation in utilization and spending has been a major concern among both researchers and health policy makers. For a political analysis of targeting variation as a policy strategy, see Tanenbaum 2012.

28. As medical ethicist Daniel Callahan observes, the relationship between physicians and the medical products industry is symbiotic: "Physicians need industry to provide the technologies and treatments to pursue their profession. Industry needs physicians as the necessary pathway to patients" (2009, 140). In addition, some doctors are de facto small businesspersons (they run and manage their own offices), and all physicians have a stake in their own careers and incomes (M. Rodwin 2011).

29. J. E. Wennberg 2010, 7.

30. J. E. Wennberg 2010.

31. The failure to give patients effective services is a serious issue, but it does not appear to be a major factor in the regional variation in Medicare utilization or spending (see J. E. Wennberg 2010, 9).

32. Makary 2012. The challenge of professional self-regulation is not unique to doctors. As journalist Megan McArdle writes,

Professionals tend to deal with some of the most sensitive and important issues that our society has, like treating illness and educating our children. It's no accident that these people generally end up being regulated by their peers—and that the rest of us are frequently unsatisfied with the results. When professional groups decide what's good for the rest of us, it usually turns out that what they think is good for the rest of us is what's best for them.

    This doesn't have to be nakedly venal, and it often isn't. College professors genuinely care about their students, lawyers about their clients, doctors about their patients, journalists about their readers, and yes, police care about the communities they serve. But when a proposal comes up that will hurt them in some way, it's very easy for the professionals to see all the reasons against it, and to convince themselves that the world will be better off without it. And when it comes time to discipline a member for some offense, unless it is straightforwardly heinous, they will naturally sympathize with the accused, thinking of all the times they made mistakes that could have landed them in the same place (2015).

33. Lyu et al. 2016.
34. Swenson n.d.
35. Callahan 2009.
36. Laugesen 2016, 24.
37. Tyssen et al. 2013, 518.
38. A. M. Garber and Skinner 2008, 46.
39. Stone 1977, 38.
40. Starr 1982, 140.
41. Skowronek, Engel, and Ackerman 2016.
42. Starr 1982, 140–2.
43. Starr 1982, 19–20 and 127–34.
44. Morone 1990, 255.
45. Starr 1982, 134.
46. Starr 1982, 140.
47. Ruger 2012a, 231.
48. D. Carpenter 2012.
49. Wilsford 1991.
50. Ruger 2011, 352.
51. Ruger 2011, 353.
52. See Wennberg International Collaborative 2011.
53. Stevens et al. 2006.
54. T. R. Marmor 2000; M. Peterson 2001.
55. According to the Centers for Medicare and Medicaid Services, "U.S. health care spending grew 5.8 percent in 2015, reaching $3.2 trillion or $9,990 per person. As a share of the nation's Gross Domestic Product, health spending accounted for 17.8 percent" (see https://www.cms.gov/research-statistics-data-and-systems/statistics-trends-and-reports/nationalhealthexpenddata/nationalhealthaccountshistorical.html; accessed March 15, 2017).
56. Ruger 2011.
57. Moe 1989, 267.
58. Bagley 2013; Abelson and Lichtblau 2014.
59. Bagley 2013, 521–22.
60. Bagley 2013, 568.
61. Tunis and Pearson 2006.
62. For an optimistic view, see Robinson 2015.
63. M. Peterson 2001.

64. Starr 1982; M. Peterson 2001.

65. For a general discussion of the power of vested interests in U.S. politics, see Moe 2015.

66. Laugesen 2016; Laugesen et al. 2012.

67. Whoriskey and Keating 2013.

68. Quoted in Whoriskey and Keating 2013.

69. Clemens and Gottlieb 2013.

70. Tuohy 1999.

71. Belkin 1998.

72. M. Peterson 2001, 1158.

73. Mechanic 2004b.

74. Blendon, Donelan, et al. 1993, 1015 (table 4).

75. D. M. Cutler 2014a, 129.

76. Mechanic 2004b; Kronebusch, Schlesinger, and Thomas 2009.

77. Mechanic 2006, 28.

78. Stevens 2001, 348–49.

79. We partnered with Medical Marketing Services (MMS), a firm that specializes in e-mail marketing within the health care industry. The firm maintains a list, derived from the AMA Physician Masterfile, of every physician in the United States (M.D. and D.O.), including both members and nonmembers of the AMA. This list of over 900,000 physicians, updated weekly, takes the AMA Masterfile, which contains demographic, education, and current practice information gleamed from over 2,100 sources, and appends to it demographic, behavioral, and psychographic data from a number of sources. We purchased a random sample of 4,000 physicians. From this list, which included 1,400 primary care and 2,600 non–primary care physicians, we called offices in a random order to verify contact information (i.e., the address at which to be mailed a survey). Once we had verified the contact information for 750 physicians, we began mailing surveys.

80. We have little information about the characteristics of the sample as a whole, but those characteristics we do have suggest that the 374 individuals who responded to our survey are relatively similar to those who did not. For example, the average age of nonrespondents and respondents is around 53 years; the average nonrespondent and respondent graduated medical school 20–21 years ago; and a similar percentage (87–88 percent) of respondents and nonrespondents were also in office-based practices. There are some regional differences between respondents and nonrespondents, but such differences are small—respondents (Midwest, 18.8 percent; South, 32.1 percent; West, 23.8 percent; Northeast, 25.2 percent) vs. nonrespondents (Midwest, 22.7 percent; South, 30.5 percent; West, 22.1 percent; Northeast, 24.6 percent). Finally, non–primary care physicians (i.e., specialists) were more likely to respond than primary care physicians—specialists constituted 65 percent of our total sample, but 72 percent of our respondents. In short, our survey respondents and nonrespondents are broadly similar for the observed characteristics we do have.

81. A response rate of 50 percent is comparable to other mail surveys of physicians (see, e.g., Keyhani, Woodward, and Federman 2010).

82. Grande et al. 2007.

83. Bonica, Rosenthal, and Rothman 2014.

84. Full question wording, for both our survey and the Pew report (see http://www .people-press.org/2014/06/26/section-10-political-participation-interest-and-knowledge/): "Some people seem to follow what's going on in government and public affairs most of the time, whether there's an election going on or not. Others aren't that interested. Would you say you follow what's going on in government and public affairs most of the time, some of the time, only now and then, or hardly at all?"

85. Full question wording: "Here is a list of federal government officials. For each one, please tell whether or not you have initiated any contacts with that type of official, or someone on the staff of such an official, in the last twelve months."

86. Unlike the political interest question, the question wording in the Pew report differed slightly from ours in that it asked generally about contacting "elected officials," rather than about specific elected officials, over a two-year, rather than one-year period.

87. See Davis et al. 2014.

88. In 2013, Americans had a life expectancy at birth of 78.8 years, compared with a median of 81.2 years in OECD nations (see: http://www.commonwealthfund.org/publications /issue-briefs/2015/oct/us-health-care-from-a-global-perspective). Most doctors recognized this. Sixty-five percent of doctors said that people in the United States have a lower life expectancy (1.5 or more years less than people in France and Germany). Six percent indicated that people in the United States had a higher life expectancy, with 29 percent saying the United States fared "about the same" to its Western European counterparts.

89. Large regional differences have been documented in the U.S. Veterans Affairs system (Ashton et al. 1999; CBO 2008; Subramanian et al. 2002), in private insurance markets (Cooper et al. 2015), and in other countries including the U.K. and Canada (McPherson et al. 1981).

90. Gawande 2009.

91. Roy 2010.

92. Skinner 2011; J. E. Wennberg 2010.

93. Cooper et al. 2015.

94. IOM 2013.

95. Baker et al. 2014.

96. J. E. Wennberg 2010, 183; also see D. Cutler et al. 2017.

97. J. E. Wennberg 2010.

98. D. Cutler et al. 2017.

99. D. M. Cutler 2014a.

100. D. Cutler et al. 2017.

101. Finkelstein et al. 2016.

102. Forsythe et al. 2015; Keyhani, Woodward, and Federman 2010.

103. In an earlier pilot study, we surveyed physicians attending a medical society meeting in the Charlottesville, Virginia, area. Many of the physicians did not report knowing anything about the regional variation literature, but of those who did self-report knowledge, most said they had learned about it from Gawande's 2009 *New Yorker* article. This suggests the limits of medical society leadership in physician education as well as the importance of outlets other than medical journals for informing rank-and-file doctors about health policy issues.

104. This analysis was conducted by estimating a regression model (table A4.1) predicting reported familiarity with studies about geographic variation in health care spending on a scale from zero (no familiarity) to four (most familiarity) with the following information about the doctors: female, region (South, Northeast, Midwest, West) indicators, political interest, partisan identification, years in practice, whether residency took place at a VA, whether their practice is affiliated with an academic medical center, specialty (medical, surgical, or primary care) indicators, income source (salary, salary plus bonus, billing only, or other) indicators, and practice type (office based, office-based specialty group, hospital based, or other) indicators.

105. All *p*-values that we report are two-tailed.

106. Hersh and Goldenberg 2016.

107. In a separate regression analysis, we also found that the more familiar doctors reported they were with the studies on regional variation, the more likely they were to say that the availability of expensive medical technologies contributed "a lot" to regional variation in Medicare spending ($p<.05$). This was the only item for which we observed a statistically significant association between reported knowledge of the studies on regional variation in Medicare spending and the items presented in figure 4.1.

108. Walker 2011. A regression analysis estimating trust in the AMA using the same predictors listed for the previous regressions discussed in this chapter reveals a statistically significant ($p<.05$) association between the longer a doctor has been in practice and *less* trust in the AMA. No other covariates were statistically significant.

109. Bagley 2013, 534–6.

110. This analysis was conducted by estimating a regression model (table A4.3) predicting beliefs about the importance of (1) protecting the clinical autonomy of physicians in the society's area of specialization and (2) identifying physicians in the society's area of specialization who are not following best medical practices and bringing them to the attention of disciplinary boards for medical societies on a scale from one (not that important) to four (extremely important) with the eight beliefs about the causes of regional variation in Medicare spending and the following information about the doctors: female, region (South, Northeast, Midwest, West) indicators, political interest, partisan identification, years in practice, whether residency took place at a VA, whether their practice is affiliated with an academic medical center, specialty (medical, surgical, or primary care) indicators, income source (salary, salary plus bonus, billing only, or other) indicators, and practice type (office based, office-based specialty group, hospital based, or other) indicators.

111. Hersh and Goldenberg 2016.

112. There are also some stark regional differences in response to this item. Specifically, doctors from the South rated discouraging clinical interventions with minor or no benefit to patients as more important than doctors from the Northeast ($p<.01$) and West ($p<.10$).

113. There were no significant differences among the medical specialties on whether medical societies should argue that individual physicians should be permitted to continue practicing as they think best or disseminate the results but not take a position on them.

114. Currie, MacLeod, and Van Parys 2016.

115. Currie, MacLeod, and Van Parys 2016.

116. A. Epstein and Nicholson 2009.

117. Lipitz-Snyderman et al. 2016.

118. Van Parys and Skinner 2016, 1549.

119. Currie, MacLeod, and Van Parys 2016.

120. Van Parys and Skinner 2016, 1550.

121. This study found that heart attack patients with more aggressive doctors who use invasive procedures consistently have better health outcomes, although also higher costs (Currie, MacLeod, and Van Parys 2016).

Notes to Chapter 5

1. Beane, Gingrich, and Kerry 2008, A31.

2. Jasanoff 2016, 383.

3. R. Cobb, Ross, and Ross 1976.

4. On the origins, goals, accomplishments, and limitations of the Progressive reform model, see Knott and Miller 1987; and Skowronek, Engel, and Ackerman 2016. On the application of this model to the rise of the medical profession, see Starr 1982.

5. Gerber and Patashnik 2006; Mayhew 1974.

6. Schumpeter 1942.

7. Mayhew 2006.

8. Mayhew 2006, 223.

9. Kingdon 2003, 122.

10. T. Oliver 2004; Sheingate 2003.

11. Posner 2003, 194.

12. See, e.g., Schumpeter 1942; Dahl 1961; Kingdon 2003; R. W. Cobb and Elder 1983; Baumgartner and Jones 1993; Schickler 2001; Sheingate 2003; Mintrom and Norman 2009; Volden and Wiseman 2014.

13. But see Schneider, Teske, and Mintrom 1995.

14. Baumol 2010.

15. Scholars have found that not only can a source influence the credibility of a message, but "messages also influence perceptions concerning the credibility of the source" (Slater and Rouner 1996, 975). For studies on how assessments of message sources are made based on the quality and content of the message, see, for example, Brehm and Lipsher 1959; Combs and Keller 2010; Eisinger and Mills 1968; Hosman and Siltanen 2011; and Reimer, Mata, and Stoecklin 2004.

16. Gerber and Patashnik 2006.

17. In their study of legislative effectiveness, Volden and Wiseman 2014 find that political entrepreneurs are critical to policy change, but that policy sectors, including health, characterized by entrepreneurial politics—diffuse benefits/concentrated costs—are more prone to gridlock.

18. Wilson 1973.

19. Derthick and Quirk 1985.

20. Arnold 1990.

21. Patashnik 2008.

22. Wilson 1973, 322–4.

23. Mayhew 1974.

24. We note that another aspect of district representation—bringing grants and projects to the district—does not rate particularly high; however, there is a partisan divide—43 percent of Democrats, 33 percent of Republicans, and only 23 percent of Independents say that this factor would make them much or a great deal more likely to vote for a representative. This pattern may reflect the anger of Republican voters about the Obama administration's economic stimulus spending. In recent years, many GOP lawmakers have declined to claim credit for projects that benefited their districts in order to inoculate themselves against primary challenges (Grimmer, Westwood, and Messing 2014).

25. Wilson 1974.

26. Both the heart disease and PSA vignette were introduced with the following text: "Please consider the following scenario based loosely on a recent medical controversy. This question is designed to understand public opinion. You should not make any health decisions based on this scenario."

27. We note that when doctors oppose the task force recommendation in the absence of political disagreement (i.e., Rep. A supports the task force recommendation, but there is no mention of Rep. B), Representative A's job approval does not decline as much (Rep. A Supports Task Force and Rep. A. Supports Task Force / Doctors Oppose Task Force are statistically indistinguishable, $p > .10$).

28. For insightful historical analyses of these developments, see Ashton and Wray 2013; Sorenson, Gusmano, and Oliver 2014.

29. Wilensky 2006.

30. As previously noted, new drugs and devices generally do not have to be shown to be superior (or even equivalent) to alternative products to gain FDA marketing approval. Pharmaceutical firms and medical device makers therefore gain little by paying for rigorous studies to determine if their products lead to superior patient outcomes. For example, the maker of a positron emission tomography (PET) scanner may be able to sell this $2.5 million machine to hospitals by marketing the PET scan's impressive ability to find areas of abnormal metabolic activity that *may* indicate malignancy. An expensive study to determine whether the PET scan actually leads to more accurate disease staging, more focused treatments, and better patient outcomes is unlikely to be worth the costs (Ashton and Wray 2013).

31. CBO 2007b, 8.

32. Wilson 1974.

33. D. Carpenter and Fendrick 2004.

34. Markman 2008.

35. Angell 2004; Rose 2013.

36. Keller and Packel 2014.

37. Different terminology has been used historically to describe activities intended to promote evidence-based medicine (EBM), including health technology assessment (HTA) and comparative effectiveness research (CER): As Sorenson, Gusmano, and Oliver note,

> Both HTA and CER address the question "Does it work?" and involve evidence synthesis. However, they can be distinguished by the fact that CER also focuses on evidence generation and is principally concerned with the comparative assessment of effectiveness of a broad range of interventions and care delivery approaches in routine settings, whereas HTA considers evidence on effectiveness, safety, cost-effectiveness, and, when broadly applied, social, ethical, and legal aspects of health technologies. Because HTA often (but not always) includes an economic dimension (cost-effectiveness), it also addresses the question "Is it worth it and should it be paid for?" and is often used to inform coverage and reimbursement decisions. As previously discussed, these are aspects that are not included in current conceptions of CER. . . . Taken together, CER can be viewed as a potential input into HTA and EBM (2014, 144).

38. Brody 1979.

39. Blumenthal 1983.

40. Perry 1982.

41. Blumenthal 1983.

42. Heritage Foundation 2005.

43. As quoted in Perry 1982, 1098.

44. Perry 1982.

45. J. Wennberg and A. M. Gittelsohn 1973; J. Wennberg and A. Gittelsohn 1982; see also Brownlee 2008; J. E. Wennberg 2010.

46. Skinner and Fisher 2010.

47. Kingdon 2003.

48. Gray 1992.

49. Gray 1992.

50. Gray, Gusmano, and Collins 2003.

51. Bimber 1996.

52. Gray, Gusmano, and Collins 2003.

53. Leary 1994.

54. Gray, Gusmano, and Collins 2003.

55. Quoted in Gray, Gusmano, and Collins 2003, W3–307.

56. Quoted in Rich 1996, A27.

57. J. Avorn 2005, 278.

58. Sorenson, Gusmano, and Oliver 2014, 150.

59. Sorenson, Gusmano, and Oliver 2014.

60. Allen 2013, 114.

61. Allen 2013, 108. Earlier in his career, as an Oregon state senator, Kitzhaber had developed a plan prioritizing the state's Medicaid spending through an explicit process of ranking medical services based on their clinical effectiveness and net benefits. The goal was to expand the access of low-income citizens to health insurance while saving money by rationing care. But the program unraveled as a result of economic and budgetary pressures and eroding political support (see Oberlander 2007).

62. Allen 2013, 116.

63. Allen 2013, 115.

64. Pear 2003.

65. Unlike the Allen-Emerson bill, the Clinton proposal did not authorize cost-effectiveness research, only comparative effectiveness studies.

66. Confidential interview with congressional staff member.

67. Congressional Record, June 25, 2003, S8529.

68. Ashton and Wray 2013.

69. In the late 1990s, pharmaceuticals were one of the fastest growing components of national health care spending (Oberlander 2003). An explosion of new drugs for treating arthritis, heart disease, and many other conditions had emerged on the market. Eight in ten seniors took medications, each getting an average of twenty prescriptions filled per year (Oberlander 2003). Yet the original Medicare benefit package did not cover outpatient prescription drugs, creating a widening gap between Medicare and the standards of private insurance plans. In the 2000 presidential campaign, all the major candidates endorsed some version of a Medicare prescription drug benefit (Oliver, Lee, and Lipton 2004). For the winning presidential candidate, George W. Bush, adding an expensive prescription drug benefit was both clever politics and good policy. By signing onto an expansion of the Medicare benefit package, the Bush administration believed it could co-opt seniors and neutralize an issue that played to the advantage of the Democratic Party. In addition, the White House believed it could use a prescription drug coverage bill as a vehicle to restructure Medicare along conservative lines by increasing the role of market competition in the program (Oberlander 2012).

70. In a memo to members of Congress, the industry group also argued that federal studies would stymie innovation, inevitably influence private insurers, and in focusing on the benefits of drugs on the average patient, overlook the value of medicines for individuals or subgroups such as racial minorities (Pear 2003).

71. Ashton and Wray 2013.

72. Wilensky 2006.

73. Heritage Lectures 2007, 13.

74. CBO 2007b.

75. Suskind 2011, 140.

76. CBO 2007b, 1.

77. Cited in Carey 2007.

78. Subcommittee on Health, "Hearing on Strategies to Increase Information on Comparative Clinical Effectiveness," June 12, 2007. Serial No. 110-46. https://www.gpo.gov/fdsys/pkg/CHRG-110hhrg45994/html/CHRG-110hhrg45994.htm.

79. Ashton and Wray 2013, 165.

80. CBO letter to Pete Stark, September 5, 2007.

81. CBO 2007b.

82. Ashton and Wray 2013.

83. Confidential interview with congressional staff member.

84. McDonough 2012, 194.

85. Reichard 2007.

Notes to Chapter 6

1. McCarty, Poole, and Rosenthal 2008.

2. Binder 2003.

3. Lee 2009.

4. Stokes 1963; Lee 2009. Our argument here is complementary to Frances Lee's (2009) insightful argument that parties strategically exploit good government issues to embarrass opponents and burnish their own party's image. Whereas Lee highlights partisan behavior on valence issues, we focus on how partisanship creates incentives to transform valence issues into position issues.

5. See Druckman, Peterson, and Slothuus 2013.

6. Polsby 1985.

7. Heclo 1996, 23. Heclo uses the term "gestation" rather than incubation.

8. Polsby 1985.

9. R. Cobb, Ross, and Ross 1976.

10. Quoted in Patel 2010, 1778.

11. Quoted in Patel 2010, 1778.

12. Daschle et al. 2008.

13. Orszag 2010, A39.

14. Orszag 2014.

15. Mooney 2005.

16. See Tierney 2016.

17. Quoted in Volsky 2009.

18. Quoted in Volsky 2009.

19. Chalkidou et al. 2009, 363.

20. Quoted in Iglehart 2010, 1759.

21. Mayhew 2006.

22. Mayhew 2006, 220.

23. Zaller 1992.

24. Zaller 1992. The Zaller model of elite opinion leadership should not be understood to suggest that citizens should never reject elite cues. As Jennifer Hochschild points out in a thoughtful essay, whether public followership is normatively desirable or undesirable depends on whether leaders' empirical claims are empirically supported and morally justified. For example, one wishes, in retrospect, that the mass public had not followed elite leadership on the need for Jim Crow laws; conversely, there are strong reasons to wish that more of the public would accept the elite scientific consensus on global warming (Hochschild 2013).

25. Lee 2009.

26. Petrocik 1996.

27. A rebuttable implication of our argument is that Republicans will soften their opposition to CER if and when the electoral incentives surrounding health reform changes. While a wholesale shift in the GOP position seems unlikely until the legislative fate of the ACA is completely settled, early signs have been interesting. When the Republicans took back the House in 2010, the new chairman of the Oversight Committee, Darrell Issa (R-CA) told the *Wall Street Journal* that Republicans should talk less about death panels and focus more on reducing the overuse of expensive medical procedures. Issa said that his own doctor told him that spine surgeons have an incentive under Medicare to implant joint and bone screws to support patients' spines, when fewer implants would be equally effective. Issa even praised having some form of CER board: "Medical panels of people who care about what's best for their patients . . . is good science and good medicine. . . . Republicans have to step back from the words 'death panels,'" he said (quoted in Mundy 2010).

28. Pear 2009b.

29. Gimpel, Lee, and Thorpe 2012, 582.

30. Alonso-Zaldivar 2008.

31. Confidential interview with Republican congressional staff member.

32. Fiorina 2006, 250.

33. Quoted in Grunwald 2012, 173.

34. Ashton and Wray 2013.

35. Quoted in Levey 2009. In fact, ambitious reform ideas for linking evidence to cost control were percolating, such as HHS secretary nominee Daschle's proposal to deny federal tax benefits to private insurers that failed to comply with a board's recommendations (Daschle et al. 2008, 179).

36. Quoted in Edney 2009. Representative Emerson, who had introduced CER legislation in previous Congresses with Tom Allen, stated that she did not support the stimulus language (Edney 2009).

37. The CBO reinforced the view that CER was unlikely to significantly increase spending on effective but underused treatments because "current incentives already favor the adoption and spread of more-expensive treatments, so new research that found those treatments to be more effective or more cost effective would probably increase their use only modestly" (2007b, 29).

38. Quoted in Ashton and Wray 2013, 193.

39. McCaughey 2009.

40. Pear 2009b.

41. The Senate Appropriations Committee even tried to address concerns that research would be used for cost-effectiveness analysis by placing the word "clinical" before every mention of comparative effectiveness research, but the final version did not include this change.

42. Quoted in Ashton and Wray 2013, 195.

43. Authors' calculations based on Lexis/Nexis data.

44. For a political history and analysis of the ACA, see L. Jacobs and Skocpol 2010; and Starr 2011.

45. Quoted in Leonhardt 2009, MM36.

46. Grunwald 2012, 442.

47. Patel 2010.

48. Quoted in McDonough 2012, 195.

49. Patel 2010, 1779–80.

50. See, e.g., Selker and Wood 2009.

51. Pew Research Center 2009.

52. Stein and Eggen 2009.

53. Ashton and Wray 2013, 202.

54. PCORI 2010.

55. Sox 2012, 2176.

56. Section 937(a)(2)(B) with the PPACA statute.

57. For an excellent discussion of PCORI's authorizing language, structure, and financing, see Ashton and Wray 2013, chapter 10.

58. Quoted in Iglehart 2010, 1759.

59. Quoted in Iglehart 2010, 1759.

60. Ashton and Wray 2013, 213.

61. Bagley 2013, 574.

62. Stokes 1963.

63. Zaller 1992.

64. Nicholson 2012; Green, Palmquist, and Schickler 2002.

65. Levendusky 2010, 114–15. In addition to cues from polarized leaders, the effort to cultivate enlightened public opinion is undermined by "motivated reasoning"—the tendency of people "to seek out information that confirms prior beliefs (i.e., a confirmation bias), view evidence consistent with prior opinions as stronger or more effective (i.e., a prior attitude effect), and spend more time arguing and dismissing evidence inconsistent with prior opinions, regardless of objective accuracy (i.e., a disconfirmation bias)" (Druckman, Peterson, and Slothuus 2013, 59).

66. Lenz 2012.

67. Fiorina and Abrams 2008, 581.

68. Or, in addition, consider net favorability ratings of Russian president Vladimir Putin. According to YouGov/Economist polls, from July 2014 to December 2016 Putin's net favorability among Republicans rose 56 points (from −66 to −10); during the same timeframe, Putin's net favorability among Democrats dropped by 8 points (from −54 to −62). During that time, Republican presidential candidate, and subsequently president-elect, Donald Trump spoke highly of Putin.

69. Dunlap and McCright 2008, 27.

70. Dunlap and McCright 2008, 27.

71. McCright and Dunlap 2011.

72. All bivariate relationships discussed in this chapter are statistically significant ($p < .05$), unless otherwise noted. The relationships we discuss are also statistically significant in multivariate analysis controlling for turnout, party identification, age, education, and race as well as income and gender. Exceptions are noted.

73. Race indicators are not jointly significant in multivariate analysis.

74. This survey was conducted as part of the 2014 Cooperative Congressional Election Study (CCES) on Yale University's private team content (Gerber 2014).

75. An alternative explanation is simply that public awareness of the CER concept, which was originally opaque to the general public and therefore led to undifferentiated survey responses among non-voters in 2010, grew by 2014 to the point that the CER concept was more understandable to the general public. We thank Mark Schlesinger for this point.

76. Interestingly, support for CER among Independents also increases with the Obamacare reference (from 54.7 to 60.1, a 10 percent increase).

77. This drop in support is even more pronounced among self-reported voters from the Republican Party (from 53.6 to 41.6, a 22 percent decrease).

Notes to Conclusion

1. This chapter discusses the political challenge of endowing EBM reforms with durability. It does not provide a policy analysis of specific reform options. For an excellent discussion of the case for the kind of reforms we believe are needed—such as strengthening the Medicare coverage process to reduce or eliminate funding on low-value treatments—see Bagley, Chandra, and Frakt 2015.

2. Amitabh Chandra states: "PCORI may do good work occasionally, but they're not cost-effective. We've not learnt much relative to the $$$ they receive." https://twitter.com/amitabhchandra2/status/798993185682821120.

3. The ACA does not explicitly prohibit the consideration of costs; rather, it forbids PCORI from using a dollar per QALY (quality-adjusted life year) metric "as a threshold" for establishing cost-effectiveness or for making recommendations.

4. Quoted in Longman 2013, 22–23.

5. Gray, Gusmano, and Collins 2003.

6. Wilensky 2006, w579.

7. McGinn 2015, 2.

8. Jerry Avorn 2011; McCulloch et al. 2013; Reames, Shubeck, and Birkmeyer 2014.

9. Schlesinger and Grob 2017, 70.

10. Goldberg et al. 2001.

11. M. Rodwin 2001; Swenson n.d.

12. Patashnik 2008.

13. Kaufman 1976, 64.

14. Berry, Burden, and Howell 2010.

15. Bimber 1996; Sorenson, Gusmano, and Oliver 2014.

16. Patashnik 2008.

17. On policy sustainability, see Heclo 1998.

18. Maltzman and Shipan 2012. Of course, it is also important to examine the direction of postenactment policy change, not merely its existence. Some amendments are friendly, while others weaken preexisting statutes.

19. Mayhew 2012, 263.

20. Skocpol 1992; Pierson 1995.

21. Mayhew 2012, 263.

22. Bagley 2013.

23. Campbell 2005.

24. Patashnik 2008.

25. Patashnik and Zelizer 2013; Oberlander and Weaver 2015.

26. This is not to suggest that diffuse-benefit reforms can never become self-reinforcing. The key point is that the direct beneficiaries of such policies will rarely develop into an effective organizational force because the per capita stakes are too small. When such policies *do* generate positive feedback, it is typically either because they bring about institutional shifts that privilege common interests or because they produce substantial resources for service providers that obtain an incentive to protect their "spoils" (Patashnik and Zelizer 2013).

27. Patashnik 2008.

28. Patashnik 2008; Moe 2015.

29. Levine 2006; Patashnik 2008.

30. Ironically, the criticisms against CER and PCORI were reinforced in 2015 when the Obama administration announced a new Precision Medicine Initiative to advance medical research that takes into account the specific characteristics of individuals, such as a person's genetic makeup or the genetic profile of an individual tumor. While CER and precision medicine *should* be mutually reinforcing—both are intended to ensure that patients receive the treatments that work best—the administration defended its new initiative by focusing on the need to avoid "one-size-fits-all" medicine. This is precisely the language that critics have used to attack CER (see http://www.whitehouse.gov/the-press-office/2015/01/30/fact-sheet-president-obama-s -precision-medicine-initiative).

31. Sedensky and Alonso-Zaldivar 2015.

32. The Independent Payment Advisory Board (IPAB) was established as an institution to constrain Medicare spending. Congress must consider Medicare reforms proposed by the board under special fast-track legislative rules, including limits on debate, designed to ensure speedy action. If Congress does not enact legislation containing those proposals or alternative policies that achieve the same savings, the IPAB's recommendations go into effect. Republicans and some Democrats have argued that IPAB represents an unacceptable delegation of legislative authority to an unelected body. Six years after the passage of the ACA, Congress had not appointed any members to IPAB's board, and President Obama had not nominated anyone. It remains to be seen whether IPAB will endure and shape health policy—or become an irrelevancy (Oberlander 2016).

33. Keller et al. 2015.

34. Keller et al. 2015.

35. Brill 2015, 139; see also Patel 2010; Longman 2013. The ACA does not prohibit Medicare from using CER, but it limits how study results can be used. Specifically, the CMS is allowed under the ACA to use CER to make a determination concerning Medicare coverage if (1) such use is through an iterative and transparent process and (2) a determination to deny Medicare coverage for a product or service is not based solely on CER. In addition, the ACA does not prohibit PCORI from considering costs. Rather, the statute forbids PCORI from using a dollar per quality-adjusted life year metric "as a threshold" for establishing cost-effectiveness or for making recommendations.

36. Orren and Skowronek 2004.

37. We avoid entering into the debate over whether agencies like the FDA were at their birth (or later became) "captured" by drug companies seeking to use government regulations to limit entry and preserve market power (Stigler 1971). Our claim here is simply that an indicator (and cause) of policy sustainability is compatibility between a policy's goals and the identities, interests, and incentives of firms subject to the policy's mandates. On theories of regulatory capture and the FDA, see D. Carpenter 2013.

38. Abrams 2012.

39. Abrams 2012.

40. Mahinka 2013, 19–20.

41. Mahinka 2013, 20.

42. Mahinka 2013, 20.

43. Temple 2012, 56.

44. Mahinka 2013, 19.

45. For a more optimistic view, see Robinson 2015.

46. Swenson n.d.

47. McCubbins, Noll, and Weingast 1989.

48. Lewis 2012.

49. Moe 1989.

50. D. P. Carpenter 2001, 359.

51. Eskridge and Ferejohn 2013, 190.

52. Moe 1989.

53. To be sure, scholars recognized during the 1980s and 1990s that political deals could be undermined by future Congresses (this risk is known as "legislative drift") as well as by the bureaucracy ("agency drift"). Nonetheless, the assumption was that the original bargain had a reasonable level of support in the enacting Congress; there was little discussion of the sustainability risks put into play when ambitious laws pass by razor-thin, partisan majorities. On legislative drift and agency drift, see Shepsle 1992.

54. Lee 2009.

55. Berry, Burden, and Howell 2010.

56. Millenson 2015.

57. Patashnik 2015.

58. Wilson 1989.

59. D. Carpenter 2010, 33.

60. D. Carpenter 2010.

61. The FDA's reputation has however been tarnished in recent years as a result of scandals, including its failure to quickly recall the arthritis drug Vioxx (Teles 2010).

62. Teles 2010, 49.

63. Tanden et al. 2014. The American Enterprise Institute had an even less forgiving assessment. "PCORI has attracted a skilled leadership team that rivals many similar private institutions. But even with its talent, and its $3.5 billion, ten-year trust fund . . . PCORI never had enough resources to fund the rigorous kinds of clinical trials that would actually inspire change in clinical practice. It never aimed to make grants on a scale to accomplish this mission. [Its] proponents and opponents alike didn't want it to. Proponents didn't really want definitive clinical answers, just policy screeds that government payers could peg decisions to. And opponents didn't really want to see it work at all" (Gottlieb 2014).

64. Tanden et al. 2014. PCORI disputed these conclusions. See http://www.pcori.org /content/statement-pcori-executive-director-joe-selby-md-mph-following-center-american -progress-event.

65. See Emanuel, Spiro, and Huelskoetter 2016.

66. Rice 2015.

67. PCORI, "Comparison of Peer-Facilitated Support Group and Cognitive Support Group and Cognitive Behavioral Therapy for Hoarding Disorder."

68. NPC 2015.

69. Quoted in Schulte 2015.

70. Ashton and Wray 2013.

71. PCORI 2013, 2.

72. Sox 2012, 2181.

73. Selby 2014.

74. Klein 2010.

75. Skocpol 2003.

76. Moore 2015. See also Carpenter's thoughtful remarks at a New America Foundation panel: https://www.youtube.com/watch?v=8vGusVXMgxY.

77. Finegold and Skocpol 1995.

78. Twedt 2016.

79. J. Avorn 2009.

80. Dayoub 2014.

81. Indeed, it is worth noting that the AHRQ back surgery study that generated such controversy was carried out through one of the agency's Patient Outcomes Research Teams (PORTs), multidisciplinary centers that focused on particular medical problems and reviews (see Gray, Gusmano, and Collins 2003). However, PORTs were fragmented and not closely tied to specific hospitals and medical centers. We are imagining locally based centers that would have stronger network ties to politicians and offer attractive credit-claiming opportunities.

Notes to Appendix to Chapter 3

1. There is a general professional consensus, supported by the findings of the Institute of Medicine (IOM), that physicians lack adequate information on the relative effectiveness of different treatment modalities (see AMA 2011). However, some doctors may be wary of CER for conceptual reasons, believing that studies focus on "average" treatment effects and miss the idiosyncratic ways in which an intervention works for a particular subgroup of patients. In addition, physicians who earn a significant portion of their income from performing a given procedure may fail to "implement the results of a study that found the procedure to be no better than a less costly or safer alternative" (J. Avorn and Fischer 2010, 1894).

These diverging possibilities are reflected in both the opinions of individual doctors and the formal statements of major physician associations. For example, a survey of physician opinion found that more than half of physicians agree that having more hard data would improve the quality of care, but that two-thirds are concerned that CER will be used to restrict their freedom to select treatments for their patients (Keyhani, Woodward, and Federman 2010; also see Ray and Sokolovsky 2009). A 2011 survey of primary care physicians and specialists found seven out of ten doctors believe that implementing CER will be made difficult by conflict between clinical effectiveness and cost-effectiveness (Deloitte 2011). And while groups such as the AMA have released official statements expressing support for CER, these endorsements are contingent on the CER agency maintaining "physician discretion in the treatment of individual patients" (AMA 2011). A 2012 letter from two former AMA presidents to the director of PCORI stated, "Physicians have always been hopeful that CER will be done in ways that actually support us in making decisions with our patients. But at the same time we've been deeply concerned that the research could easily be skewed towards a government cost-cutting agenda and misused in ways that come between doctors and patients" (Coalition to Protect Patients' Rights 2011).

Similar concerns that CER will lead to government interference with the doctor-patient relationship were raised in a statement from a Tennessee oncologist: "Comparative effectiveness research done right is a good thing for our country's health care system. However, when the government begins telling physicians what medicines they should or should not prescribe, ultimately it's the patient who suffers" (Patton 2013). The American Academy of Orthopaedic Surgeons (AAOS) and other doctors' groups have given CER similarly qualified endorsements (AAOS 2009). Because levels of support for the implementation of CER among both individual doctors and medical associations remain in flux, it is important to understand how changes in the public positions such actors and groups adopt—including whether they adopt a position at all—may affect public support for CER.

2. The outcome measure was respondents' support for a policy that would "allow the government and insurance companies to refuse payment for treatments or procedures if their effectiveness has not been demonstrated by rigorous scientific evidence" and was measured using a 100-point sliding scale ranging from "strongly oppose" (0) to "strongly support" (100) where the midpoint of the scale indicated that respondents "neither support nor oppose this policy."

3. These nine conditions were randomly assigned with equal probability, except that 20 percent of respondents were randomly assigned to receive no group cue and every other condition (e.g., leading doctors oppose) was assigned to 10 percent of respondents.

4. In this experiment we did assign respondents to the condition in which neither a political cue nor a group cue was provided.

5. The 5.4 net difference between leading doctors support (48.1) and leading doctors oppose (42.7) in column F is also statistically significant ($p=.07$).

6. The difference between the support and opposition of high-level government administrators is also statistically significant in column F ($p=.07$), whereas the difference between the support and opposition of top drug companies in column F is not ($p=.32$).

7. Aggregate public support for the proposal is also not significantly affected by the support of both parties ($p=.30$) or the support of Republicans and opposition of Democrats ($p=.48$).

BIBLIOGRAPHY

AAOS (American Academy of Orthopaedic Surgeons). 2002. "Arthroscopic Surgery and Osteoarthritis of the Knee." Decision memo for arthroscopy for the osteoarthritic knee (CAG-00167N). A report for the Centers for Medicare and Medicaid Services, Coverage Analysis Group. https://www.cms.gov/medicare-coverage-database/details/nca-decision-memo.aspx?NCAId=7&fromdb=true.

———. 2009. "American Academy of Orthopaedic Surgeons Position Statement 1178." June. http://www6.aaos.org/news/PDFopen/PDFopen.cfm?page_url=http://www.aaos.org/about/papers/position/1178.asp. Accessed September 13, 2012.

———. 2013a. "Five Things Physicians and Patients Should Question." Choosing Wisely, An Initiative of the ABIM Foundation. September 11. http://www.choosingwisely.org/societies/american-academy-of-orthopaedic-surgeons/.

———. 2013b. "We Cannot Recommend Performing Arthroscopy with Lavage and/or Debridement in Patients with a Primary Diagnosis of Symptomatic Osteoarthritis of the Knee." https://aaos.webauthor.com/go/cpg/detail.cfm?id=1217.

AAPOR Executive Council Task Force. 2010. "Research Synthesis: AAPOR Report on Online Panels." *Public Opinion Quarterly* 74 (4): 711–81.

Aaron, Henry J., and Paul B. Ginsburg. 2009. "Is Health Spending Excessive? If So, What Can We Do about It?" *Health Affairs* 28 (5): 1260–75. doi:10.1377/hlthaff.28.5.1260.

Abbott, Andrew Delano. 1988. *The System of Professions: An Essay on the Division of Expert Labor*. Chicago: University of Chicago Press.

Abelson, Reed, and Eric Lichtblau. 2014. "Pervasive Medicare Fraud Proves Hard to Stop." *New York Times*, August 15. https://www.nytimes.com/2014/08/16/business/uncovering-health-care-fraud-proves-elusive.html?_r=0.

ABIM Foundation. 2005. "Medical Professionalism in the New Millennium: A Physician Charter." http://abimfoundation.org/wp-content/uploads/2015/12/Medical-Professionalism-in-the-New-Millenium-A-Physician-Charter.pdf.

Ablin, Richard J. 2010. "The Great Prostate Mistake." *New York Times*, March 9. http://www.nytimes.com/2010/03/10/opinion/10Ablin.html.

Abrams, Michael N. 2012. "Pharma's Stake in Comparative Effectiveness Research." *Pharmaceutical Commerce*, December 30. http://pharmaceuticalcommerce.com/opinion/pharmas-stake-in-comparative-effectiveness-research/.

Abramson, J. 2008. *Overdosed America: The Broken Promise of American Medicine*. New York: HarperCollins.

Acemoglu, Daron, and James A. Robinson. 2012. *Why Nations Fail: The Origins of Power, Prosperity, and Poverty*. New York: Crown.

AETNA. 2003. "Osteoarthritis of the Knee: Selected Treatments." Last modified January 25, 2017. http://www.aetna.com/cpb/medical/data/600_699/0673.html.

Allen, Tom. 2013. *Dangerous Convictions: What's Really Wrong with the U.S. Congress.* Oxford: Oxford University Press.

Alonso-Zaldivar, Ricardo. 2008. "The Bean Counter Will See You Now." *Los Angeles Times*, June 9. http://articles.latimes.com/2008/jun/09/nation/na-costs9.

AMA (American Medical Association). 2011. "Comparative Effectiveness Research." http://www.ama-assn.org/ama1/pub/upload/mm/399/hsr-comparative-effectiveness.pdf. Accessed August 1, 2011.

Angell, Marcia. 2004. *The Truth about the Drug Companies: How They Deceive Us and What to Do about It.* New York: Random House.

Ansolabehere, Stephen, Shigeo Hirano, James M. Snyder, and Michiko Ueda. 2006. "Party and Incumbency Cues in Voting: Are They Substitutes?" *Quarterly Journal of Political Science* 1 (2): 119–37.

Anthony, Denise L., M. Brooke Herndon, Patricia M. Gallagher, Amber E. Barnato, Julie P. W. Bynum, Daniel J. Gottlieb, Elliott S. Fisher, and Jonathan S. Skinner. 2009. "How Much Do Patients' Preferences Contribute to Resource Use?" *Health Affairs* 28 (3): 864–73. doi:10.1377/hlthaff.28.3.864.

Arnold, R. Douglas. 1990. *The Logic of Congressional Action.* New Haven, CT: Yale University Press. http://www.jstor.org/stable/j.ctt32bm5b.

Arrow, Kenneth Joseph. 1963. "Uncertainty and the Welfare Economics of Medical Care." *American Economic Review* 53 (5): 941–73.

"Arthroscopic Surgery for Osteoarthritis of the Knee." Multiple letters: Jackson, Robert W.; Ewing, Whit; Ewing, John W.; Chambers, Keith G.; Schulzer, Michael; Blacher, Richard S.; Morse, Leonard J.; Wray, Nelda P.; Moseley, J. Bruce; O'Malley, Kimberly; Horng, Sam; Miller, Franklin G. 2002. *New England Journal of Medicine* 347 (21): 1717–19.

Ashton, Carol M., Nancy J. Petersen, Julianne Souchek, Terri J. Menke, Hong-Jen Yu, Kenneth Pietz, Marsha L. Eigenbrodt, Galen Barbour, Kenneth W. Kizer, and Nelda P. Wray. 1999. "Geographic Variations in Utilization Rates in Veterans Affairs Hospitals and Clinics." *New England Journal of Medicine* 340 (1): 32–39.

Ashton, Carol M., and Nelda P. Wray. 2013. *Comparative Effectiveness Research: Evidence, Medicine, and Policy.* Oxford: Oxford University Press.

Avorn, J. 2005. *Powerful Medicines: The Benefits, Risk and Costs of Prescription Drugs.* New York: Vintage.

———. 2009. "Debate about Funding Comparative Effectiveness Research." *New England Journal of Medicine* 360 (19): 1927–29.

Avorn, J., and M. Fischer. 2010. "'Bench to Behavior': Translating Comparative Effectiveness Research into Improved Clinical Practice." *Health Affairs* 29 (10): 1891–900.

Avorn, Jerry. 2005. "FDA Standards—Good Enough for Government Work?" *New England Journal of Medicine* 353 (10): 969–72. doi:10.1056/NEJMp058174.

———. 2011. "Teaching Clinicians about Drugs—50 Years Later, Whose Job Is It?" *New England Journal of Medicine* 364 (13): 1185–87.

Avorn, Jerry, and Aaron S. Kesselheim. 2015. "The 21st Century Cures Act—Will It Take Us Back in Time?" *New England Journal of Medicine* 372 (26): 2473–75.

Avorn, Jerry, and Aaron S. Kesselheim. 2017. "The 21st Century Cures Legislation: Speed and Ease vs. Science." *JAMA* 317 (6): 581–82.

Azvolinsky, Anna. 2015. "PSA Screening for Prostate Cancer Declined in Men Over 50." *Cancer Network*, June 15. http://www.cancernetwork.com/prostate-cancer/psa-screening-prostate-cancer-declined-men-over-50.

Bach, Peter B. 2012. "The Trouble with 'Doctor Knows Best.'" *New York Times*, June 4. http://www.nytimes.com/2012/06/05/health/views/essay-urging-doctors-to-do-less-may-fall-on-deaf-ears.html.

Bagley, Nicholas. 2013. "Bedside Bureaucrats: Why Medicare Reform Hasn't Worked." *Georgetown Law Journal* 101 (3): 519–80.

Bagley, Nicholas, Amitabh Chandra, and Austin Frakt. 2015. "Correcting Signals for Innovation in Health Care. Hamilton Project. http://www.hamiltonproject.org/assests/files/correcting _signals_for_innovation_in_health care_bagley.pdf.

Bahr, Daniel, and Thomas Huelskoetter. 2014. "Comparing the Effectiveness of Prescription Drugs: The German Experience." *Center for American Progress*, May 21. https://www .americanprogress.org/issues/healthcare/reports/2014/05/21/90120/comparing-the -effectiveness-of-prescription-drugs-the-german-experience/.

Baker, Laurence C., M. Kate Bundorf, and Daniel P. Kessler. 2014. "Patients' Preferences Explain a Small but Significant Share of Regional Variation in Medicare Spending." *Health Affairs* 33 (6): 957–63. doi:10.1377/hlthaff.2013.1184.

Balas, E. Andrew. 1998. "From Appropriate Care to Evidence-Based Medicine." *Pediatric Annals* 27 (9): 581–4.

Barabas, Jason, and Jennifer Jerit. 2010. "Are Survey Experiments Externally Valid?" *American Political Science Review* 104 (2): 226–42.

Baumgartner, Frank R., and Bryan D. Jones. 1993. *Agendas and Instability in American Politics.* American Politics and Political Economy Series. Chicago: University of Chicago Press.

Baumol, William J. 2010. *The Microtheory of Innovative Entrepreneurship.* Kauffman Foundation Series on Innovation and Entrepreneurship. Princeton, NJ: Princeton University Press.

Beane, Billy, Newt Gingrich, and John Kerry. 2008. "How to Take American Health Care from Worst to First." *New York Times*, October 24. http://www.nytimes.com/2008/10/24 /opinion/24beane.html.

Belkin, Gary S. 1997. "The Technocratic Wish: Making Sense and Finding Power in the "Managed" Medical Marketplace." *Journal of Health Politics, Policy and Law* 22 (2): 509–32.

———. 1998. "The Technocratic Wish: Making Sense and Finding Power in the "Managed" Medical Marketplace." In *Healthy Markets? The New Competition in Medicare Care*, ed. Mark A. Peterson, 140–60. Durham, NC: Duke University Press.

Belluck, Pam. 2013. "Common Knee Surgery Does Very Little for Some, Study Suggests." *New York Times*, December 25. http://www.nytimes.com/2013/12/26/health/common-knee -surgery-does-very-little-for-some-study-suggests.html?pagewanted=all.

Benen, Steve. 2010. "Brains on Drugs." *Washington Monthly*, April 28. http://washingtonmonthly .com/2010/04/28/brains-on-drugs/.

Bernstein, J., and T. Quach. 2003. "A Perspective on the Study of Moseley et al.: Questioning the Value of Arthroscopic Knee Surgery for Osteoarthritis." *Cleveland Clinic Journal of Medicine*, 401, 405–6, 408–10. http://www.ncbi.nlm.nih.gov/pubmed/12779130.

Berry, Christopher R., Barry C. Burden, and William G. Howell. 2010. "After Enactment: The Lives and Deaths of Federal Programs." *American Journal of Political Science* 54 (1): 1–17. doi:10.1111/j.1540-5907.2009.00414.x.

Berwick, D. M., and A. D. Hackbarth. 2012. "Eliminating Waste in US Health Care." *JAMA* 307 (14): 1513–16. doi:10.1001/jama.2012.362.

Bevan, Gillian, and Michelle Brown. 2014. "Interventions in Exclusive Breastfeeding: A Systematic Review." *British Journal of Nursing* 23 (2): 86–89. doi:10.12968/bjon.2014.23.2.86.

Bhatia, Sanjeev. 2014. "Arthroscopic Meniscectomy 'Sham Surgery' Paper Presentation Spurs Debate at AAOS." *Healio Orthopedicstoday*, March 17. http://www.healio.com/orthopedics /sports-medicine/news/online/%7B7a7cb3aa-e09d-4ecd-9cc5-40cf100d6cad%7D /arthroscopic-meniscectomy-sham-surgery-paper-presentation-spurs-debate-at-aaos.

Bimber, Bruce Allen. *The Politics of Expertise in Congress: The Rise and Fall of the Office of Technology Assessment.* Albany: State University of New York Press, 1996.

Binder, Sarah A. 2003. *Stalemate: Causes and Consequences of Legislative Gridlock*. Washington, DC: Brookings Institution Press.

Blendon, Robert J., John M. Benson, Michael D. Botta, Deborah Zeldow, and Minah Kang Kim. 2012. "A Four-Country Survey of Public Attitudes towards Restricting Healthcare Costs by Limiting the Use of High-Cost Medical Interventions." *British Medical Journal Open* 2: e001087. doi:10.1136/bmjopen-2012-001087.

Blendon, Robert J., John M. Benson, Gillian K. SteelFisher, and John M. Connolly. 2010. "Americans' Conflicting Views about the Public Health System, and How to Shore Up Support." *Health Affairs* 29 (11): 2033–40. doi:10.1377/hlthaff.2010.0262.

Blendon, Robert J., Mollyann Brodie, John Benson, and Drew E. Altman. 2010. *American Public Opinion and Health Care*. CQ Press.

Blendon, Robert J., Mollyann Brodie, John M. Benson, Drew E. Altman, and Tami Buhr. 2006. "Americans' Views of Health Care Costs, Access, and Quality." *Milbank Quarterly* 84 (4): 623–57.

Blendon, Robert J., Karen Donelan, Robert Leitman, Arnold Epstein, Joel C. Cantor, Alan B. Cohen, Ian Morrison, Thomas Moloney, Christian Koeck, and Samuel W. Levitt. 1993. "Physicians' Perspectives on Caring for Patients in the United States, Canada, and West Germany." *New England Journal of Medicine* 328 (14): 1011–16.

Blendon, Robert J., Tracey Stelzer Hyams, and John M. Benson. 1993. "Bridging the Gap between Expert and Public Views on Health Care Reform." *Journal of the American Medical Association* 269 (19): 2573–78.

Blendon, Robert J., Minah Kim, and John M. Benson. 2001. "The Public versus the World Health Organization on Health System Performance." *Health Affairs* 20 (3): 10–20. doi:10.1377/hlthaff.20.3.10.

Blumenthal, David. 1983. "Federal Policy toward Health Care Technology: The Case of the National Center." *Milbank Memorial Fund Quarterly: Health and Society* 61 (4): 584–612.

———. 2014. "Realizing the Rewards of a Medical Career in a Changing Health Care System." *Commonwealth Fund Blog*, June 13. http://www.commonwealthfund.org/publications/blog/2014/jun/medical-career.

Blumenthal, David, and David Squires. 2014. "Drugs and Dollars." *Commonwealth Fund Blog*, July 28. http://www.commonwealthfund.org/publications/blog/2014/jul/drugs-and-dollars.

Bonica, Adam, Howard Rosenthal, and David J. Rothman. 2014. "The Political Polarization of Physicians in the United States: An Analysis of Campaign Contributions to Federal Elections, 1991 through 2012." *JAMA Internal Medicine* 174 (8): 1308–17.

Bradley, Elizabeth H., Jeph Herrin, Jennifer A. Mattera, Eric S. Holmboe, Yongfei Wang, Paul Frederick, Sarah A. Roumanis, Martha J. Radford, and Harlan M. Krumholz. 2005. "Quality Improvement Efforts and Hospital Performance: Rates of Beta-Blocker Prescription after Acute Myocardial Infarction." *Medical Care* 43 (3): 282–92.

Brehm, Jack W., and David Lipsher. 1959. "Communicator-Communicatee Discrepancy and Perceived Communicator Trustworthiness." *Journal of Personality* 27 (3): 352–61.

Brill, Steven. 2015. *America's Bitter Pill: Money, Politics, Backroom Deals, and the Fight to Fix Our Broken Healthcare System*. New York: Random House.

Brody, Jane. 1979. "Consensus Program Praised by Doctors; Panels Evaluate Technologies and Practices That Affect Health of Millions of Americans." *New York Times*, September 23. http://www.nytimes.com/1979/09/23/archives/consensus-program-praised-by-doctors-panels-evaluate-technologies.html.

Brown, David. 1995. "Small Agency Is a Target in Budgeting." *New York Times*, April 16, p. 17.

———. 2011. "'Comparative Effectiveness Research' Tackles Medicine's Unanswered Questions." *Washington Post Blog*, August 15. https://www.washingtonpost.com/national/health

-science/comparative-effectiveness-research-tackles-medicines-unanswered-questions
/2011/08/01/gIQA7RJSHJ_story.html.

Brownlee, Shannon. 2008. *Overtreated: Why Too Much Medicine Is Making Us Sicker and Poorer.* New York: Bloomsbury USA.

Brownlee, Shannon, Christine Cassel, and Vikas Saini. 2014. "When More Is Less: Overuse of Medical Services Harms Patients." In *Meeting the Needs of Older Adults with Serious Illness,* edited by Amy S. Kelley and Diane E. Meier, 3–18. New York: Springer.

Buchbinder, Rachelle, Richard H. Osborne, Peter R. Ebeling, John D. Wark, Peter Mitchell, Chris Wriedt, Stephen Graves, Margaret P. Staples, and Bridie Murphy. 2009. "A Randomized Trial of Vertebroplasty for Painful Osteoporotic Vertebral Fractures." *New England Journal of Medicine* 361 (6): 557–68. doi:10.1056/NEJMoa0900429.

Buhr, Tami, and Robert J. Blendon. 2011. "Trust in Government and Health Care Institutions." In *American Public Opinion and Health Care,* edited by R. J. Blendon, M. Brodie, J. M. Benson, and D. E. Altman, 15–38. Washington, DC: CQ Press.

Bunker, J. P., D. Hinkley, and W. V. McDermott. 1978. "Surgical Innovation and Its Evaluation." *Science* 200 (4344): 937–41. doi:10.1126/science.347581.

Burling, Stacey. 2002. "Is a Knee Operation Worth It? A Fake Surgery Did as Well for Patients with Arthritis." Philly.com, July 11. http://articles.philly.com/2002-07-11/news/25357065_1 _knee-replacement-placebo-surgery-fake-surgery.

Burman, M. S., Harry Finkelstein, and Leo Mayer. 1934. "Arthroscopy of the Knee Joint." *Journal of Bone and Joint Surgery* 16 (2): 255–68.

Callahan, Daniel. 2009. *Taming the Beloved Beast: How Medical Technology Costs Are Destroying Our Health Care System.* Princeton, NJ: Princeton University Press.

Campbell, Andrea Louise. 2005. *How Policies Make Citizens: Senior Political Activism and the American Welfare State.* Princeton, NJ: Princeton University Press.

Carey, John. 2006. "Medical Guesswork: From Heart Surgery to Prostate Care, the Health Industry Knows Little about Which Common Treatments Really Work." *Bloomberg Businessweek,* May 28. https://www.bloomberg.com/news/articles/2006-05-28/medical-guesswork.

Carey, Mary Agnes. 2007. "Allen, Emerson Introduce Comparative Effectiveness Bill." *Washington Health Policy Week in Review,* May 21. http://www.commonwealthfund.org/publications /newsletters/washington-health-policy-in-review/2007/may/washington-health-policy -week-in-review-may-21-2007/allen-emerson-introduce-comparative-effectiveness-bill.

Carman, Kristin L., Maureen Maurer, Jill Mathews Yegian, Pamela Dardess, Jeanne McGee, Mark Evers, and Karen O. Marlo. 2010. "Evidence That Consumers Are Skeptical about Evidence-Based Health Care." *Health Affairs* 29 (7): 1400–1406.

Carpenter, Daniel. 2010. *Reputation and Power: Organization Image and Pharmaceutical Regulation at the FDA.* Princeton, NJ: Princeton University Press.

———. 2012. "Is Health Politics Different?" *Annual Review of Political Science* 15: 287–311.

———. 2013. *Reputation and Power: Organizational Image and Pharmaceutical Regulation at the FDA.* Princeton, NJ: Princeton University Press.

Carpenter, Daniel, and A. M. Fendrick. 2004. "Accelerating Approval Times for New Drugs in the U.S." *Regulatory Affairs Journal—Pharma* 15 (6): 411–17.

Carpenter, Daniel P. 2001. *The Forging of Bureaucratic Autonomy: Reputations, Networks, and Policy Innovation in Executive Agencies, 1862–1928.* Princeton, NJ: Princeton University Press.

Carroll, Aaron E. 2014. "The Placebo Effect Doesn't Apply Just to Pills." Upshot, *New York Times,* October 6. https://www.nytimes.com/2014/10/07/upshot/the-placebo-effect-doesnt-apply -just-to-pills.html.

CBO (Congressional Budget Office). 2007a. "Letter to Honorable Pete Stark." *Congress of the United States, Congressional Budget Office,* September 5. https://www.cbo.gov/sites/default /files/110th-congress-2007-2008/reports/09-05-comparativeeffectiveness.pdf.

CBO (Congressional Budget Office). 2007b. "Research on the Comparative Effectiveness of Medical Treatments: Issues and Options for an Expanded Federal Role." *Congress of the United States, Congressional Budget Office*, December. https://www.cbo.gov/sites/default /files/110th-congress-2007-2008/reports/12-18-comparativeeffectiveness.pdf.

———. 2008. "Geographic Variation in Health Care Spending." *Congress of the United States, Congressional Budget Office*, February. https://www.cbo.gov/sites/default/files/110th . . . 2007 -2008/ . . . /02-15-geoghealth_0.pdf.

Chalkidou, Kalipso, Sean Tunis, Ruth Lopert, Lise Rochaix, Peter T Sawicki, Mona Nasser, and Bertrand Xerri. 2009. "Comparative Effectiveness Research and Evidence-Based Health Policy: Experience from Four Countries." *Milbank Quarterly* 87 (2): 339–67. doi:10.1111/j.1468-0009.2009.00560.x.

Chambers, James D., Matthew Chenoweth, Michael J. Cangelosi, Junhee Pyo, Joshua T. Cohen, and Peter J. Neumann. 2015. "Medicare Is Scrutinizing Evidence More Tightly for National Coverage Determinations." *Health Affairs* 34 (2): 253–60.

Chambers, James D., Matthew Chenoweth, Teja Thorat, and Peter J. Neumann. 2015. "Private Payers Disagree with Medicare over Medical Device Coverage about Half the Time." *Health Affairs* 34 (8): 1376–82. doi:10.1377/hlthaff.2015.0133.

Chandra, Amitabh, Amy Finkelstein, Adam Sacarny, and Chad Syverson. 2016. "Health Exceptionalism? Performance and Allocation in the US Health Care Sector." *American Economic Review* 106 (8): 2110–44. doi:10.1257/aer.20151080.

Chandra, Amitabh, Jonathan Holmes, and Jonathan Skinner. 2013. "Is This Time Different? The Slowdown in Health Care Spending." *Brookings Papers on Economic Activity* 2: 261–323.

Chandra, Amitabh, Anupam B. Jena, and Jonathan S. Skinner. 2011. "The Pragmatist's Guide to Comparative Effectiveness Research." *Journal of Economic Perspectives* 25 (2): 27–46.

CIGNA. 2004. "Cigna HealthCare Coverage Position 0032: Arthroscopic Lavage and Debridement of the Knee for the Treatment of Osteoarthritis." April 15. http://www.cigna .com/health/provider/medical/procedural/coverage_positions/medical/mm_0032 _coveragepositioncriteria_arthroscopic_lavage_and_debridement_for_knees.pdf.

Clemens, Jeffrey, and Joshua D. Gottlieb. 2013. "In the Shadow of a Giant: Medicare's Influence on Private Physician Payments." National Bureau of Economic Research. doi:10.3386/ w19503.

Clifton, Guy L. 2009. *Flatlined: Resuscitating American Medicine*. New Brunswick, NJ: Rutgers University Press.

CMS (Centers for Medicare and Medicaid Services). 2003. "Decision Memo for Arthroscopy for the Osteoarthritic Knee (CAG-00167N)." July 3. https://www.cms.gov/medicare-coverage -database/details/nca-decision-memo.aspx?NCAId=7&bc=ACAAAAAACAAAAA%3D %3D&.

Coalition to Protect Patients' Rights. 2011. "Letter from Former Presidents of the American Medical Association to PCORI Executive Director Joe Selby." February 27. http://www .protectpatientsrights.org/the-news/259-letter-from-former-presidents-of-the-american -medical-association-to-pcori-executive-directot-joseph-selby. Accessed September 17, 2012.

Cobb, Leonard A., George I. Thomas, David H. Dillard, K. Alvin Merendino, and Robert A. Bruce. 1959. "An Evaluation of Internal-Mammary-Artery Ligation by a Double-Blind Technic." *New England Journal of Medicine* 260 (22): 1115–18.

Cobb, Roger, Jennie-Keith Ross, and Marc Howard Ross. 1976. "Agenda Building as a Comparative Political Process." *American Political Science Review* 70 (1): 126–38.

Cobb, Roger W., and Charles D. Elder. 1983. *Participation in American Politics: The Dynamics of Agenda-Building*. 2nd ed. Baltimore: Johns Hopkins University Press.

Coburn, Tom, Joseph R. Antos, Grace-Marie Turner. 2007. "Competition: A Prescription for Health Care Transformation." Lecture 1030 on Health Care. Heritage Foundation, June 13. http://www.heritage.org/research/lecture/competition-a-prescription-for-health-care -transformation.

Cohen, Alan B., and Ruth S. Hanft, William E. Encinsoa, Stephanie M. Spernak, Shirley A. Stewart, and Catherine C. White. 2004. *Technology in American Health Care: Policy Directions for Effective Evaluation and Management*. Ann Arbor: University of Michigan Press.

Cohen, Joshua, Ashley Malins, and Zainab Shahpurwala. 2013. "Compared to US Practice, Evidence-Based Reviews in Europe Appear to Lead to Lower Prices for Some Drugs." *Health Affairs* 32 (4): 762–70.

Combs, David J. Y., and Peggy S. Keller. 2010. "Politicians and Trustworthiness: Acting Contrary to Self-Interest Enhances Trustworthiness." *Basic and Applied Social Psychology* 32 (4): 328–39.

Cooper, Zack, Stuart V. Craig, Martin Gaynor, and John Van Reenen. 2015. "The Price Ain't Right? Hospital Prices and Health Spending on the Privately Insured." No. w21815. National Bureau of Economic Research. http://www.nber.org/papers/w21815.

Cruess, Sylvia R., and Richard L Cruess. 2004. "Professionalism and Medicine's Social Contract with Society." *AMA Journal of Ethics* 6 (4). http://journalofethics.ama-assn.org/2004/04 /msoc1-0404.html.

Currie, Janet W., Bentley MacLeod, and Jessica Van Parys. 2016. "Provider Practice Style and Patient Health Outcomes: The Case of Heart Attacks." *Journal of Health Economics* 47 (May): 64–80. doi:10.1016/j.jhealeco.2016.01.013.

Cutler, David. 2013. "Why Does Health Care Cost So Much in America? Ask Harvard's David Cutler." *PBS NewsHour*, November 19. http://www.pbs.org/newshour/rundown/why-does -health-care-cost-so-much-in-america-ask-harvards-david-cutler/.

Cutler, David M. 2005. *Your Money or Your Life*. New York: Oxford University Press.

———. 2014a. *The Quality Cure: How Focusing on Health Care Quality Can Save Your Life and Lower Spending Too*. Berkeley: University of California Press.

———. 2014b. "Who Benefits from Health System Change?" *JAMA* 312 (16): 1639–41. doi:10.1001/jama.2014.13491.

Cutler, David, Jonathan Skinner, Ariel Dora Stern, and David Wennberg. 2017. "Physician Beliefs and Patient Preferences: A New Look at Regional Variation in Health Care Spending." NBER Working Paper no. 19320. http://www.nber.org/papers/w19320.

Cutler, David M., and Dan P. Ly. 2011. "The (Paper)Work of Medicine: Understanding International Medical Costs." *Journal of Economic Perspectives* 25 (2): 3–25.

Dahl, Robert A. 1961. *Who Governs? Democracy and Power in an American City*. New Haven, CT: Yale University Press.

Daschle, Tom, Scott S. Greenberger, and Jeanne M. Lambrew. 2008. *Critical: What We Can Do about the Health-Care Crisis*. New York: Thomas Dunne Books.

Davis, Karen, Kristof Stremikis, David Squires, and Cathy Schoen. 2014. "Mirror, Mirror on the Wall, 2014 Update: How the U.S. Health Care System Compares Internationally." *Commonwealth Fund*, June. http://www.commonwealthfund.org/publications/fund-reports/2014 /jun/mirror-mirror.

Dawes, P. T., C. Kirlew, and I. Haslock. 1987. "Saline Washout for Knee Osteoarthritis: Results of a Controlled Study." *Clinical Rheumatology* 6 (1): 61–63. doi:10.1007/BF02201002.

Dayoub, Elias. 2014. "Lessons from Abroad and at Home: How PCORI Can Improve Quality of Care (and Prove It) by 2019." *Health Affairs Blog*, May 2. http://healthaffairs.org/blog /2014/05/02/lessons-from-abroad-and-at-home-how-pcori-can-improve-quality-of-care -and-prove-it-by-2019/.

Delli Carpini, Michael X., and Scott Keeter. 1996. *What Americans Know about Politics and Why It Matters*. New Haven, CT: Yale University Press.

Deloitte. 2011. "Physician Perspectives about Health Care Reform and the Future of the Medical Profession." December. http://www.deloitte.com/assets/Dcom-UnitedStates/Local%20 Assets/Documents/us_lshc_PhysicianPerspectives_121211.pdf. Accessed September 13, 2012.

Department of Justice. 2012. "GlaxoSmithKline to Plead Guilty and Pay $3 Billion to Resolve Fraud Allegations and Failure to Report Safety Data." *Justice News*, July 2. https://www.justice.gov/opa/pr/glaxosmithkline-plead-guilty-and-pay-3-billion-resolve-fraud-allegations-and-failure-report. Accessed March 15, 2017.

Derthick, Martha. 2005. *Up in Smoke: From Legislation to Litigation in Tobacco Politics*. Washington, DC: CQ Press.

Derthick, Martha, and Paul J. Quirk. 1985. *The Politics of Deregulation*. New York: Brookings Institution Press.

Dervin, Geoffrey F., Ian G. Stiell, Kelly Rody, and Jenny Grabowski. 2003. "Effect of Arthroscopic Débridement for Osteoarthritis of the Knee on Health-Related Quality of Life." *Journal of Bone and Joint Surgery* 85 (1): 10–19.

De Vries, Raymond, and Trudo Lemmens. 2006. "The Social and Cultural Shaping of Medical Evidence: Case Studies from Pharmaceutical Research and Obstetric Science." *Social Science and Medicine* 62 (11): 2694–706.

Deyo, Richard A. 2014. *Watch Your Back! How the Back Pain Industry Is Costing Us More and Giving Us Less—and What You Can Do to Inform and Empower Yourself in Seeking Treatment*. Ithaca, NY: Cornell University Press.

Deyo, Richard A., Alf Nachemson, and Sohail K. Mirza. 2004. "Spinal-Fusion Surgery—The Case for Restraint." *The Spine Journal* 4 (5): S138–42.

Deyo, Richard A., and Donald L. Patrick. 2005. *Hope or Hype: The Obsession with Medical Advances and the High Cost of False Promises*. New York: AMACOM.

Drazer, Michael W., Dezheng Huo, and Scott E. Eggener. 2015. "National Prostate Cancer Screening Rates after the 2012 US Preventive Services Task Force Recommendation Discouraging Prostate-Specific Antigen–Based Screening." *Journal of Clinical Oncology* 33 (22): 2416–23.

Drossman, Susan R., Elisa R. Port, and Emily B. Sonnenblick. 2015. "Why the Annual Mammogram Matters." *New York Times*, October 28. http://www.nytimes.com/2015/10/29/opinion/why-the-annual-mammogram-matters.html.

Druckman, James N., Cari Lynn Hennessy, Kristi St. Charles, and Jonathan Webber. 2010. "Competing Rhetoric over Time: Frames versus Cues." *Journal of Politics* 72 (1): 136–48.

Druckman, James N., Erik Peterson, and Rune Slothuus. 2013. "How Elite Partisan Polarization Affects Public Opinion Formation." *American Political Science Review* 107 (1): 57–79.

Dunlap, Riley E., and Aaron M. McCright. 2008. "A Widening Gap: Republican and Democratic Views on Climate Change." *Environment: Science and Policy for Sustainable Development* 50 (5): 26–35.

Dutton, Paul V. 2007. *Differential Diagnoses: A Comparative History of Health Care Problems and Solutions in the United States and France*. Ithaca, NY: ILR Press/Cornell University Press.

Dzur, Albert W. 2002. "Democratizing the Hospital: Deliberative-Democratic Bioethics." *Journal of Health Politics, Policy and Law* 27 (2): 177–211.

———. 2008. *Democratic Professionalism: Citizen Participation and the Reconstruction of Professional Ethics, Identity, and Practice*. University Park: Penn State University Press.

Eagly, Alice H., and Shelly Chaiken. 1993. *The Psychology of Attitudes*. Fort Worth, TX: Harcourt Brace.

Eddy, David M. 1990. "The Challenge." *Journal of the American Medical Association* 263 (2): 287–90.

———. 2005. "Evidence-Based Medicine: A Unified Approach." *Health Affairs* 24 (1): 9–17.

Edney, Anna, 2009. "Medical Treatment Amendment Leads to Consternation Wednesday." *Congress Daily*, January 28. https://www.nationaljournal.com/s/492637/medical-treatment-amendment-leads-consternation.

Eisenberg, John M. 2001. "What Does Evidence Mean? Can the Law and Medicine Be Reconciled?" *Journal of Health Politics, Policy and Law* 26 (2): 369–81.

———. 2002a. "Globalize the Evidence, Localize the Decision: Evidence-Based Medicine and International Diversity." *Health Affairs* 21 (3): 166–68.

———. 2002b. "Physician Utilization: The State of Research about Physicians' Practice Patterns." *Medical Care* 40 (11): 1016–35.

Eisinger, Richard, and Judson Mills. 1968. "Perception of the Sincerity and Competence of a Communicator as a Function of the Extremity of His Position." *Journal of Experimental Social Psychology* 4 (2): 224–32.

Elattrache, Neal, Christian Lattermann, Michael Hannon, and Brian Cole. 2014. "*New England Journal of Medicine* Article Evaluating the Usefulness of Meniscectomy Is Flawed. *Arthroscopy* 30 (5): 542–43.

Emanuel, Zeke, Topher Spiro, and Thomas Huelskoetter. 2016. "Re-Evaluating the Patient-Centered Outcomes Research Institute." *Center for American Progress*, May 31. https://www.americanprogress.org/issues/healthcare/reports/2016/05/31/138242/re-evaluating-the-patient-centered-outcomes-research-institute/.

Emery, Gene. 2013. "Common Knee Surgery Ineffective in Study." *Reuters*, December 25. http://www.reuters.com/article/us-common-knee-idUSBRE9BO0BV20131225.

Englund, Martin, Ali Guermazi, Daniel Gale, David J. Hunter, Piran Aliabadi, Margaret Clancy, and David T. Felson. 2008. "Incidental Meniscal Findings on Knee MRI in Middle-Aged and Elderly Persons." *New England Journal of Medicine* 359 (11): 1108–15. doi:10.1056/NEJMoa0800777.

Epstein, David. 2017. "When Evidence Says No, but Doctors Say Yes." *Atlantic*, February 22. https://www.theatlantic.com/health/archive/2017/02/when-evidence-says-no-but-doctors-say-yes/517368/. Accessed March 15, 2017.

Epstein, Andrew J., and Sean Nicholson. 2009. "The Formation and Evolution of Physician Treatment Styles: An Application to Cesarean Sections" *Journal of Health Economics* 28 (6): 1126–40.

Epstein, Robert S., and J. Russell Teagarden. 2010. "Comparative Effectiveness Research and Personalized Medicine: Catalyzing or Colliding?" *Health Affairs* 28 (10): 905–13.

Eskridge, William N., and John A. Ferejohn. 2013. *A Republic of Statutes: The New American Constitution*. New Haven, CT: Yale University Press.

Fairbrother, Gerry, Ellen O'Brien, Rosina Pradhananga, and Kalipso Chalkidou. 2014. "Improving Quality and Efficiency in Health Care through Comparative Effectiveness Analyses." Academy Health, 1–16. https://www.academyhealth.org/files/publications/2014CERImprovingQuality.pdf.

Feldstein, Paul J. 2011. *Health Policy Issues: An Economic Perspective*, 5th edition. Chicago, IL: Health Administration Press.

Felson, David T. 2010. "Arthroscopy as a Treatment for Knee Osteoarthritis." *Best Practice and Research Clinical Rheumatology* 24 (1): 47–50.

Felson, David T., and Joseph Buckwalter. 2002. "Débridement and Lavage for Osteoarthritis of the Knee." *New England Journal of Medicine* 347 (2): 132–33.

Ferguson, John H., Michael Dubinsky, and Peter J. Kirsch. 1993. "Court-ordered Reimbursement for Unproven Medical Technology: Circumventing Technology Assessment." *JAMA* 269 (16): 2116–21.

Finegold, Kenneth, and Theda Skocpol. 1995. *State and Party in America's New Deal.* Madison: University of Wisconsin Press.

Finkelstein, Amy, Matthew Gentzkow, and Heidi Williams. 2016. "Sources of Geographic Variation in Health Care: Evidence from Patient Migration." *Quarterly Journal of Economics* 131 (4): 1681–726.

Fiorina, Morris P. 2006. "Parties as Problem Solvers." In *Promoting the General Welfare: New Perspectives on Government Performance*, edited by Alan S. Gerber and Eric M. Patashnik, 237–55. Washington, DC: Brookings Institution Press.

Fiorina, Morris P., and Samuel J. Abrams. 2008. "Political Polarization in the American Public." *Annual Review of Political Science* 11: 563–88.

Fiorina, Morris P., with Samuel J. Abrams and Jeremy Pope. 2006. *Culture War? The Myth of a Polarized America.* 2nd ed. New York: Pearson Education.

Fisher, Elliot S., John-Erik Bell, Ivan M. Tomek, Amos R. Esty, and David C. Goodman. 2010. "Trends and Regional Variation in Hip, Knee, and Shoulder Replacement." *Dartmouth Institute for Health Policy and Clinical Practice*, April 6. http://www.dartmouthatlas.org/downloads/reports/Joint_Replacement_0410.pdf.

Fisher, Elliott S., David E. Wennberg, Thrse A. Stukel, Daniel J. Gottlieb, F. L. Lucas, and Étoile L. Pinder. 2003. "The Implications of Regional Variations in Medicare Spending. Part 2: Health Outcomes and Satisfaction with Care." *Annals of Internal Medicine* 138 (4): 288–98. doi:10.7326/0003-4819-138-4-200302180-00007.

Foote, Sandra M. 2003. "Population-Based Disease Management under Fee-for-Service Medicare." *Health Affairs Web Exclusives*, July 30. http://content.healthaffairs.org/cgi/content/abstract/hlthaff.w3.342v1.

Foote, Susan Bartlett. 2002. "Why Medicare Cannot Promulgate a National Coverage Rule: A Case of Regula Mortis." *Journal of Health Politics, Policy and Law* 27 (5): 707–30. doi:10.1215/03616878-27-5-707.

Foote, Susan Bartlett, and Lynn A. Blewett. 2003. "Politics of Prevention: Expanding Prevention Benefits in the Medicare Program." *Journal of Public Health Policy* 24 (1): 26–40. doi:10.2307/3343175.

Forsythe, Laura P., Lori Frank, Kara Odom Walker, Ayodola Anise, Natalie Wegener, Harlan Weisman, Gail Hunt, and Anne Beal. 2015. "Patient and Clinician Views on Comparative Effectiveness Research and Engagement in Research." *Journal of Comparative Effectiveness Research* 4 (1): 11–25.

Frakt, Austin. 2015a. "Coverage of Health Care Technology: Medicare vs. Commercial Market." *The Incidental Economist*, August 7. http://theincidentaleconomist.com/wordpress/coverage-of-health-care-technology-medicare-vs-commercial-market/.

Frakt, Austin. 2015b. "Your New Medical Team Algorithms and Physicians." *New York Times*, December 7. http://www.nytimes.com/2015/12/08/upshot/your-new-medical-team-algorithms-and-physicians.html?_r=1.

Freidson, Eliot 1970. *Profession of Medicine: A Study of the Sociology of Applied Knowledge.* New York: Dodd, Mead.

———. 1988. *Profession of Medicine: A Study of the Sociology of Applied Knowledge.* Chicago: University of Chicago Press.

———. 2001. *Professionalism, the Third Logic.* Chicago: University of Chicago Press.

Fuchs, Victor R. 1974. *Who Shall Live? Health, Economics, and Social Choice.* New York: Basic Books.

Fuchs, Victor R., and Arnold Milstein. 2011. "The $640 Billion Question—Why Does Cost-Effective Care Diffuse So Slowly?" *New England Journal of Medicine* 364 (21): 1985–87.

Gallo, Nick, and David E. Lewis. 2011. "The Consequences of Presidential Patronage for Federal Agency Performance." *Journal of Public Administration Research and Theory*, May. doi:10.1093/jopart/mur010.

Gallup. 2009. "On Healthcare, Americans Trust Physicians over Politicians." June 17. http://www.gallup.com/poll/120890/healthcare-americans-trust-physicians-politicians.aspx. Accessed February 23, 2012.

Garber, Alan M. 2005. "Evidence-Based Guidelines as a Foundation for Performance Incentives." *Health Affairs* 24 (1): 174–79.

Garber, Alan M., and Jonathan Skinner. 2008. "Is American Health Care Uniquely Inefficient?" *Journal of Economic Perspectives : A Journal of the American Economic Association* 22 (4): 27–50. doi:10.1257/jep.22.4.27.

Garber, Alan M., and Sean R. Tunis. 2009. "Does Comparative-Effectiveness Research Threaten Personalized Medicine?" *New England Journal of Medicine* 360 (19): 1925–27.

Gaus, C. R. 1995. "The Outcome for AHCPR: Interview by Laura Lynn Brown." *Health Systems Review* 28 (4): 41–43.

Gawande, Atul. 2009. "The Cost Conundrum." *New Yorker*, June 1. http://www.newyorker.com/magazine/2009/06/01/the-cost-conundrum.

———. 2015. "Overkill." *New Yorker*, May 11. http://www.newyorker.com/magazine/2015/05/11/overkill-atul-gawande.

Gerber, Alan S. 2014. Cooperative Congressional Election Study, 2014: Yale University Content. [Computer File] Release: February 2015. New Haven, CT. [producer] http://cces.gov.harvard.edu.

Gerber, Alan S., and Eric M. Patashnik. 2006. "Sham Surgery: The Problem of Inadequate Medical Evidence." In *Promoting the General Welfare: New Perspectives on Government Performance*, edited by Alan S. Gerber and Eric M. Patashnik, 43–73. Washington, DC: Brookings Institution Press.

———. 2010. "Problem Solving in a Polarized Age: Comparative Effectiveness Research and the Politicization of Evidence-Based Medicine." *Forum* 8 (1): Article 3. https://doi.org/10.2202/1540-8884.1353.

———. 2011. "The Politicization of Evidence-Based Medicine: The Limits of Pragmatic Problem Solving in an Era of Polarization." *California Journal of Politics and Policy* 3 (4). doi:10.2202/1944-4370.1188.

Gerber, Alan S., Eric M. Patashnik, David Doherty, and Conor Dowling. 2010a. "The Public Wants Information, Not Board Mandates, from Comparative Effectiveness Research." *Health Affairs* 29 (10): 1872–81.

———. 2010b. "A National Survey Reveals Public Skepticism about Research-Based Treatment Guidelines." *Health Affairs* 29 (10): 1882–84.

———. 2014. "Doctor Knows Best: Physician Endorsements, Public Opinion, and the Politics of Comparative Effectiveness Research." *Journal of Health Politics, Policy and Law* 39 (1): 171–208.

Gilens, Martin. 2012. *Affluence and Influence: Economic Inequality and Political Power in America*. Princeton, NJ: Princeton University Press.

Gimpel, James G., Frances E. Lee, and Rebecca U. Thorpe. 2012. "The Distributive Politics of the Federal Stimulus: The Geography of the American Recovery and Reinvestment Act of 2009." *Political Science Quarterly* 127 (4): 567–95.

Glied, Sherry, and Adam Sacarny. 2017. "Is the U.S. Healthcare System Wasteful and Inefficient? A Review of the Evidence?" Paper presented at "Challenging the Conventional Wisdom: Is the US Healthcare System as Bad as Critics Contend?" Columbia University, June 19–20.

Glied, Sherry A., and Richard G. Frank. 2017. "Care for the Vulnerable vs. Cash for the Powerful—Trump's Pick for HHS." *New England Journal of Medicine* 376: 103–5.

Gogineni, Keerthi, Katherine Shuman, Derek Chinn, Anita Weber, Carol Cosenza, Mary Ellen Colten, and Ezekiel J. Emanuel. 2015. "Making Cuts to Medicare: The Views of Patients, Physicians, and the Public." *Journal of Clinical Oncology* 33 (8): 846–53. doi:10.1200/JCO.2014.56.3262.

Goldberg, H. I., R. A. Deyo, V. M. Taylor, A. D. Cheadle, D. A. Conrad, J. D. Loeser, P. J. Heagerty, and P. Diehr. 2001. "Can Evidence Change the Rate of Back Surgery? A Randomized Trial of Community-Based Education." *Effective Clinical Practice* 4 (3): 95–104.

Goldhill, David. 2013. *Catastrophic Care: Why Everything We Think We Know about Health Care Is Wrong.* New York: Vintage Books.

Gollust, S., and J. Lynch. 2011. "Who Deserves Health Care? The Effects of Causal Attributions and Group Cues on Public Attitudes about Responsibility for Health Care Costs." *Journal of Health Politics, Policy and Law* 36 (6): 1061–95.

Gottlieb, Scott. 2014. "PCORI's Efforts Could Leave Obamacare Boosters Stressed Out." *Morning Consult*, July 31. https://morningconsult.com/opinions/pcoris-efforts-leave-obamacare-boosters-stressed/.

Grady, Denise. 2015. "American Cancer Society, in a Shift, Recommends Fewer Mammograms." *New York Times*, October 20. http://www.nytimes.com/2015/10/21/health/breast-cancer-screening-guidelines.html.

Grande, David, David A. Asch, and Katrina Armstrong. 2007. "Do Doctors Vote?" *Journal of General Internal Medicine* 22 (5): 585–89.

Gray, Bradford H. 1992. "The Legislative Battle over Health Services Research." *Health Affairs* 11 (4): 38–66.

Gray, Bradford H., Michael K. Gusmano, and Sara R. Collins. 2003. "AHCPR and the Changing Politics of Health Services Research." *Health Affairs Web Exclusives*, June 25, W3-283–W3-307. http://content.healthaffairs.org/content/early/2003/06/25/hlthaff.w3.283.full.pdf+html.

Green, Donald P., Bradley Palmquist, and Eric Schickler. 2002. *Partisan Hearts and Minds: Political Parties and the Social Identities of Voters.* New Haven, CT: Yale University Press.

Grimmer, Justin, Sean J. Westwood, and Solomon Messing. 2014. *The Impression of Influence: Legislator Communication, Representation, and Democratic Accountability.* Princeton, NJ: Princeton University Press.

Groopman, Jerome. 2007. *How Doctors Think.* Boston: Houghton Mifflin.

———. 2010. "Health Care: Who Knows 'Best'?" *New York Review of Books*, February 11. http://www.nybooks.com/articles/2010/02/11/health-care-who-knows-best/.

Gruber, Jonathan. 2011. "Health Care Reform without the Individual Mandate: Replacing the Individual Mandate Would Significantly Erode Coverage Gains and Raise Premiums for Health Care Consumers." Center for American Progress, February. http://www.americanprogress.org/wp-content/uploads/issues/2011/02/pdf/gruber_mandate.pdf.

Grunwald, Michael. 2012. *The New New Deal: The Hidden Story of Change in the Obama Era.* New York: Simon and Schuster.

Hacker, Jacob S. 1997. *The Road to Nowhere: The Genesis of President Clinton's Plan for Health Security.* Princeton, NJ: Princeton University Press.

———. 1998. "The Historical Logic of National Health Insurance: Structure and Sequence in the Development of British, Canadian, and U.S. Medical Policy." *Studies in American Political Development* 12 (1): 57–130.

Hadler, Nortin M. 2008. *Worried Sick: A Prescription for Health in an Overtreated America.* Chapel Hill: University of North Carolina Press.

Hall, Mark A. 2003. "State Regulation of Medical Necessity: The Case of Weight-Reduction Surgery." *Duke Law Journal* 53: 653.

Hanssen, Arlen D., Michael J. Stuart, Richard D. Scott, and Giles R. Scuderi. 2000. "Surgical Options for the Middle-Aged Patient with Osteoarthritis of the Knee Joint." *Journal of Bone and Joint Surgery* 82 (12): 1767–81.

Harris, Gardiner. 2011. "U.S. Panel Says No to Prostate Screening for Healthy Men." *New York Times*, October 6. http://www.nytimes.com/2011/10/07/health/07prostate.html.

Harris, Ian. 2016. *Surgery, the Ultimate Placebo: A Surgeon Cuts through the Evidence*. Sydney: University of New South Wales Press.

"Health Policy Brief: Comparative Effectiveness Research." 2010. *Health Affairs*, October 5. https://www.healthaffairs.org/healthpolicybriefs/brief.php?brief_id=27.

"Health Policy Brief: Geographic Variation in Medicare Spending." 2014. *Health Affairs*, March 6. https://www.healthaffairs.org/healthpolicybriefs/brief.php?brief_id=109.

"Health Policy Brief: Reducing Waste in Health Care." 2012. *Health Affairs*, December 13. https://www.healthaffairs.org/healthpolicybriefs/brief.php?brief_id=82.

Health Quality Ontario. 2005. "Arthroscopic Lavage and Debridement for Osteoarthritis of the Knee: An Evidence-Based Analysis." *Ontario Health Technology Assessment Series* 5 (12): 1–37.

Heclo, Hugh. 1996. "Clinton's Health Reform in Historical Perspective." In *The Problem That Won't Go Away: Reforming U.S. Health Care Financing*, edited by Henry J. Aaron, 15–33. Washington, DC: Brookings Institution Press.

———. 1998. "A Political Science Perspective on Social Security Reform." In *Framing the Social Security Debate: Values, Politics, and Economics*, edited by R. Douglas Arnold, Michael J. Graetz, and Alicia H. Munnell, 65–88. Washington, DC: Brookings Institution Press.

Heritage Foundation, ed. 2005. *Mandate for Leadership: Principles to Limit Government, Expand Freedom, and Strengthen America*. Washington, DC: Heritage Foundation.

Heritage Lectures. 2007. "Competition: A Prescription for Health Care Transformation." Washington, DC: Heritage Foundation. April 13. http://www.heritage.org/health-care-reform/report/competition-prescription-health-care-transformation.

Herrlin, Sylvia, Maria Hållander, Peter Wange, Lars Weidenhielm, and Suzanne Werner. 2007. "Arthroscopic or Conservative Treatment of Degenerative Medial Meniscal Tears: A Prospective Randomised Trial." *Knee Surgery, Sports Traumatology, Arthroscopy* 15 (4): 393–401. doi:10.1007/s00167-006-0243-2.

Herrlin, Sylvia V., Peter O. Wange, Gunilla Lapidus, Maria Hållander, Suzanne Werner, and Lars Weidenhielm. 2013. "Is Arthroscopic Surgery Beneficial in Treating Non-traumatic, Degenerative Medial Meniscal Tears? A Five Year Follow-Up." *Knee Surgery, Sports Traumatology, Arthroscopy* 21 (2): 358–64.

Hersh, Eitan, and Matthew Goldenberg. 2016. "Democratic and Republican Physicians Provide Different Care on Politicized Health Issues." *Proceedings of the National Academy of Sciences* 113 (42): 11811–16.

Hetherington, Marc J. 2005. *Why Trust Matters: Declining Political Trust and the Demise of American Liberalism*. Princeton, NJ: Princeton University Press.

Hochschild, Jennifer L. 2013. "Should the Mass Public Follow Elite Option? It Depends . . ." *Critical Review: A Journal of Politics and Society* 24 (4): 527–43. doi:10.1080/08913811.2012.788280.

Hochschild, Jennifer L., and Katherine Levine Einstein. 2015. "Do Facts Matter? Information and Misinformation in American Politics." *Political Science Quarterly* 130 (4): 585–624. doi:10.1002/polq.12398.

Hosman, Lawrence A., and Susan A. Siltanen. 2011. "Hedges, Tag Questions, Message Processing, and Persuasion." *Journal of Language and Social Psychology* 30 (3): 341–49.

Howard, David, Robert Brophy, and Stephen Howell. 2012. "Evidence of No Benefit from Knee Surgery for Osteoarthritis Led to Coverage Changes and Is Linked to Decline in Procedures." *Health Affairs* 31 (10): 2242–49. doi:10.1377/hlthaff.2012.0644.

Howard, David H., Florence K. Tangka, Gery P. Guy, Donatus U. Ekwueme, and Joseph Lipscomb. 2013. "Prostate Cancer Screening in Men Ages 75 and Older Fell by 8 Percentage Points after Task Force Recommendation." *Health Affairs* 32 (3): 596–602. doi:10.1377/hlthaff.2012.0555.

Iglehart, John K. 2010. "The Political Fight over Comparative Effectiveness Research." *Health Affairs* 29 (10): 1757–60.

IOM (Institute of Medicine). 2000. *To Err Is Human: Building a Safer Health System.* Washington, DC: National Academies Press. doi:10.17226/9728.

———. 2007. "Learning What Works Best: The Nations Need for Evidence on Comparative Effectiveness in Health Care." http://www.iom.edu/~/media/Files/Activity%20Files/Quality/VSRT/ComparativeEffectivenessWhitePaperESF.pdf. Accessed June 6, 2012.

———. 2009. "Initial National Priorities for Comparative Effectiveness Research." http://www.iom.edu/~/media/Files/Report%20Files/2009/ComparativeEffectivenessResearchPriorities/CER%20report%20brief%2008-13-09.ashx. Accessed June 6, 2012.

———. 2011. *Learning What Works: Infrastructure Required for Comparative Effectiveness Research—Workshop Summary.* Washington, DC: National Academies Press.

———. 2013. *Best Care at Lower Cost: The Path to Continuously Learning Health Care in America.* Washington, DC: National Academies Press. doi:10.17226/13444.

Jackson, Robert W. 2002. "Letter to the Editor." *New England Journal of Medicine* 347: 1717.

Jacobs, Lawrence, and Theda Skocpol. 2010. *Health Care Reform and American Politics: What Everyone Needs to Know.* New York: Oxford University Press.

Jacobs, Lawrence R. 1993. *The Health of Nations: Public Opinion and the Making of Health Policy in the U.S. and Britain.* Ithaca, NY: Cornell University Press.

Jacobs, Lawrence R., and Robert Y. Shapiro. 1994. "Questioning the Conventional Wisdom on Public Opinion toward Health Reform." *PS: Political Science and Politics* 27 (2): 208–14.

Järvinen, Teppo L. N., Raine Sihvonen, and Martin Englund. 2014. "Arthroscopy for Degenerative Knee—a Difficult Habit to Break?" *Acta Orthopaedica* 85 (3): 215–17.

Järvinen, Teppo L. N., Raine Sihvonen, and Antti Malmivaara. 2014. "Arthroscopy for Degenerate Meniscal Tears of the Knee." *British Medical Journal* 348: g2382. https://doi.org/10.1136/bmj.g2382.

Jasanoff, Sheila. 2016. "A Century of Reason: Experts and Citizens in the Administrative State." In *The Progressives' Century: Political Reform, Constitutional Government, and the Modern American State*, edited by Stephen Skowronek, Stephen M. Engel, and Bruce Ackerman, 382–404. New Haven, CT: Yale University Press.

Jaslow, Ryan. 2012. "Panel's PSA Test Recommendations Spark Debate among Doctors, Cancer Survivors." *CBS News*, May 22. http://www.cbsnews.com/news/panels-psa-test-recommendations-spark-debate-among-doctors-cancer-survivors/.

———. 2013. "Urologists No Longer Recommend Routine PSA Testing for Prostate Cancer." *CBS News*, May 3. http://www.cbsnews.com/news/urologists-no-longer-recommend-routine-psa-testing-for-prostate-cancer/.

Jemal, Ahmedin, Stacey A. Fedewa, Jiemin Ma, Rebecca Siegel, Chun Chieh Lin, Otis Brawley, and Elizabeth M. Ward. 2015. "Prostate Cancer Incidence and PSA Testing Patterns in Relation to USPSTF Screening Recommendations." *JAMA* 314 (19): 2054–61. doi:10.1001/jama.2015.14905.

Jennings, Jerome E. 1986. "Arthroscopic Debridement as an Alternative to Total Knee Replacement." *Arthroscopy* 2 (2): 123–4.

Kallmes, David F., Bryan A. Comstock, Patrick J. Heagerty, Judith A. Turner, David J. Wilson, Terry H. Diamond, Richard Edwards, et al. 2009. "A Randomized Trial of Vertebroplasty for Osteoporotic Spinal Fractures." *New England Journal of Medicine* 361 (6): 569–79.

Kalunian, K. C, L. W. Moreland, D. J. Klashman, P. H. Brion, A. L. Concoff, S. Myers, R. Singh, et al. 2000. "Visually-Guided Irrigation in Patients with Early Knee Osteoarthritis: A Multicenter Randomized, Controlled Trial." *Osteoarthritis and Cartilage* 8 (6): 412–18. doi:10.1053/joca.1999.0316.

Kam, Cindy D. 2005. "Who Toes the Party Line? Cues, Values, and Individual Differences." *Political Behavior* 27 (2): 163–82.

Katz, Jeffrey N., Robert H. Brophy, Christine E. Chaisson, Leigh de Chaves, Brian J. Cole, Diane L. Dahm, Laurel A. Donnell-Fink, et al. 2013. "Surgery versus Physical Therapy for a Meniscal Tear and Osteoarthritis." *New England Journal of Medicine* 368 (18): 1675–84. doi:10.1056/NEJMoa1301408.

Katz, Jeffrey N., Sarah A. Brownlee, and Morgan H. Jones. 2014. "The Role of Arthroscopy in the Management of Knee Osteoarthritis." *Osteoarthritis: Moving from Evidence to Practice* 28 (1): 143–56. doi:10.1016/j.berh.2014.01.008.

Kaufman, Herbert. 1976. *Are Government Organizations Immortal?* Washington, DC: Brookings Institution.

Keller, Ann C., Robin Flagg, Justin Keller, and Suhasini Ravi. 2015. "Impossible Politics? PCORI and the Search for Publicly Funded Comparative Effectiveness Research in the United States." Paper prepared for presentation at the Annual Meeting of the American Political Science Association, September 3–6, San Francisco.

Keller, Ann C., and Laura Packel. 2014. "Going for the Cure: Patient Interest Groups and Health Advocacy in the United States." *Journal of Health Politics, Policy and Law* 39 (2): 331–67.

Keyhani, Salomeh, Mark Woodward, and Alex D. Federman. 2010. "Physician Views on the Use of Comparative Effectiveness Research: A National Survey." *Annals of Internal Medicine* 153 (8): 551–52.

Kim, Minah, Robert J. Blendon, and John M. Benson. 2001. "How Interested Are Americans in New Medical Technologies? A Multicountry Comparison." *Health Affairs* 20 (5): 194–201.

Kim, Sunny, J. Bosque, J. P. Meehan, A. Jamali, and R. Marder. 2011. "Increase in Outpatient Knee Arthroscopy in the United States: A Comparison of National Surveys of Ambulatory Surgery, 1996 and 2006." *Journal of Bone and Joint Surgery* 93 (11): 994–1000.

Kingdon, John W. 2003. *Agendas, Alternatives, and Public Policies.* Longman Classics in Political Science. Boston: Longman. https://books.google.com/books?id=hSolAQAAIAAJ.

Kirkley, Alexandra, Trevor B. Birmingham, Robert B. Litchfield, J. Robert Giffin, Kevin R. Willits, Cindy J. Wong, Brian G. Feagan, et al. 2008. "A Randomized Trial of Arthroscopic Surgery for Osteoarthritis of the Knee." *New England Journal of Medicine* 359 (11): 1097–107. doi:10.1056/NEJMoa0708333.

Klein, Rudolph. 2010. *The New Politics of the NHS: From Creation to Reinvention.* 6th ed. Oxon, UK: Radcliffe.

Kliff, Sarah. 2013. "It's Tough to Get Cervical Cancer without a Cervix." *Washington Post*, January 7. https://www.washingtonpost.com/news/wonk/wp/2013/01/07/its-tough-to-get-cervical-cancer-without-a-cervix/.

Knott, Jack H., and Gary J. Miller. 1987. *Reforming Bureaucracy: The Politics of Institutional Choice.* Englewood Cliffs, NJ: Prentice Hall.

Knox, Richard. 2012. "Doctors Urge Their Colleagues to Quit Doing Worthless Tests." *NPR*, April 4. http://m.npr.org/story/149978690?url=/blogs/health/2012/04/04/149978690/doctors-urge-their-colleagues-to-quit-doing-worthless-tests. Accessed June 6, 2012.

Kolata, Gina. 2002a. "Arthritis Surgery in Ailing Knees Is Cited as Sham." *New York Times*, July 11. http://www.nytimes.com/2002/07/11/us/arthritis-surgery-in-ailing-knees-is-cited-as-sham.html.

———. 2002b. "Study Casts Doubt on Value of Popular Knee Surgery." *New York Times*, July 10. http://www.nytimes.com/2002/07/10/health/study-casts-doubt-on-value-of-popular-knee-surgery.html.

———. 2002c. "V.A. Suggests Halt to Kind of Knee Surgery." *New York Times*, August 24. http://www.nytimes.com/2002/08/24/us/va-suggests-halt-to-kind-of-knee-surgery.html.

———. 2008. "A Study Revives a Debate on Arthritis Knee Surgery." *New York Times*, September 10. http://www.nytimes.com/2008/09/11/health/research/11knee.html.

———. 2009. "Panel Urges Mammograms at 50, Not 40." *New York Times*, November 16. http://www.nytimes.com/2009/11/17/health/17cancer.html.

———. 2017. "Lower Back Ache? Be Active and Wait It Out, New Guidelines Say." *New York Times*, February 13. https://www.nytimes.com/2017/02/13/health/lower-back-pain-surgery-guidelines.html?_r=0.

Kowalczyk, Liz. 2002. "Sham Surgery Aids Patients' Knees Woes, Study Finds." *Boston Globe*, July 11. https://www.highbeam.com/doc/1P2-7736369.html.

Krause, Elliott A. 1996. *Death of the Guilds: Professions, States and the Advance of Capitalism: 1930 to the Present*. New Haven, CT: Yale University Press.

Kronebusch, Karl, Mark Schlesinger, and Tracey Thomas. 2009. "Managed Care Regulation in the States: The Impact on Physicians' Practices and Clinical Autonomy." *Journal of Health Politics, Policy and Law* 34 (2): 219–59.

Krueger, Anne O. 1974. "The Political Economy of the Rent-Seeking Society." *American Economic Review* 64 (3): 291–303.

LaBorde Thomas C. 1993. "Reimbursement for Unproven Therapies: The Case of Thermography." *JAMA* 270 (21): 2558. doi:10.1001/jama.1993.03510210044019.

Langreth, Robert. 2003. "Operation! Do You Really Need to Go Under the Knife? Read this First." *Forbes*, October 27, 172 (9): 246.

Laugesen, Miriam J. 2009. "Siren Song: Physicians, Congress, and Medicare Fees." *Journal of Health Politics, Policy and Law* 34 (2): 157–79. doi:10.1215/03616878-2008-043.

———. 2016. *Fixing Medical Prices: How Physicians Are Paid*. Cambridge, MA: Harvard University Press.

Laugesen, Miriam J., and Sherry A. Glied. 2011. "Higher Fees Paid To US Physicians Drive Higher Spending For Physician Services Compared To Other Countries." *Health Affairs* 30 (9): 1647–56.

Laugesen, Miriam J., and Thomas Rice. 2003. "Is the Doctor In? The Evolving Role of Organized Medicine in Health Policy." *Journal of Health Politics, Policy and Law* 28 (2–3): 289–316. doi:10.1215/03616878-28-2-3-289.

Laugesen, Miriam J., Roy Wada, and Eric M. Chen. 2012. "In Setting Doctors' Medicare Fees, CMS Almost Always Accepts the Relative Value Update Panel's Advice on Work Values." *Health Affairs* 31 (5): 965–72. doi:10.1377/hlthaff.2011.0557.

Leary, Warren E. 1994. "U.S. Guidelines for Back Pain Reject Some Common Notions." *New York Times*, December 9. http://www.nytimes.com/1994/12/09/us/us-guidelines-for-back-pain-reject-some-common-notions.html.

Lee, Frances E. 2009. *Beyond Ideology: Politics, Principles, and Partisanship in the U.S. Senate*. Chicago: University of Chicago Press.

Lenz, Gabriel S. 2012. *Follow the Leader? How Voters Respond to Politician's Policies and Performance*. Chicago: University of Chicago Press.

Lenzer, Jeanne. 2015. "Choosing Wisely: Setbacks and Progress." *British Medical Journal* 351: 6760.

Leonhardt, David. 2009. "After the Great Recession." *New York Times*, April 28. http://www
.nytimes.com/2009/05/03/magazine/03Obama-t.html?pagewanted=all.

Levendusky, Matthew S. 2010. "Clearer Cues, More Consistent Voters: A Benefit of Elite Polarization." *Political Behavior* 32 (1): 111–31.

Levey, Noam N. 2009. "A Warning Shot in the Healthcare Fight." *Los Angeles Times*, February 24. http://latimes.com/news/nation-world/nation/la-na-healthcare24-2009feb24,0
,5706385.story.

Levine, Michael E. 2006. "Why Weren't the Airlines Reregulated?" *Yale Journal on Regulation* 23
(2): Article 5. http://digitalcommons.law.yale.edu/yjreg/vol23/iss2/5/.

Lewis, David E. 2012. "Policy Durability and Agency Design." In *Living Legislation: Durability,
Change, and the Politics of American Lawmaking*, edited by Jeffery A. Jenkins and Eric M.
Patashnik, 175–96. Chicago: University of Chicago Press.

Lillis, M. 2010. "Doctors' Lobby Urges Congress to Prevent Steep Medicare Cut." *Healthwatch: The
Hill's Healthcare Blog*, November 8. http://thehill.com/blogs/healthwatch/medicare/128207
-doctors-lobby-urges-congress-to-prevent-steep-medicare-cut. Accessed June 6, 2012.

Lipitz-Snyderman, Allison, Camilia S. Sima, and Coral L. Atoria. 2016. "Physician-Driven Variation in Nonrecommended Services among Older Adults Diagnosed with Cancer." *JAMA Internal Medicine* 176 (10): 1541–48. doi:10.1001/jamainternmed.2016.4426.

Longman, Phillip. 2013. "The Republican Case for Waste in Health Care." *Washington Monthly*,
March/April: 20–26.

Lupia, Arthur. 1994. "Shortcuts versus Encyclopedias." *American Political Science Review* 88 (1):
63–76.

Lupia, Arthur, and Mathew D. McCubbins. 1998. *The Democratic Dilemma: Can Citizens Learn
What They Need to Know?* Political Economy of Institutions and Decisions. Cambridge:
Cambridge University Press.

Lyu, Heather, Michol Cooper, Kavita Patel, Michael Daniel, and Martin A. Makary. 2016. "Preva-
lence and Data Transparency of National Clinical Registries in the United States." *Journal for
Healthcare Quality* 38 (4): 223–34.

Mahinka, Stephen Paul. 2013. "Imperative: Comparative Effectiveness Research." *LMG Life Sciences Guide*, August, 18–21.

Makary, Marty. 2012. *Unaccountable: What Hospitals Won't Tell You and How Transparency Can
Revolutionize Health Care*. New York: Bloomsbury.

Maltzman, Forrest, and Charles R. Shipan. 2012. "Beyond Legislative Productivity: Enactment
Conditions, Subsequent Conditions, and the Shape and Life of the Law." In *Living Legislation: Durability, Change, and the Politics of American Lawmaking*, edited by Jeffrey A. Jenkins and Eric M. Patashnik, 111–34. Chicago: University of Chicago Press.

Markman, Maurie. 2008. "The Increasingly Complex World of Cancer Patient Advocacy Organizations." *Current Oncology Reports* 10 (1): 1–2.

Marmor, Theodore, Jonathan Oberlander, and Joseph White. 2009. "The Obama Administration's Options for Health Care Cost Control: Hope versus Reality." *Annals of Internal Medicine* 150 (7): 485–89.

Marmor, Theodore R. 1973. *The Politics of Medicare*. Chicago: Aldine.

———. 2000. *The Politics of Medicare*. 2nd ed. Social Institutions and Social Change. New York:
A. de Gruyter.

Marshall, Eliot. 2012. "Prostate Cancer Test Gets a Failing Grade." *Science*, May 21. http://www
.sciencemag.org/news/2012/05/prostate-cancer-test-gets-a-failing-grade.

Mayes, Rick, and Robert A. Berenson. 2006. *Medicare Prospective Payment and the Shaping of
U.S. Health Care*. Baltimore: Johns Hopkins University Press.

Mayhew, David R. 1974. *Congress: The Electoral Connection*. 2nd ed. New Haven, CT: Yale University Press.

Mayhew, David R. 2006. "Congress as a Problem Solver." In *Promoting the General Welfare: New Perspectives on Government Performance*, edited by Alan S. Gerber and Eric M. Patashnik, 219–36. Washington, DC: Brookings Institution Press.

———. 2012. "Lawmaking as Cognitive Enterprise." In *Living Legislation: Durability, Change, and the Politics of American Lawmaking*, edited by Jeffrey A. Jenkins and Eric M. Patashnik, 255–64. Chicago: University of Chicago Press.

Maynard, Alan, and Karen Bloor. 2003. "Trust and Performance Management in the Medical Marketplace." *Journal of the Royal Society of Medicine* 96 (11): 532–39.

Mazer, Deborah, and Gregory Curfman. 2017. "21st Century Cures Act Lowers Confidence in FDA-Approved Drugs." *Health Affairs Blog*, February 14. http://healthaffairs.org/blog/2017/02/14/21st-century-cures-act-lowers-confidence-in-fda-approved-drugs-and-devices/.

McArdle, Megan. 2015. "Regulation? Great idea. For someone else." *Bloombergview*, July 2. https://www.bloomberg.com/view/articles/2015-07-02/regulation-great-idea-for-someone-else-.

McCarty, Nolan M., Keith T. Poole, and Howard Rosenthal. 2008. *Polarized America: The Dance of Ideology and Unequal Riches*. Cambridge, MA: MIT Press.

McCaughey, Betsy. 2009. "Ruin Your Health with the Obama Stimulus Plan: Betsy McCaughey." Bloomberg.com, February 9. http://www.bloomberg.com/apps/news?pid=newsarchive&sid=aLzfDxfbwhzs.

McCrae, Cynthia, Eva Cherin, Gayle Yamazaki, Gretchen Diem, Alexander H. Vo, Dan Russell, J. Heiner Ellgring, Stanley Fahn, Paul Greene, Sandra Dillon, Hal Winfield, Kimberly B. Bjugstad, and Curt R. Freed. 2004. "Effects of Perceived Treatment on Quality of Life and Medical Outcomes in a Double-Blind Placebo Surgery Trial." *Archives of General Psychiatry* 61 (4): 412–20.

McCright, Aaron M., and Riley E. Dunlap. 2011. "The Politicization of Climate Change and Polarization in the American Public's Views of Global Warming, 2001–2010." *Sociology Quarterly* 52 (2): 155–94.

McCubbins, Mathew D., Roger G. Noll, and Barry R. Weingast. 1987. "Administrative Procedures as Instruments of Political Control." *Journal of Law, Economics, and Organization* 3 (2): 243–77.

———. 1989. "Structure and Process, Politics and Policy: Administrative Arrangements and the Political Control of Agencies." *Virginia Law Review* 75 (2): 431–82. doi:10.2307/1073179.

———. 1992. "Positive Canons: The Role of Legislative Bargains in Statutory Interpretation." *Georgetown Law Journal* 80: 705–42.

McCulloch, Peter, Myura Nagendran, W. Bruce Campbell, Andrew Price, Anant Jani, John D. Birkmeyer, and Muir Gray. 2013. "Strategies to Reduce Variation in the Use of Surgery." *Lancet* 382 (9898): 1130–39.

McDonough, John E. 2012. *Inside National Health Reform*. Berkeley: University of California Press.

McGinn, Thomas. 2015. "CDS, UX, and System Redesign—Promising Techniques and Tools to Bridge the Evidence Gap." *eGEMs* 3 (2): 1–4.

McGinty, J. B., L. L. Johnson, R. W. Jackson, A. M. McBryde, and J. W. Goodfellow. 1992. "Uses and Abuses of Arthroscopy: A Symposium." *Journal of Bone and Joint Surgery* 74 (10): 1563–77.

McGlynn, Elizabeth A. 2004. "There Is No Perfect Health System." *Health Affairs* 23 (3): 100–102. doi:10.1377/hlthaff.23.3.100.

McGlynn, Elizabeth A., Steven M. Asch, John Adams, John Keesey, Jennifer Hicks, Alison DeCristofaro, and Eve A. Kerr. 2003. "The Quality of Health Care Delivered to Adults in the United States." *New England Journal of Medicine* 348 (26): 2635–45.

McGlynn, Elizabeth A., David Meltzer, and Jacob S. Hacker. 2008. "Just How Good *Is* American Medical Care?" In *Health at Risk: America's Ailing Health System—And How to Heal It*, edited by Jacob S. Hacker, 88–105. New York: Columbia University Press.

McGlynn, Elizabeth A., Paul G. Shekelle, Susan Chen, Martha Timmer, Dana Goldman, John Romley, Peter Hussey, Han de Vries, Margaret Wang, Jason Carter, Carlo Tringale, and Roberta Shanman. 2008. "Health Care Efficiency Measures: Identification, Categorization, and Evaluation." AHRQ Publication 08-0030. Accessed September 16, 2008. http://www.ahrq .gov/qual/efficiency/index.html.

McKee, Selina. 2016. "Janssen Drops Price of Imbruvica to secure NICE nod." *PharmaTimes*, November 25. http://www.pharmatimes.com/news/janssen_drops_price_of_imbruvica _to_secure_nice_nod_1178544.

McNollgast. 1994. "Legislative Intent: The Use of Positive Political Theory in Statutory Interpretation." *Law and Contemporary Problems* 57 (1): 3–37.

McPherson, Klim, P. M. Strong, Arnold Epstein, and Lesley Jones. 1981. "Regional Variations in the Use of Common Surgical Procedures: Within and between England and Wales, Canada and the United States of America." *Social Science and Medicine: Part A; Medical Psychology and Medical Sociology* 15 (3): 273–88.

Mechanic, David. 1998a. "Public Trust and Initiatives for New Health Care Partnerships." *Milbank Quarterly* 76 (2): 281–302.

———. 1998b. "The Functions and Limitations of Trust in the Provision of Medical Care." *Journal of Health Politics, Policy and Law* 23 (4): 661–86.

———. 2004a. "In My Chosen Doctor I Trust." *British Medical Journal* 329 (7480): 1418–19.

———. 2004b. "The Rise and Fall of Managed Care." *Journal of Health and Social Behavior* 45 (extra issue): 76–86.

———. 2006. *The Truth about Health Care: Why Reform Is Not Working in America*. New Brunswick, NJ: Rutgers University Press. http://site.ebrary.com/id/10167786.

Mello, Michelle M., and Troyen A. Brennan. 2001. "The Controversy over High-Dose Chemotherapy with Autologous Bone Marrow Transplant for Breast Cancer." *Health Affairs* 20 (5): 101–17.

Mello, Michelle M., Amitabh Chandra, Atul Gawande, and David M. Studdert. 2010. "National Costs of the Medical Liability System." *Health Affairs* 29 (9): 1569–77.

Millenson, Michael. 2015. "Averting the Ax at AHRQ." *Health Care Blog*, June 21. http:// thehealthcareblog.com/blog/2015/06/21/averting-the-ax-at-ahrq/.

Miller, Franklin G. 2004 "Sham Surgery: An Ethical Analysis." *American Journal of Bioethics* 3 (4): 42.

Miller, Jake. 2014. "$1.9 Billion in Medicare Waste: 'Tip of the Iceberg.'" *Harvard Medical School News*, May 12. https://hms.harvard.edu/news/health-care-policy/19-billion-medicare-waste -tip-iceberg-5-12-14.

Mintrom, Michael, and Phillipa Norman. 2009. "Policy Entrepreneurship and Policy Change." *Policy Studies Journal* 37 (4): 649–67. doi:10.1111/j.1541-0072.2009.00329.x.

Moe, Terry M. 1984. "The New Economics of Organization." *American Journal of Political Science* 28 (4): 739–77. doi:10.2307/2110997.

———. 1989. "The Politics of Bureaucratic Structure." In *Can the Government Govern*, edited by John E. Chubb and Paul E. Peterson, 267–329. Washington, DC: Brookings Institution Press.

———. 2011. *Special Interest: Teachers Unions and America's Public Schools*. Washington, DC: Brookings Institution Press.

———. 2012. "Teachers Unions and American Education Reform: The Politics of Blocking." *Forum* 10 (1). doi:10.1515/1540-8884.1494.

———. 2015. "Vested Interests and Political Institutions." *Political Science Quarterly* 130 (2): 277–318. doi:10.1002/polq.12321.

Mooney, Chris. 2005. *The Republican War on Science*. New York: Basic Books.

Moore, Colin D. 2015. "Innovation without Reputation: How Bureaucrats Saved the Veterans' Health Care System." *Perspectives on Politics* 13 (2): 327–44.

Morone, James A. 1990. *The Democratic Wish: Popular Participation and the Limits of American Government.* Rev. ed. New Haven, CT: Yale University Press.

Morone, James A., and Gary S. Belkin. 1995. "The Science Illusion and the Triumph of Medical Capitalism." Paper presented at the American Political Science Association Annual Meeting, Chicago, September 2.

Morris, Zoë Slote, Steven Wooding, and Jonathan Grant. 2011. "The Answer Is 17 Years, What Is the Question: Understanding Time Lags in Translational Research." *Journal of the Royal Society of Medicine* 104 (12): 510–20.

Moseley, J. Bruce, Kimberly O'Malley, Nancy J. Petersen, Terri J. Menke, Baruch A. Brody, David H. Kuykendall, John C. Hollingsworth, Carol M. Ashton, and Nelda P. Wray. 2002. "A Controlled Trial of Arthroscopic Surgery for Osteoarthritis of the Knee." *New England Journal of Medicine* 347 (2): 81–88.

Moseley, J. Bruce, Nelda P. Wray, David Kuykendall, Kelly Willis, and Glenn Landon. 1996. "Arthroscopic Treatment of Osteoarthritis of the Knee: A Prospective, Randomized, Placebo-Controlled Trial Results of a Pilot Study." *American Journal of Sports Medicine* 24 (1): 28–34.

Mundy, Alicia. 2010. "Republican Targets Use of Costly Medical Devices." *Wall Street Journal*, December 9. http://www.wsj.com/articles/SB1000142405274870444760457600771265 5552694.

National Cancer Institute Division of Cancer Prevention. "Prostate, Lung, Colorectal, and Ovarian Cancer Screening Trial (PLCO)." http://prevention.cancer.gov/major-programs /prostate-lung-colorectal.

NPC (National Pharmaceutical Council). 2015. "NPC Highlight Stakeholder Views on Comparative Effectiveness Research and the Environment for Health Care Decision-Making." National Pharmaceutical Council, March 26. http://www.npcnow.org/newsroom/press-releases/npc -highlights-stakeholder-views-comparative-effectiveness-research-and-environment.

Neumann, Peter J. 2006. "Emerging Lessons from the Drug Effectiveness Review Project." *Health Affairs* 25 (4): W262–71. doi:10.1377/hlthaff.25.w262.

Neumann, Peter J., and James Chambers. 2013. "Medicare's Reset on 'Coverage with Evidence Development.'" *Health Affairs Blog*, April 1. http://healthaffairs.org/blog/2013/04/01 /medicares-reset-on-coverage-with-evidence-development/.

Neumann, Peter J., and Milton C. Weinstein. 2010. "Legislating against Use of Cost-Effectiveness Information." *New England Journal of Medicine* 363 (16): 1495–97.

Newhouse, Joseph P. 1992. "Medical Care Costs: How Much Welfare Loss?" *Journal of Economic Perspectives* 6 (3): 3–21.

Nicholson, Stephen P. 2012. "Polarizing Cues." *American Journal of Political Science* 56 (1): 52–66. doi:10.1111/j.1540-5907.2011.00541.x.

North American Spine Society. 2009. "Position Statement on Comparative Effectiveness Research (CER)." http://www.spine.org/Documents/Position_Statement_CER.pdf. Accessed February 4, 2013.

Oberlander, Jonathan. 2003. *The Political Life of Medicare.* American Politics and Political Economy. Chicago: University of Chicago Press.

———. 2007. "Health Reform Interrupted: The Unraveling of the Oregon Health Plan." *Health Affairs* 26 (1): w96–w105.

———. 2012. "The Bush Administration and Politics of Medicare Reform." In *Building Coalitions, Making Policy: The Politics of the Clinton, Bush & Obama Presidencies*, edited by Martin A. Levin, Daniel DiSalvo, and Martin M. Shapiro, 150-80. Baltimore: Johns Hopkins University Press.

———. 2016. "The $40 Trillion Question: Can Congress Control Health Care Spending." In *Congress and Policymaking in the 21st Century*, edited by Jeffrey A. Jenkins and Eric M. Patashnik, 211–41. Cambridge: Cambridge University Press.

Oberlander, Jonathan, and Miriam J. Laugesen. 2015. "Leap of Faith—Medicare's New Physician Payment System." *New England Journal of Medicine* 373 (13): 1185–87. doi:10.1056/NEJMp1509154.

Oberlander, Jonathan, and R. Kent Weaver. 2015. "Unraveling from Within? The Affordable Care Act and Self-Undermining Policy Feedbacks." *Forum* 13 (1): 37–62.

Okie, Susan. 2002. "Knee Surgery for Arthritis Is Ineffective, Study Finds." *Washington Post*, July 11. https://www.washingtonpost.com/archive/politics/2002/07/11/knee-surgery-for-arthritis-is-ineffective-study-finds/68c3a82e-86eb-4632-bfe8-7eea47bc4662/?utm_term=.07076c1f8d36.

Oliver, Michael J., and Hugh Pemberton. 2004. "Learning and Change in 20th-Century British Economic Policy." *Governance* 17 (3): 415–41.

Oliver, Thomas R. 2004. "Policy Entrepreneurship in the Social Transformation of American Medicine: The Rise of Managed Care and Managed Competition." *Journal of Health Politics, Policy and Law* 29 (4–5): 701–33.

Oliver, Thomas R., Philip R. Lee, and Helene L. Lipton. 2004. "A Political History of Medicare and Prescription Drug Coverage." *Milbank Quarterly* 82 (2): 283–354.

Olsen, LeighAnne, Claudia Grossman, and J. Michael McGinnis, eds. 2011. *Learning What Works: Infrastructure Required for Comparative Effectiveness Research: Workshop Summary*. Washington, DC: National Academies Press.

Olson, Mary K. 2014. "The Food and Drug Administration." In *The Guide to U.S. Health and Health Care Policy*, edited by Thomas Oliver, 65–77. Thousand Oaks, CA: Sage; London: CQ Press.

Orren, Karen, and Stephen Skowronek. 2004. *The Search for American Political Development*. Cambridge: Cambridge University Press.

Orszag, Peter. 2010. "Malpractice Methodology." *New York Times*, October 20. http://www.nytimes.com/2010/10/21/opinion/21orszag.html.

———. 2014. "A Better Fix for Medical Malpractice." *BloombergView*, February 25. https://www.bloomberg.com/view/articles/2014-02-25/a-better-fix-for-medical-malpractice.

Page, Benjamin I., and Robert Y. Shapiro. 1992. *The Rational Public: Fifty Years of Trends in Americans' Policy Preferences*. Chicago: University of Chicago Press.

Parker-Pope, Tara. 2012a. "Older Men Still Being Screened for Prostate Cancer." *New York Times*, April 24. http://well.blogs.nytimes.com/2012/04/24/older-men-still-being-\screened-for-prostate-cancer/.

———. 2012b. "Questioning Surgery for Early Prostate Cancer." *New York Times*, July 18. http://well.blogs.nytimes.com/2012/07/18/questioning-surgery-for-early-prostate-cancer/.

Parsons, Talcott. 1939. "The Professions and Social Structure." *Social Forces* 17 (4): 457–67.

Patashnik, Eric M. 2008. *Reforms at Risk: What Happens after Major Policy Changes Are Enacted*. Princeton, NJ: Princeton University Press.

———. 2015. "Here are the 5 Reasons Republicans Are Trying to Cut Research on Evidence-Based Medicine." *Washington Post*, June 22. https://www.washingtonpost.com/news/monkey-cage/wp/2015/06/22/here-are-the-5-reasons-republicans-are-trying-to-cut-research-on-evidence-based-medicine/?utm_term=.c050ee81be1b.

Patashnik, Eric M., and Julian E. Zelizer. 2013. "The Struggle to Remake Politics: Liberal Reform and the Limits of Policy Feedback in the Contemporary American State." *Perspectives on Politics* 11 (4): 1071–87.

Patel, K. 2010. "Health Reform's Tortuous Route to the Patient-Centered Outcomes Research Institute." *Health Affairs* 29 (10): 1777–82.

Patton, J. 2013. "One-Size-Fits-All Approach to Health Care Is Bad for Patients." *Tennessean*, January 10. http://www.tennessean.com/apps/pbcs.dll/article?AID=2013301110059&gcheck=1. Accessed January 23, 2013.

PCORI (Patient-Centered Outcomes Research Institute). 2013. "Strategic Plan," PCORI, November 18. http://www.pcori.org/assets/2013/11/PCORI-Board-Meeting-Strategic-Plan -111813.pdf.

PCORI (Patient-Centered Outcomes Research Institute). 2010. "Compilation of Patient Protection and Affordable Care Act," PCORI, June 9. http://www.pcori.org/sites/default/files /PCORI_Authorizing_Legislation.pdf.

PCORI (Patient-Centered Outcomes Research Institute). 2017. "Comparison of Peer-Facilitated Support Group and Cognitive Behavioral Therapy for Hoarding Disorder," PCORI, accessed June 6. http://www.pcori.org/research-results/2013/comparison-peer-facilitated -support-group-and-cognitive-behavioral-therapy.

Pear, Robert. 1991. "New Cost Control Asked on Medicare." *New York Times*, June 9. http:// www.nytimes.com/1991/06/09/us/new-cost-control-asked-on-medicare.html.

———. 2003. "Congress Weighs Drug Comparisons." *New York Times*, August 24. http://www .nytimes.com/2003/08/24/us/congress-weighs-drug-comparisons.html.

———. 2009a. "Obama Push to Cut Health Costs Faces Tough Odds." *New York Times*, May 11. http://www.nytimes.com/2009/05/12/us/politics/12health.html.

———. 2009b. "U.S. to Study Effectiveness of Treatments." *New York Times*, February 15. http:// www.nytimes.com/2009/02/16/health/policy/16health.html.

Pearson, Steven D., and Peter B. Bach. 2010. "How Medicare Could Use Comparative Effectiveness Research in Deciding on New Coverage and Reimbursement." *Health Affairs* 29 (10): 1796–804.

Perlroth, Daniella J., Dana P. Goldman, and Alan M. Garber. 2010. "The Potential Impact of Comparative Effectiveness Research on U.S. Health Care Expenditures." *Demography* 47 (1): S173–S190.

Perry, Seymour. 1982. "The Brief Life of the National Center for Health Care Technology." *New England Journal of Medicine* 307 (17): 1095–100.

Peterson, Mark A. 1993. "Political Influence in the 1990s: From Iron Triangles to Policy Networks." *Journal of Health Politics, Policy and Law* 18 (2): 395–438.

———. 2001. "From Trust to Political Power: Interest Groups, Public Choice, and Health Care Markets." Special Issue on Kenneth Arrow and the Changing Economics of Health Care. *Journal of Health Politics, Policy and Law* 26: 1145–63.

———. 2003. "From Trust to Political Power: Interest Groups, Public Choice, and Health Care Markets." In *Uncertain Times: Kenneth Arrow and the Changing Economics of Health Care*, edited by Peter J. Hammer, Deborah Haas-Wilson, Mark A. Peterson, and William M. Sage, 272–89. Durham, NC: Duke University Press.

Peterson, Paul E., and Martin R. West. 2003. *No Child Left Behind? The Politics and Practice of School Accountability*. Washington, DC: Brookings Institution Press.

Petrocik, John R. 1996. "Issue Ownership in Presidential Elections, with a 1980 Case Study." *American Journal of Political Science* 40 (3): 825–50.

Pew Research Center. 2009. "Surprise, Disagreement over Mammogram: Guidelines Strong Interest in Health Care, Little Interest in Palin." *For The People and the Press*, November 25. http://www.people-press.org/files/legacy-pdf/567.pdf.

———. 2014. "Section 10: Political Participation, Interest and Knowledge." *Beyond Red vs. Blue: The Political Typology*, June 26. http://www.people-press.org/2014/06/26/section-10 -political-participation-interest-and-knowledge/.

Phurrough, Steve, Anthony Norris, Shamiram Feinglass, Tanisha Carino, Lawrence Schott. 2003. "National Coverage Determination Memorandum for Arthroscopy for the Knee." *Centers for Medicare and Medicaid Services*, July 3. https://www.cms.gov/medicare-coverage -database/details/nca-decision memo.aspx?NCAId=7&NCDId=285&ncdver=1&IsPopup =y&bc=AAAAAAAAgAAAA%3D%3D&.

Pierson, Paul. 1995. *Dismantling the Welfare State? Reagan, Thatcher and the Politics of Retrenchment*. Cambridge: Cambridge University Press.

———. 2000. "Increasing Returns, Path Dependence, and the Study of Politics." *American Political Science Review* 94 (2): 251–67.

———, ed. 2001. *The New Politics of the Welfare State*. Oxford: Oxford University Press.

Pollack, Andrew. 2013. "Looser Guidelines Issued on Prostate Screening." *New York Times*, May 3. http://www.nytimes.com/2013/05/04/business/prostate-screening-guidelines-are-loosened.html.

Polsby, Nelson W. 1985. *Political Innovation in America: The Politics of Policy Initiation*. New Haven, CT: Yale University Press.

Popkin, Samuel L. 1994. *The Reasoning Voter*. 2nd ed. Chicago: University of Chicago Press.

Posner, Richard A. 2003. *Law, Pragmatism, and Democracy*. Cambridge, MA: Harvard University Press.

Quirk, Paul J. 2010. "Politicians Do Pander: Mass Opinion, Polarization, and Law Making." *Forum* 7 (4). https://doi.org/10.2202/1540-8884.1343.

Rahn, W. 1993. "The Role of Partisan Stereotypes in Information Processing about Political Candidates." *American Journal of Political Science* 37 (2): 472–96.

Rasmussen Reports. 2010. "79% Trust Their Doctor." August 24. http://www.rasmussenreports.com/public_content/lifestyle/general_lifestyle/august_2010/79_trust_their_doctor. Accessed February 23, 2012.

Ravaud, Philippe, Laurence Moulinier, Bruno Giraudeau, Xavier Ayral, Corinne Guerin, Eric Noel, Philippe Thomas, Bruno Fautrel, Bernard Mazieres, and Maxime Dougados. 1999. "Effects of Joint Lavage and Steroid Injection in Patients with Osteoarthritis of the Knee: Results of a Multicenter, Randomized, Controlled Trial." *Arthritis and Rheumatism* 42 (3): 475–82. doi:10.1002/1529-0131(199904) 42:3<475::AID-ANR12>3.0.CO;2-S.

Ray, N., and J. Sokolovsky. 2009. "Comparative Effectiveness: Ongoing Initiatives and Physician Perspectives." *Medpac*, September 18. http://www.medpac.gov/transcripts/comparative%20effectiveness.pdf. Accessed September 13, 2012.

Reames, Bradley N., Sarah P. Shubeck, and John D. Birkmeyer. 2014. "Strategies for Reducing Regional Variation in the Use of Surgery: A Systematic Review." *Annals of Surgery* 259 (4): 616–27.

Reichard, John. 2007. "Consensus Emerging on Need for New Board to Determine 'What Works' in Medicine." *Washington Health Policy Week in Review*, June 18. http://authoring.commonwealthfund.org/publications/newsletters/washington-health-policy-in-review/2007/jun/washington-health-policy-week-in-review-june-18-2007/consensus-emerging-on-need-for-new-board-to-determine-what-works-in-medicine.

Reimer, Torsten, Rui Mata, and Markus Stoecklin. 2004. "The Use of Heuristics in Persuasion: Deriving Cues on Source Expertise from Argument Quality." *Current Research in Social Psychology* 10 (6): 69–83.

Reinhardt, Uwe E., Peter S. Hussey, and Gerard F. Anderson. 2002. "Cross-National Comparisons of Health Systems Using OECD Data, 1999." *Health Affairs* 21 (3): 169–81.

Reuben, David B., and Christine K. Cassel. 2011. "Physician Stewardship of Health Care in an Era of Finite Resources." *Journal of the American Medical Association* 306 (4): 430–31.

Rice, Sabriya. 2015. "First PCORI studies on improving care are done, but where are the results?" *Modern Healthcare*, May 1. http://www.modernhealthcare.com/article/20150501/NEWS/150429915/first-pcori-studies-on-improving-care-are-done-but-where-are-the.

Rich, Spencer. 1996. "Citing Duplication, Private Sector Effort, GOP Moves to Cut Health Cost Research." *Washington Post*, June 27. https://www.washingtonpost.com/archive/politics/1996/06/27/citing-duplication-private-sector-effort-gop-moves-to-cut-health-cost-research/783434e2-369b-4a7f-9b9c-650742ab8613/?utm_term=.4ff6ec831d45.

Robinson, James C. 2001. "The End of Managed Care." *JAMA* 285 (20): 2622–8.

Robinson, James C. 2015. *Purchasing Medical Innovation: The Right Technology, for the Right Patient, at the Right Price*. Berkeley: University of California Press.

Rodwin, Marc A. 2001. "The Politics of Evidence-Based Medicine." *Journal of Health Politics, Policy and Law* 26 (2): 439–46.

Rodwin, Marc A. 2011. *Conflicts of Interest and the Future of Medicine: The United States, France and Japan*. New York: Oxford University Press.

Roman, Benjamin R., and David A. Asch. 2014. "Faded Promises: The Challenge of Deadopting Low-value Care." *Annals of Internal Medicine* 161 (2): 149–50.

Rose, Susannah L. 2013. "Patient Advocacy Organizations: Institutional Conflicts of Interest, Trust, and Trustworthiness." *Journal of Law, Medicine and Ethics* 41 (3): 680–87.

Rosenberg, Alan, Abiy Agiro, Marc Gottlieb, John Barron, Peter Brady, Ying Liu, Cindy Li, and Andrea DeVries. 2015. "Early Trends among Seven Recommendations from the Choosing Wisely Campaign." *JAMA Internal Medicine* 175 (12): 1913–20. doi:10.1001/jamainternmed.2015.5441.

Rosenthal, Elisabeth. 2014. "Patients' Costs Skyrocket; Specialists' Incomes Soar." *New York Times*, January 18. https://www.nytimes.com/2014/01/19/health/patients-costs-skyrocket-specialists-incomes-soar.html?_r=1.

Roy, Avik. 2010. "The Dartmouth Atlas and Obamacare." *National Review*, June 9. http://www.nationalreview.com/article/229919/dartmouth-atlas-and-obamacare-avik-roy.

Ruger, Theodore W. 2011. "Plural Constitutionalism and the Pathologies of American Health Care." *Yale Law Journal Online* 120: 347–65. http://lawlib.wlu.edu/CLJC/index.aspx?mainid=1409&issuedate=2011-05-09.

———. 2012a. "Of Icebergs and Glaciers: The Submerged Constitution of American Healthcare." *Law and Contemporary Problems* 75 (3): 215–35.

———. 2012b. "Failure by Obsolescence: Regulatory Challenges for the DFA in the Twenty-First Century." In *Regulatory Breakdown: The Crisis of Confidence in U.S. Regulation*, edited by Cary Coglianese, 245–58. Philadelphia: University of Pennsylvania Press.

Saad, Lydia. 2009. "On Healthcare, America Trusts Physicians over Politicians." *Gallup*, June 17. http://www.gallup.com/poll/120890/healthcare-americans-trust-physicians-politicians.aspx.

Sackett, David L., William M. C. Rosenberg, J. A. Muir Gray, R. Brian Haynes, and W. Scott Richardson. 1996. "Evidence Based Medicine: What It Is and What It Isn't." *British Journal of Medicine* 312: 71–72. http://www.ncbi.nlm.nih.gov/pmc/articles/PMC2349778/.

Sammon, Jesse D., Firas Abdollah, Toni K. Choueiri, Philip W. Kantoff, Paul L. Nguyen, Mani Menon, and Quoc-Dien Trinh. 2015. "Prostate-Specific Antigen Screening after 2012 US Preventive Services Task Force Recommendations." *JAMA* 314 (19): 2077–79. doi:10.1001/jama.2015.7273.

Sanger-Katz, Margot. 2012. "Why We Trust Doctors." *National Journal*, April 21, 24–28.

Schaffner, Brian F., Matthew Streb, and Gerald Wright. 2001. "Teams without Uniforms: The Nonpartisan Ballot in State and Local Elections." *Political Research Quarterly* 54: 7–30.

Schickler, Eric. 2001. *Disjointed Pluralism: Institutional Innovation and the Development of the U.S. Congress*. Princeton Studies in American Politics. Princeton, NJ: Princeton University Press.

Schlesinger, Mark. 2002. "A Loss of Faith: The Sources of Reduced Political Legitimacy for the American Medical Profession." *Milbank Quarterly* 80 (2): 185–235.

Schlesinger, Mark, and Bradford H. Gray. 2016. "Incomplete Markets and Imperfect Institutions: Some Challenges Posed by Trust for Contemporary Health Care and Health Policy." *Journal of Health Politics, Policy and Law* 41 (4): 717–42.

Schlesinger, Mark, and Rachel Grob. 2017. "Treating, Fast and Slow: Americans' Understanding of and Responses to Low-Value Care." *Milbank Quarterly* 95 (1): 70–116.

Schneider, Mark, Paul Teske, with Michael Mintrom. 1995. *Public Entrepreneurs: Agents for Change in American Government*. Princeton, NJ: Princeton University Press.

Schoen, Cathy, Robin Osborn, Michelle M. Doty, Meghan Bishop, Jordon Peugh, and Nandita Murukutla. 2007. "Toward Higher-Performance Health Systems: Adults' Health Care Experiences in Seven Countries." *Health Affairs* 26 (6): w717–w734.

Schoen, Cathy, Robin Osborn, David Squires, Michelle M. Doty, Roz Pierson, and Sandra Applebaum. 2010. "How Health Insurance Design Affects Access to Care and Costs, by Income, in Eleven Countries. *Health Affairs* 29 (12): 2323–34.

Schulte, Fred. 2015. "Is Obamacare's Research Institute Worth the Billions?" *NPR*. August 4. http://www.npr.org/sections/health-shots/2015/08/04/428164731/is-obamacares-research-institute-worth-the-billions.

Schumpeter, Joseph A. 1942. *Capitalism, Socialism, and Democracy*. New York: Harper Perennial Modern Thought.

Sedensky, Matt, and Ricardo Alonso-Zaldivar. 2015. "Once Politically Toxic, Medicare Plans to Cover End-of-Life Counseling." *PBS Newshour*. July 9. http://www.pbs.org/newshour/rundown/politically-toxic-medicare-plans-cover-end-life-counseling/.

Selby, Joe. 2014. "PCORI's Research Will Answer Patients' Real-World Questions." *Health Affairs Blog*, March 25. http://healthaffairs.org/blog/2014/03/25/pcoris-research-will-answer-patients-real-world-questions/.

Selker, Harry P., and Alastair J. J. Wood. 2009. "Industry Influence on Comparative-Effectiveness Research Funded through Health Care Reform." *New England Journal of Medicine* 361 (27): 2595–97. doi:10.1056/NEJMp0910747.

Sheingate, Adam D. 2003. "Political Entrepreneurship, Institutional Change, and American Political Development." *Studies in American Political Development* 17 (2): 185–203. doi:10.1017/S0898588X03000129.

Shepsle, Kenneth A. 1992 "Bureaucratic Drift, Coalitional Drift, and Time Consistency: A Comment on Macey." *Journal of Law, Economics, and Organization* 8 (1): 111–18.

Sihvonen, Raine, Mika Paavola, Antti Malmivaara, Ari Itälä, Antti Joukainen, Heikki Nurmi, Juha Kalske, and Teppo L. N. Järvinen. 2013. "Arthroscopic Partial Meniscectomy versus Sham Surgery for a Degenerative Meniscal Tear." *New England Journal of Medicine* 369 (26): 2515–24. doi:10.1056/NEJMoa1305189.

Sirovich, Brenda, Patricia M. Gallagher, David E. Wennberg, and Elliott S. Fisher. 2008. "Discretionary Decision Making by Primary Care Physicians and the Cost of U.S. Health Care." *Health Affairs* 27 (3): 813–23. doi:10.1377/hlthaff.27.3.813.

Sirovich, Brenda E., and H. Gilbert Welch. 2004. "Cervical Cancer Screening among Women without a Cervix." *JAMA* 291 (24): 2990–93.

Sirovich, Brenda E., Steven Woloshin, and Lisa M. Schwartz. 2011. "Too Little? Too Much? Primary Care Physicians' Views on US Health Care: A Brief Report." *Archives of Internal Medicine* 171 (17): 1582–85.

Skinner, Jonathan. 2011. "Causes and Consequences of Geographic Variation in Health Care." In *Handbook of Health Economics*, edited by Mark V. Pauly, Thomas G. McGuire, and Pedro P. Barros, 2: 45–93. Oxford: North Holland.

Skinner, Jonathan. 2006. "Geography and the Use of Effective Health Care in the United States." In *Health Care Issues in the United States and Japan*, edited by David A. Wise and Jaohiro Yashiro, 195–208. Chicago: University of Chicago Press.

Skinner, Jonathan, Amitabh Chandra, David Goodman, and Elliott S. Fisher. 2009. "The Elusive Connection between Health Care Spending and Quality." *Health Affairs* 28 (1): w119–23.

Skinner, Jonathan, and Elliott S. Fisher. 2010. "Reflections on Geographic Variations in U.S. Health Care." The Dartmouth Institute for Health Policy and Clinical Practice. http://www.dartmouthatlas.org/downloads/press/Skinner_Fisher_DA_05_10.pdf.

Skinner, Jonathan S., Elliott S. Fisher, and John Wennberg. 2005. "The Efficiency of Medicare." In *Analyses in the Economics of Aging*, edited by David A. Wise, 129–60. Chicago: University of Chicago Press.

Skinner, Jonathan S., David Goodman, and Elliott Fisher. 2015. "Making Sense of Price and Quantity Variations in U.S. Health Care." *Health Affairs Blog*, December 30. http://healthaffairs.org/blog/2015/12/30/making-sense-of-price-and-quantity-variations-in-u-s-health-care/.

Skocpol, Theda. 1992. "The Narrow Vision of Today's Experts on Social Policy." *Chronicle of Higher Education*, April 15. http://chronicle.com/article/The-Narrow-Vision-of-Todays/82174/.

———. 2003. *Diminished Democracy: From Membership to Management in American Civic Life*. Norman, OK: University of Oklahoma Press.

Skowronek, Stephen, Stephen M. Engel, and Bruce Ackerman. 2016. *The Progressives' Century: Political Reform, Constitutional Government, and the Modern American State*. New Haven, CT: Yale University Press.

Slater, Michael D., and Donna Rouner. 1996. "How Message Evaluation and Source Attributes May Influence Credibility Assessment and Belief Change." *Journalism and Mass Communication Quarterly* 74 (4): 974–91.

Sorenson, Corinna. 2015. *Toward Effective Health Technology Regulation*. PhD dissertation, London School Economics and Political Science.

Sorenson, Corinna, Michael K. Gusmano, and Adam Oliver. 2014. "The Politics of Comparative Effectiveness Research: Lessons from Recent History." *Journal of Health Politics, Policy and Law* 39 (1): 139–70. doi:10.1215/03616878-2395199.

Sox, Harold. 2012. "The Patient-Centered Outcomes Research Institute Should Focus on High-Impact Problems That Can Be Solved Quickly." *Health Affairs* 31 (10): 2176–82. doi:10.1377/hlthaff.2012.0171.

Spodick, David H. 1975. "Numerators without Denominators: There Is No FDA for the Surgeon." *JAMA* 232 (1): 35–36. doi:10.1001/jama.1975.03250010017015.

Sprague, Norman F. 1981. "Arthroscopic Debridement for Degenerative Knee Joint Disease." *Clinical Orthopaedics and Related Research* 160: 118–23.

Squires, David A. 2011. "The U.S. Health System in Perspective: A Comparison of Twelve Industrialized Nations." *Issue Brief (The Commonwealth Fund)* 16: 1–14.

Stabile, Mark, Sarah Thomson, Sara Allin, Seán Boyle, Reinhard Busse, Karine Chevreul, Greg Marchildon, and Elias Mossialos. 2013. "Health Care Cost Containment Strategies Used in Four Other High-Income Countries Hold Lessons for the United States." *Health Affairs* 32 (4): 643–52.

Stafford, Randall S., Todd H. Wagner, and Philip W. Lavori. 2009. "New, but Not Improved? Incorporating Comparative-Effectiveness Information into FDA Labeling." *New England Journal of Medicine* 361 (13): 1230–33.

Starr, Paul. 1982. *The Social Transformation of American Medicine*. New York: Basic Books.

———. 2011. *Remedy and Reaction*. New Haven, CT: Yale University Press.

Stein, Rob, and Dan Eggen. 2009. "White House Backs off Cancer Test Guidelines." *Washington Post*, November 19. http://www.washingtonpost.com/wp-dyn/content/article/2009/11/18/AR2009111802545.html. Accessed March 16, 2010.

Steinbrook, Robert. 2008. "Saying No Isn't NICE—the Travails of Britain's National Institute for Health and Clinical Excellence." *New England Journal of Medicine* 359 (19): 1977–81.

Stevens, Rosemary A. 2001. "Public Roles for the Medical Profession in the United States: Beyond Theories of Decline and Fall." *Milbank Quarterly* 79 (3): 327–53.

Stevens, Rosemary, Charles E. Rosenberg, and Lawton R. Burns. 2006. *History and Health Policy in the United States: Putting the Past Back In*. New Brunswick, NJ: Rutgers University Press.

Stigler, George J. 1971. "The Theory of Economic Regulation." *Bell Journal of Economics and Management Science* 2 (1): 3–21.

Stokes, Donald E. 1963. "Spatial Models of Party Competition." *American Political Science Review* 57 (2): 368–77.

Stone, Deborah A. 1977. "Professionalism and Accountability. Controlling Health Services in the United States and West Germany." *Journal of Health Politics, Policy and Law* 2 (1): 32–47.

Stone, Deborah. 2011. *Policy Paradox: The Art of Political Decision Making.* 3rd ed. New York: W. W. Norton.

Subramanian, Usha, Morris Weinberger, George J. Eckert, Gilbert J. L'Italien, Pablo Lapuerta, and William Tierney. 2002. "Geographic Variation in Health Care Utilization and Outcomes in Veterans with Acute Myocardial Infarction." *Journal of General Internal Medicine* 17 (8): 604–11.

Sung, Daniel H. 2003. "Orthopaedics Responds as Medicare Questions Arthroscopy for Osteoarthritis of the Knee." *American Academy of Orthopedic Surgeons Bulletin* 51 (4). http://www2.aaos.org/bulletin/aug03/fline2.htm.

Suskind, Ron. 2011. *Confidence Men: Wall Street, Washington, and the Education of a President.* New York: Harper Collins.

Swenson, Peter. n.d. "The Political Transformation of American Medicine: Doctors, Democracy, and Disease in the Progressive Era." Unpublished book manuscript. Yale University Department of Political Science.

Tanden, Neera, Zeke Emanuel, Topher Spiro, Emily Oshima Lee, and Thomas Huelskoetter. 2014. "Comparing the Effectiveness of Health Care." *Center for American Progress*, January 24. https://www.americanprogress.org/issues/healthcare/reports/2014/01/24/82775/comparing-the-effectiveness-of-health-care/.

Tanenbaum, Sandra J. 2012. "Reducing Variation in Health Care: The Rhetorical Politics of a Policy Idea." *Journal of Health Politics, Policy and Law* 37 (6): 5–26.

Teles, Steven. 2010. "Brains on Drugs." *Washington Monthly*, May/June, 48–52.

Temple, Robert. 2012. "A Regulator's View of Comparative Effectiveness Research." *Clinical Trials* 9 (1): 56–65.

Tenery, Robert, Herbert Rakatansky, Frank A. Riddick, Jr., Michael S. Goldrich, Leonard J. Morse, John M. O'Bannon, III, Priscilla Ray, et al. 2002. "Surgical 'Placebo' Controls." *Annals of Surgery* 235 (2): 303–7.

Thorlund, Jonas Bloch, Carsten Bogh Juhl, Ewa M. Roos, and L. S. Lohmander. 2015. "Arthroscopic Surgery for Degenerative Knee: Systematic Review and Meta-analysis of benefits and harms." *British Medical Journal* 350: h2747, 1–7.

Tierney, John. 2016. "The Real War on Science." *City Journal*, Autumn. https://www.city-journal.org/html/real-war-science-14782.html.

Tilburt, Jon C., Matthew K. Wynia, Robert D. Sheeler, Bjord Thorsteinsdottir, Katherine M. James, Jason S. Egginton, Mark Liebow, Samia Hurst, Marion Danis, and Susan Dorr Goold. 2013. "Views of US Physicians about Controlling Health Care Costs." *JAMA* 310 (4): 380–89. doi:10.1001/jama.2013.8278.

Timbie, Justin W., D. Steven Fox, Kristin Van Busum, and Eric C. Schneider. 2012. "Five Reasons That Many Comparative Effectiveness Studies Fail to Change Patient Care and Clinical Practice." *Health Affairs* 31 (10): 2168–75. doi:10.1377/hlthaff.2012.0150.

Timmermans, Stefan, and Marc Berg. 2003. "The Practice of Medical Technology." *Sociology of Health and Illness* 25 (3): 97–114.

———. 2010. *The Gold Standard: The Challenge of Evidence-Based Medicine and Standardization in Health Care.* Philadelphia: Temple University Press.

Tuohy, Carolyn Hughes. 1999. *Accidental Logics: The Dynamics of Change in the Health Care Arena in the United States, Britain, and Canada.* Oxford: Oxford University Press.

Tunis, Sean R., Robert A. Berenson, Steve E. Phurrough, and Penny E. Mohr. 2011. "Improving the Quality and Efficiency of the Medicare Program through Coverage Policy." Princeton, NJ: Robert Wood Johnson Foundation.

Tunis, Sean R., and Steven D. Pearson. 2006. "Coverage Options for Promising Technologies: Medicare's Coverage with Evidence Development.'" *Health Affairs* 25 (5): 1218–30.

———. 2010. "US Moves to Improve Health Decisions." *British Medical Journal* 341 (1): 431–33.

Twedt, Steve. 2016. "Medicare Part B Proposal Draws Physician Protests." *Pittsburgh Post-Gazette*, March 10. http://www.post-gazette.com/business/healthcare-business/2016/03/11/Medicare-Part-B-proposal-draws-physician-protests/stories/201603110131.

Tyssen, Reidar, Karen S. Palmer, Ingunn B. Solberg, Edgar Voltmer, and Erica Frank. 2013. "Physicians' Perceptions of Quality of Care, Professional Autonomy, and Job Satisfaction in Canada, Norway, and the United States." *BioMed Central Health Services Research* 13: 516–25.

Ubel, Peter A. 2015. "Why It's Not Time for Health Care Rationing." *Hastings Center Report* 45 (2): 15–19. doi:10.1002/hast.427.

Ubel, Peter A., and David A. Asch. 2015. "Creating Value in Health by Understanding and Overcoming Resistance to De-innovation." *Health Affairs* 34 (2): 239–44.

U.S. Congress. Congressional Record. 108th Cong., 1st sess., 2003. Vol. 149, no. 95—daily edition.

USPSTF (U.S. Preventive Services Task Force). 2008. "Screening for Prostate Cancer: U.S. Preventive Services Task Force Recommendation Statement." *Annals of Internal Medicine* 149: 185–91.

———. 2012. "Final Recommendation Statement: Colorectal Cancer; Screening." http://www.uspreventiveservicestaskforce.org/Page/Document/RecommendationStatementFinal/colorectal-cancer-screening.

———. 2012. "Draft Recommendation Statement: Prostate Cancer; Screening." https://www.uspreventiveservicestaskforce.org/Page/Document/draft-recommendation-statement/prostate-cancer-screening1.

Van Parys, Jessica, and Jonathan Skinner. 2016. "Physician Practice Style Variation—Implications for Policy." *JAMA Internal Medicine* 176 (10): 1549–50.

Vavreck, Lynn, and Douglas Rivers. 2008. "The 2006 Cooperative Congressional Election Study." *Journal of Elections, Public Opinion and Parties* 18 (4): 355–66.

Volden, Craig, and Alan E. Wiseman. 2014. *Legislative Effectiveness in the United States Congress: The Lawmakers*. New York: Cambridge University Press.

Volsky, Igor. 2009. "Thomas Scully: 'Medicare Makes Decisions on Coverage All the Time, I Made Decisions on Coverage All the Time.'" *Think Progress*, April 2. http://thinkprogress.org/health/2009/04/02/170731/scully-cer/.

Walker, Emily P. 2011. "AMA: One Again Fewer Doctors Choose AMA." *MedPage*, June 20. http://www.medpagetoday.com/meetingcoverage/ama/27147.

Weaver, R. K. 1986. "The Politics of Blame Avoidance." *Journal of Public Policy* 6 (4): 371–98.

Weimer, David L. 2010. *Medical Governance: Values, Expertise, and Interests in Organ Transplantation*. Washington, DC: Georgetown University Press.

Welch, H. Gilbert. 2015. "Responding to the Challenge of Overdiagnosis." *Academic Radiology* 8 (22): 945–46. doi:10.1016/j.acra.2014.08.019.

Welch, H. Gilbert, Lisa Schwartz, and Steve Woloshin. 2011. *Overdiagnosed: Making People Sick in the Pursuit of Health*. Boston: Beacon.

Wennberg, John, and Alan Gittelsohn. 1982. "Variations in Medical Care among Small Areas." *Scientific American* 246 (4): 120–34.

Wennberg, John, and Alan M. Gittelsohn. 1973. "Small Area Variations in Health Care Delivery." *Science* 182 (117): 1102–8.

Wennberg, John E. 2010. *Tracking Medicine: A Researcher's Quest to Understand Health Care*. Oxford: Oxford University Press.

Wennberg, John E., Elliot S. Fisher, and Jonathan S. Skinner. 2002. "Geography and the Debate over Medicare Reform." *Health Affairs*, February. doi:10.1377/hlthaff.w2.96.

Wennberg International Collaborative. 2011. "Report of the Second Annual Conference." http://wennbergcollaborative.org/uploads/documents/WIC2011Report.pdf.

Westfall, John M., James Mold, and Lyle Fagnan. 2007. "Practice-Based Research—'Blue Highways' on the NIH Roadmap." *JAMA* 297 (4): 403–6. doi:10.1001/jama.297.4.403.

Whoriskey, Peter, and Dan Keating. 2013. "How a Secretive Panel Uses Data That Distorts Doctors' Pay." *Washington Post*, July 20. https://www.washingtonpost.com/business/economy/how-a-secretive-panel-uses-data-that-distorts-doctors-pay/2013/07/20/ee134e3a-eda8-11e2-9008-61e94a7ea20d_story.html.

Wildavsky, Aaron. 1977. "Doing Better and Feeling Worse: The Political Pathology of Health Policy." *Daedalus* 106 (1): 105–23.

Wilensky, Gail R. 2006. "Developing a Center for Comparative Effectiveness Information." *Health Affairs* 25 (6): w572–w585.

———. 2008. "Cost-Effectiveness Information: Yes, It's Important, but Keep It Separate, Please!" *Annals of Internal Medicine* 148 (12): 967–68.

———. 2009. "The Policies and Politics of Creating a Comparative Clinical Effectiveness Research Center." *Health Affairs* 28 (4): w719–w729.

———. 2010a. "Comparative Effectiveness Research: So Far, So Good." *Healthcare Financial Management* 64 (11): 34–36.

———. 2010b. "The Mammography Guidelines and Evidence-Based Medicine." *Health Affairs Blog*, January 12. http://healthaffairs.org/blog/2010/01/12/the-mammograpy-guidelines-and-evidence-based-medicine/. Accessed June 6, 2012.

Wilsford, David. 1991. *Doctors and the State: The Politics of Health Care in France and the United States*. Durham, NC: Duke University Press.

Wilson, James Q. 1973. *Political Organizations*. Princeton, NJ: Princeton University Press.

———. 1989. *Bureaucracy: What Government Agencies Do and Why They Do It*. New York: Basic Books.

Wray, Nelda P., J. Bruce Moseley, and Kimberly O'Malley. 2003. "Arthroscopic Treatment of Osteoarthritis of the Knee." *Journal of Bone and Joint Surgery* 85 (2): 381.

Wulff, Katherine Cooper, Franklin G. Miller, and Steven D. Pearson. 2011. "Can Coverage Be Rescinded When Negative Trial Results Threaten a Popular Procedure? The Ongoing Saga of Vertebroplasty." *Health Affairs* 30 (12): 2269–76.

Yang, S. Steven, and Barton Nisonson. 1995. "Arthroscopic Surgery of the Knee in the Geriatric Patient." *Clinical Orthopaedics and Related Research* 316: 50–58.

Yim, Ji-Hyeon, Jong-Keun Seon, Eun-Kyoo Song, Jun-Ik Choi, Min-Cheol Kim, Keun-Bae Lee, and Hyoung-Yeon Seo. 2013. "A Comparative Study of Meniscectomy and Nonoperative Treatment for Degenerative Horizontal Tears of the Medial Meniscus. *American Journal of Sports Medicine* 41 (7): 1565–70.

Zaller, J. R. 1992. *The Nature and Origins of Mass Opinion*. Cambridge: Cambridge University Press.

INDEX

A NOTE ON THE TYPE

This book has been composed in Adobe Text and Gotham. Adobe Text, designed by Robert Slimbach for Adobe, bridges the gap between fifteenth- and sixteenth-century calligraphic and eighteenth-century Modern styles. Gotham, inspired by New York street signs, was designed by Tobias Frere-Jones for Hoefler & Co.